THE **BabyCenter**

ESSENTIAL

GUIDE TO

PREGNANCY

AND BIRTH

36 - Anthony
34 1/2 - Annabelle

THE BabyCenter® ESSENTIAL GUIDE TO PREGNANCY AND BIRTH

EXPERT ADVICE
AND REAL-WORLD WISDOM
FROM THE TOP
PREGNANCY AND PARENTING
RESOURCE

RODALE®

© 2005 by BabyCenter

All photographs and illustrations by BabyCenter, except for the following:
Photograph on page 2 © Digital Vision, Getty Images
Photograph on page 122 © Photodisc Blue, Getty Images
Photograph on page 256 © John Slater, Getty Images
Photograph on page 368 © Photodisc Green, Getty Images
Photograph on page 446 © Digital Vision, Getty Images
Photograph on page 484 © Stockbyte, Getty Images

Book design by Joanna Williams

Library of Congress Cataloging-in-Publication Data

Murray, Linda, date.
The Babycenter essential guide to pregnancy and birth : expert advice and
real-world wisdom from the top pregnancy and parenting resource /
Linda Murray, Leah Hennen, Jim Scott, with the BabyCenter Editorial Team.
p.   cm.
Includes index.
ISBN-13 978–1–59486–211–3 paperback
ISBN-10 1–59486–211–7 paperback
1. Pregnancy—Popular works. 2. Labor (Obstetrics)—Popular works. I. Hennen, Leah.
II. Scott, Jim, date. III. Title.
RG525.M865 2005
618.2—dc22   2005006691

Distributed to the book trade by Holtzbrinck Publishers

2   4   6   8   10   9   7   5   3   1   paperback

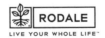

LIVE YOUR WHOLE LIFE™

We inspire and enable people to improve their lives and the world around them
For more of our products visit **rodalestore.com** or call 800-848-4735

CONTENTS

PREFACE

The BabyCenter© Essential Guide to Pregnancy and Birth collects and distills the best and latest thinking about pregnancy to help you enjoy a healthy, happy pregnancy. It thoroughly explores the amazing changes you'll experience—not only the "what," but the "why"—and provides a close look into the fascinating world of fetal development. As medical reviewers, we (and a team of other professionals) worked with the BabyCenter editorial team to ensure that this volume contains accurate information about the entire birth cycle, including the 40 (and sometimes more!) weeks of pregnancy, labor and birth, and the postpartum period. This book also addresses many important aspects of everyday life—such as relationships, sex, nutrition, exercise, and work—from the vantage point of a pregnant woman. In addition to advice from professionals, the words of pregnant women themselves, drawn from the vast online BabyCenter community, are woven throughout the book. Their voices speak to both the highs and lows you may feel—and everything in between—and give you a real sense of the diverse ways in which other women experience pregnancy.

Writing a comprehensive pregnancy book that's helpful for *all* women—but not needlessly scary—requires a delicate balancing act. And we, along with the authors, have tried mightily to achieve that balance. In addition to an in-depth look at the normal progress of pregnancy, this book also includes several separate chapters about issues that only a minority of women will encounter. These sections provide a useful resource if you're diagnosed with medical problems or pregnancy complications. They're not meant to frighten, only to arm you with essential information so you can be a more knowledgeable and active participant in your own care.

As the two of us are, respectively, a midwife and an obstetrician, our professional education, training, and experiences inform our perspectives. While we share the common (and overriding) goal of helping women have healthy babies, we sometimes approach issues from different points of view. Nevertheless, we're united in our belief that you need complete and accurate information to help you decide—in partnership with your caregiver—what's best for you, your baby, and your family. We believe that *The BabyCenter Essential Guide to Pregnancy and Birth* offers a comprehensive, up-to-date, and trustworthy resource that will serve you well as you make the wondrous journey to parenthood.

Ann Linden, C.N.M.
Natan Haratz-Rubinstein, M.D.

MEET OUR EXPERTS

Carol Archie, M.D., is an associate clinical professor of maternal-fetal medicine at the University of California at Los Angeles School of Medicine and an associate professor at the UCLA School of Public Health.

Raul Artal, M.D., is chair of the department of obstetrics, gynecology, and women's health at the St. Louis University School of Medicine in Missouri.

Thomas Bader, M.D., is an assistant professor in the department of obstetrics and gynecology at the University of Pennsylvania in Philadelphia.

Pennelope Morrison Bosarge, M.S.N., C.R.N.P., is a women's healthcare nurse-practitioner at the University of Alabama School of Nursing in Birmingham.

Gerald Briggs, B. Pharm., is a clinical professor of pharmacy at the School of Pharmacy, University of California at San Francisco, and chairman of the research committee for the Organization of Teratology Information Services (OTIS).

Gina Brown, M.D., is a maternal-fetal medicine and critical-care obstetrics specialist in New York City.

Trudy Brown is a board-certified electrologist and licensed electrology instructor in High Point, North Carolina and a member of the Society of Clinical and Medical Electrologists and the American Society of Laser & Surgery Medicine.

Christina Chambers, Ph.D., M.P.H., is an assistant professor in the department of pediatrics and family and preventive medicine at the University of California, San Diego and the director of the California Teratogenic Information Service.

Julie Daniels, Ph.D., is an assistant professor of epidemiology and maternal and child health at the University of North Carolina at Chapel Hill's School of Public Health.

Kay Daniels, M.D., is an associate clinical professor of obstetrics and gynecology at Stanford University in Stanford, California.

Thomas Easterling, M.D., is an associate professor of maternal-fetal medicine at the University of Washington School of Medicine.

Deborah Ehrenthal, M.D., is a women's-health specialist and clinical assistant professor of medicine at Thomas Jefferson University Medical School in Philadelphia.

Bruce Flamm, M.D., is a clinical professor of obstetrics and gynecology at the University of California at Irvine. He's the author of four books, including *Birth After Cesarean: The Medical Facts.*

Will Forest, M.P.H., is a toxicologist at the Hazard Evaluation System and Information Service of the California Department of Health Services in Oakland.

Meredith Goodwin, M.D., practices the full range of family practice, including prenatal care and delivery, well-child care, and well-woman care.

Joyce and Marshall Gottesfeld, M.D.s, are obstetricians in Denver, Colorado.

Cornelia Graves, M.D., is an associate professor of maternal-fetal medicine at Vanderbilt University in Nashville.

Edward (Ned) Groth III, Ph.D., is an independent food safety and environmental health consultant and a former senior scientist at Consumers Union.

Jeanne-Marie Guise, M.D., is an assistant professor of obstetrics and gynecology at the Oregon Health Services Center in Portland.

Debra Gussman, M.D., is an ob-gyn at the Jersey Shore Medical Center in Neptune, New Jersey, and a fellow of the American College of Obstetricians and Gynecologists.

Jeff Hampl, R.D., is registered dietitian and associate professor of nutrition at Arizona State University in Mesa.

M. J. Hanafin, C.N.M., is a certified nurse-midwife in London, England.

Natan Haratz-Rubinstein, M.D., is an associate clinical professor of Obstetrics and Gynecology at SUNY Downstate Medical Center in New York City. He is also the director of the Obstetrical and Gynecological Ultrasound Center at Long Island College Hospital in Brooklyn, New York.

Lewis Holmes, M.D., is a professor of pediatrics at Harvard University Medical School and chief of genetics and teratology at MassGeneral Hospital for Children in Boston.

Michael Ignelzi, D.D.S., Ph.D., is an associate professor of orthodontics and pediatric dentistry at the University of Michigan School of Dentistry and former chair of the Council on Scientific Affairs for the American Academy of Pediatric Dentistry.

Sandra Johnson, M.D., is an assistant professor of dermatology at the University of Arkansas for Medical Sciences in Little Rock.

Kristina Kahl, M.S., is a board-certified genetic counselor at Sacramento Maternal Fetal Medicine in California.

Tekoa L. King, C.N.M., M.P.H., is a certified nurse-midwife in the department of obstetrics, gynecology, and reproductive sciences at the University of California at San Francisco.

Karen Kleiman, M.S.W., is the executive director of the Postpartum Stress Center near Philadelphia and the author of *This Isn't What I Expected: Overcoming Postpartum Depression.*

Lisa Lamson, M.S., is a doctor of audiology at the University of California, San Francisco Medical Center.

John Larsen, M.D., is chairman of obstetrics and gynecology at The George Washington University in Washington, D.C.

Yiming Li, D.D.S., is a professor of dentistry and director of the research laboratory at Loma Linda University's School of Dentistry in California.

Ann Linden, C.N.M., M.P.H, is a certified nurse-midwife with more than 20 years experience and is a member of the Midwifery Service of the Columbia campus of the New York-Presbyterian Hospital.

Christine Loomis has written several books about family travel, including *Simplify Family Travel* and *Fodor's Family Adventures.*

Catherine Lynch, M.D., is director of the division of general obstetrics and gynecology at the University of South Florida.

Morgan Martin, N.D., L.M., is chair of the naturopathic midwifery department at Bastyr University in Kenmore, Washington.

Marguerite McDonald, M.D., is the founder of the Eye Give Foundation, director of the Southern Vision Institute, and a clinical professor of ophthalmology at Tulane University in New Orleans.

Laura Fijolek McKain, M.D., is a board-certified obstetrician in private practice in Wilmington, North Carolina and a teacher at the Coastal Area Health Education Center.

George Mussalli, M.D., is a board-certified maternal-fetal medicine specialist and director of obstetrics at North Central Bronx Hospital and Jacobi Medical Center and associate professor of clinical obstetrics and gynecology at Albert Einstein College of Medicine in New York City.

Mary O'Malley, M.D., is an attending psychiatrist and sleep medicine consultant at Norwalk Hospital in Connecticut.

Wendy Page-Echols, D.O., is an osteopath in East Lansing, Michigan.

Larry Pickering, M.D., is senior advisor to the director of the National Immunization Program at the Centers for Disease Control and Prevention and a professor of pediatrics at Emory University School of Medicine in Atlanta.

Mary Lake Polan, M.D., is chair of the department of gynecology and obstetrics at Stanford University School of Medicine in Stanford, California.

Suzanne Sherwood Powell is a certified childbirth educator, doula, and monitrice in the Atlanta, Georgia, area.

Robert Price, Ph.D., is an extension specialist with the food science and technology department at the University of California, Davis.

Ronald Ruggiero, M.D., is a clinical professor and pharmacist specialist in women's health with the departments of clinical pharmacy and obstetrics, gynecology and reproductive sciences at the medical center at the University of California at San Francisco.

Jack Schneider, M.D., is the medical director of women's and children's services at the Mary Birch Hospital for Women in San Diego, California.

Sherman Silber, M.D., is a fertility specialist at St. Luke's Hospital in St. Louis, Missouri and the author of four books, including *How to Get Pregnant with the New Technology*.

Jill Stovsky, R.D., L.D., M.Ed., is an exercise physiologist and registered dietitian in Cleveland, Ohio. Stovsky is also an aerobics instructor and personal trainer, as well as a writer and speaker on nutrition and fitness.

Bridget Swinney, R.D., is a clinical dietician specializing in prenatal nutrition in El Paso, Texas, and the author of *Eating Expectantly: The Practical and Tasty Guide to Prenatal Nutrition*.

Russell Turk, M.D., is the founder Riverside Obstetrics & Gynecology in Riverside, Connecticut.

Toni Weschler, M.P.H., is a fertility educator and founder of Fertility Awareness Counseling and Training Seminars (FACTS) in Seattle. She's the author of *Taking Charge of Your Fertility*.

Craig Winkel, M.D., is former chair of the department of obstetrics and gynecology at Georgetown University School of Medicine in Washington, D.C.

ACKNOWLEDGMENTS

The authors wish to thank all of the people who contributed their time and talent to making this book a reality:

• Our medical reviewers: Ann Linden, C.N.M., and Natan Haratz-Rubinstein, M.D., who put their heart and soul into this project and scrutinized every sentence in the book for medical accuracy. This book is immeasurably better for their efforts. And our other reviewers: George Mussalli, M.D.; Bridget Swinney, R.D.; Jodi Mindell, Ph.D.; Diane Sanford, Ph.D.; Gerald Briggs; Kathleen Huggins, IBCLC; and Raul Artal, M.D.

• The small army of talented writers and editors who contributed in ways great and small: Topping the list is Holly Hanke, who did her work with unfailing good humor and grace. Heidi Kotansky, copy puller, fact finder, doctor tracker, proofreader, and overall "Girl Wednesday" extraordinaire. And (in alphabetical order) Sara Bethell, Emily Bloch, Julia Bourland, Dawn Margolis, Kate Marple, Bonnie Monte, Catherine Newman, Karen Ohlson, and Mary VanClay.

• The millions of women and men who visit BabyCenter each month—and who constantly tell us, in great and inspiring detail, about their pregnancies, children, and lives.

• Our intrepid photographer, Judi Swinks, and our ever-blossoming model, Charro Knight-Lilly. And our medical illustrator, Peg Gerrity, who created the breathtaking fetal development illustrations within.

• Everyone at Rodale who helped bring this book to life. Most notably, our editor, Heather Jackson, who believed in this project from the start and nurtured it every step of the way, our project manager, Lois Hazel, our designer, Joanna Williams, and layout designer, Jennifer Giandomenico.

• Our agent Jeff Kleinman, a loyal BabyCenter reader whose enthusiasm, patience, and passion were instrumental in translating the online world of BabyCenter into the book you hold today.

• Finally, the people who perhaps taught us the most about pregnancy and birth—our children: Alessandra, Austin and Laurel, and Chris and Alec.

—Linda Murray, Leah Hennen, and Jim Scott
January 2005

PART I

THE FIRST TRIMESTER: 0 TO 13 WEEKS

You're Pregnant!

Congratulations—and welcome to the beginning of an incredible journey. In the next three months, an amazing amount of change will take place in your body and in your life.

In the coming weeks, you'll likely feel surprise, panic, relief, worry, and joy (perhaps all at the same time). You'll have questions— lots of 'em—about everything from how to find a pregnancy caregiver and what kinds of prenatal tests you might need, to why they call it morning sickness if it lasts *all day*, to how to break the news to your loved ones, get through the days at work, and prepare for the financial, emotional, and practical considerations of pregnancy and parenthood.

Fear not. In this section, you'll find everything you need to know about what's happening in your belly—and what's on your mind.

First-Trimester Highlights

Congratulations, you're pregnant!

During this trimester, your baby will:

▶ Start out the size of a poppy seed and grow to the size of a jumbo shrimp

▶ Form all the necessary organs and body parts, including the heart and eyes

▶ Start moving (but you won't be able to feel it until later)

▶ Be most vulnerable during weeks 4 to 10—so take extra care of yourself

You will:

▶ Most likely experience nausea, fatigue, sore breasts, mood swings, and frequent urination

▶ Gain about 5 pounds

▶ Probably feel bloated and uncomfortable in your clothes within weeks

▶ Grow one cup size

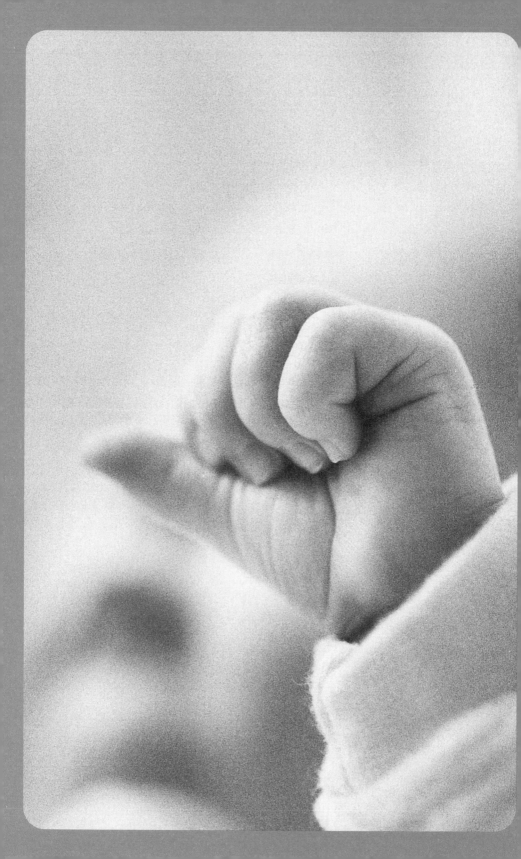

YOUR PREGNANCY WEEK BY WEEK

Just the Facts: Your Due Date and the Timing of Your Pregnancy

Strange as it may seem, your doctor or midwife calculates your pregnancy starting from the first day of your last menstrual period (LMP). Pregnancy lasts about 38 weeks from conception to birth, but because it's often hard to pin down exactly when the egg and sperm did their mating dance, practitioners count 40 weeks (280 days) of pregnancy, beginning with the start of your LMP. That's why you're already considered "two weeks pregnant" when you conceive.

Here's how the timing breaks down in your first trimester.

Your Pregnancy: 0 through 3 Weeks

Your Changing Body

During the first two weeks or so of your cycle, your body's like an anxious host anticipating the arrival of an important houseguest: First, your uterus sheds its old, unneeded lining when your period starts. Then, prompted by a surge in the

HOT TOPICS

- The first signs of pregnancy (page 5)
- Symptoms you should never ignore (page 21)
- Tips for tender breasts (page 47)
- Coping with fatigue (page 52)
- Why you have to pee so much now (page 52)
- Getting enough folic acid (page 64)

What's Your Due Date?

To calculate your due date, find the first day of your last menstrual period (LMP) in bold. The date directly below it is your estimated date of delivery (EDD). If your last period started on January 11, for instance, then your EDD is October 18. Be aware, though , that a normal, full-term baby can arrive anywhere between three weeks before and two weeks after your due date.

January	1	2	3	4	5	6	7	8	9	10	11	12	13	14	15	16	17	18	19	20	21	22	23	24	25	26	27	28	29
Oct/Nov	8	9	10	11	12	13	14	15	16	17	18	19	20	21	22	23	24	25	26	27	28	29	30	31	1	2	3	4	5
February	1	2	3	4	5	6	7	8	9	10	11	12	13	14	15	16	17	18	19	20	21	22	23	24	25	26	27	28	
Nov/Dec	8	9	10	11	12	13	14	15	16	17	18	19	20	21	22	23	24	25	26	27	28	29	30		1	2	3	4	5
March	1	2	3	4	5	6	7	8	9	10	11	12	13	14	15	16	17	18	19	20	21	22	23	24	25	26	27	28	29
Dec/Jan	6	7	8	9	10	11	12	13	14	15	16	17	18	19	20	21	22	23	24	25	26	27	28	29	30	31	1	2	3
April	1	2	3	4	5	6	7	8	9	10	11	12	13	14	15	16	17	18	19	20	21	22	23	24	25	26	27	28	29
Jan/Feb	6	7	8	9	10	11	12	13	14	15	16	17	18	19	20	21	22	23	24	25	26	27	28	29	30	31	1	2	3
May	1	2	3	4	5	6	7	8	9	10	11	12	13	14	15	16	17	18	19	20	21	22	23	24	25	26	27	28	29
Feb/Mar	5	6	7	8	9	10	11	12	13	14	15	16	17	18	19	20	21	22	23	24	25	26	27	28	1	2	3	4	5
June	1	2	3	4	5	6	7	8	9	10	11	12	13	14	15	16	17	18	19	20	21	22	23	24	25	26	27	28	29
Mar/Apr	8	9	10	11	12	13	14	15	16	17	18	19	20	21	22	23	24	25	26	27	28	29	30	31	1	2	3	4	5
July	1	2	3	4	5	6	7	8	9	10	11	12	13	14	15	16	17	18	19	20	21	22	23	24	25	26	27	28	29
Apr/Mar	7	8	9	10	11	12	13	14	15	16	17	18	19	20	21	22	23	24	25	26	27	28	29	30	1	2	3	4	5
August	1	2	3	4	5	6	7	8	9	10	11	12	13	14	15	16	17	18	19	20	21	22	23	24	25	26	27	28	29
May/June	8	9	10	11	12	13	14	15	16	17	18	19	20	21	22	23	24	25	26	27	28	29	30	31	1	2	3	4	5
September	1	2	3	4	5	6	7	8	9	10	11	12	13	14	15	16	17	18	19	20	21	22	23	24	25	26	27	28	29
June/July	8	9	10	11	12	13	14	15	16	17	18	19	20	21	22	23	24	25	26	27	28	29	30		1	2	3	4	5	6
October	1	2	3	4	5	6	7	8	9	10	11	12	13	14	15	16	17	18	19	20	21	22	23	24	25	26	27	28	29
July/Aug	8	9	10	11	12	13	14	15	16	17	18	19	20	21	22	23	24	25	26	27	28	29	30	31	1	2	3	4	5
November	1	2	3	4	5	6	7	8	9	10	11	12	13	14	15	16	17	18	19	20	21	22	23	24	25	26	27	28	29
Aug/Sept	8	9	10	11	12	13	14	15	16	17	18	19	20	21	22	23	24	25	26	27	28	29	30	31	1	2	3	4	5
December	1	2	3	4	5	6	7	8	9	10	11	12	13	14	15	16	17	18	19	20	21	22	23	24	25	26	27	28	29
Sept/Oct	7	8	9	10	11	12	13	14	15	16	17	18	19	20	21	22	23	24	25	26	27	28	29	30	1	2	3	4	5

hormones estrogen and progesterone coursing through your bloodstream, your womb begins priming itself to shelter a growing baby by building up a lush lining of blood-rich tissue. Meanwhile, several eggs race to mature in your ovaries, until the heartiest of the bunch bursts out and is swept into a fallopian tube to meet its suitors. Though many will try, only one of the awaiting army of sperm will successfully fertilize your egg. After its trip down your fallopian tube is complete, the fertilized egg nestles into your womb and sets up residence for the next nine months or so. You won't know

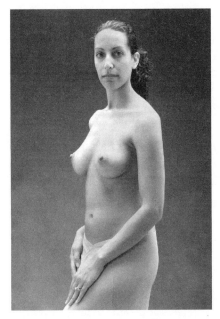

Within a few weeks, small clues will start hinting at the miraculous events unfolding inside your body. Among the first: painfully tender breasts, exhaustion, and a seemingly constant need to pee.

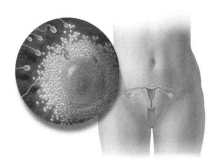

Several hours or even days after you and your mate make love, nearly 250 million sperm have fallen by the wayside, leaving just a few hundred battling it out to gain entrance into your egg. Only one will succeed.

that you've conceived, but you may soon start to notice the early signs of pregnancy: fatigue, frequent urination, and tender, swollen breasts. You may also have a little spotting a few days before your period is due. Some women confuse this implantation bleeding with menstruation—but only a small portion notice it at all. Even though you're still waiting to find out for sure if you're pregnant, don't forget to take your folic acid!

Your Growing Baby

Just after ovulation, a momentous meeting takes place: A microscopic sperm cell breaks through the protective barrier surrounding your egg and fertilizes it. A baby is in the making! Over the next day or so, you and your mate's DNA will do the tango within the fertilized egg, merging their genetic material into the blueprint for your baby-to-be. All the while, the fertilized egg is traveling down your fallopian tube toward your uterus, dividing and multiplying into a ball of 16 identical cells. By the time it reaches your uterus, three or four days later, and begins burrowing into the lining there a day or two after that, this ball will be stretched like a double-layered water balloon. The outer layer of cells will form the placenta, the organ that delivers life-sustaining oxygen and nutrients to your baby; the inner layer will become your baby; and the fluid-filled center will become the amniotic sac that cushions her as she grows. The ball of cells is also producing the pregnancy hormone human chorionic gonadotropin (hCG), which tells your ovaries to stop releasing eggs and triggers a boost in the production of estrogen and progesterone, which prevents your uterus from shedding its lining—and its tiny passenger. Right now, your baby is getting her oxygen and nutrients (and discarding her waste products) through microscopic tunnels that connect the developing ball of cells to the blood vessels in your uterine wall because the placenta won't be ready to take over this task until the end of week 4. All this, and your baby-in-the-making (now technically called an embryo) is still no bigger than a poppy seed.

Your Pregnancy: 4 Weeks
Your Changing Body

Now that 28 days have passed since you last menstruated, the period that you've been expecting may be a no-show. If it's still MIA in a few days, take a trip to the drugstore—a home pregnancy test may be able to confirm your news! If the test is positive, let out a celebratory whoop (or indulge in a few private tears)—false positives are much less common than false negatives. Then call your practitioner and set up your first prenatal checkup. Don't be surprised when she says she won't see you for a month or more—most initial prenatal visits are scheduled for around week eight. If you haven't had a recent preconception visit or if you have any medical problems, don't be shy about pressing for an earlier appointment. And be sure to ask about starting a prenatal vitamin if you're not already taking one. Also give your caregiver a rundown of any medications—prescription *and* over-the-counter—you're

> ### HOT TOPICS
>
> - Determining your due date (page 4)
> - Choosing a pregnancy caregiver (page 22)
> - Tests in early pregnancy (page 31)
> - Prenatal vitamins (page 64)
> - When you and your mate have different reactions to the pregnancy (page 97)
> - Medicine safety guide (page 551)

BabyCenter Buzz

What Other Women Say at 4 Weeks

"I just found out that we're pregnant! I was only 12 days past ovulation but decided to test after I noticed some discharge the color of light coffee. Never in 20 years did I get my period that early. I thought, 'Wow—maybe this is that implantation spotting everyone talks about.'"   —Holly

"I just tested positive, and I'm finding that I'm more scared than happy. I'm just thinking of all the changes to be made in my life. I've been trying for 8 years, so this is pretty unbelievable."   —Kim

"I took a pregnancy test and got a negative, but I just *knew* I was pregnant. So I waited a few days and took another test at a different time of day. Sure enough, this time it was positive."   —Anonymous

taking; the next six weeks are critical to your baby's development, and some drugs aren't safe now.

Your Growing Baby

The embryo has nestled into the soft lining of your uterus and will derive its nourishment from the yolk sac—yes, human eggs have them, too—until your placenta starts functioning next week.

The big news this week: The microscopic cells that will become your baby are multiplying and dividing at a dizzying rate, and a tiny, primitive heart is forming. From now until week 10, all of your baby's organs will start to develop, and some will actually start to work. The next six weeks are the time when your baby is most vulnerable to anything that might interfere with his development—and the time when you need to be most careful about anything that might harm him. Meanwhile, the placenta is weaving its way into your uterine lining, gearing up for its job of siphoning oxygen and nutrients from your bloodstream to your baby's and, in turn, dumping your baby's waste back into your blood to be flushed from your body. Also present now: the amniotic sac, which surrounds your baby; the amniotic fluid, which cushions him; and the yolk sac, which churns out red blood cells and helps nourish your baby until the placenta is up and running.

Your Pregnancy: 5 Weeks

Your Changing Body

Pregnancy symptoms may make their debut this week. If you're like most women, you'll soon experience nausea and perhaps vomiting (and not just in the morning), sore breasts, fatigue, and a more frequent need to pee. All are normal, all are annoying, but the upside is that these complaints are all a part of being pregnant and won't last forever. (If you're one of the lucky few who has a symptomless or near-symptomless pregnancy, don't fret about it—just enjoy it!) The outside world won't see any sign of the dramatic developments taking place inside you—except maybe that you're suddenly taking better care of yourself.

HOT TOPICS

- Morning sickness survival guide (page 54)
- What to eat—and what to avoid (page 64)
- Breaking the news to friends and family (page 103)
- Dealing with pregnancy symptoms at work (page 108)
- Protecting your baby-to-be from environmental hazards (page 110)
- Red flags for ectopic pregnancy (page 546)

Your Growing Baby

Big news: Your baby's heart, which has started to divide into chambers, begins beating this week, and cells for vital organs like her kidneys and liver are forming. Even so, your tiny embryo—no bigger than a sesame seed—is still very much a work in progress. She looks more like a tadpole than a

BabyCenter Buzz

What Other Women Say at 5 Weeks

"I'm having all these symptoms already: My breasts are sore, I'm having terrible migraines, and I'm so bloated that I can barely put on a pair of my loosest pants. How could this be, so early in the pregnancy?"   —Jessica

"I feel tired all the time, and my breasts feel like they weigh 12 pounds each!" —Anonymous

"If I have to pee one more time, I'm going to scream! It's making sleeping really difficult, since I have to keep getting up."   —Steffie

human being, and her body is made up of three layers—the ectoderm, the mesoderm, and the endoderm—that will later form organs and tissues. The neural tube—from which your baby's brain, spinal cord, and nerves will sprout—develops in the ectoderm, or top layer. This layer will also give rise to your baby's skin, hair, nails, mammary and sweat glands, and tooth enamel. The heart and circulatory system appear in the mesoderm, or middle layer. The mesoderm will also form your baby's muscles, cartilage, bone, and under-skin tissue. The endoderm, or third layer, will give rise to parts of your baby's lungs, intestines, and urinary system, as well as her thyroid, liver, and pancreas. Primitive versions of the placenta and the umbilical cord are already hard at work.

Your Pregnancy: 6 Weeks

Your Changing Body

You may find yourself developing a bit of a split personality—feeling moody one day and joyful the next. Disturbing as this is (especially if you pride yourself on being in control), what you're going through is normal and may even get more intense as your pregnancy progresses. Ricocheting emotions are caused partly by fluctuating hormones. But hormones aside, your entire life is about to change—and who *wouldn't* feel emotional about that?

HOT TOPICS

- Pregnancy symptoms you should never ignore (page 21)
- Food aversions (page 68)
- First-trimester weight gain (page 76)
- First-trimester emotions (page 90)
- Which beauty treatments to avoid now (page 575)
- What to know about a *lack* of symptoms (opposite page)

Your Growing Baby

This week's major developments: The nose, mouth, and ears that you'll be spending so much time kissing in eight months are beginning to take shape. If you could see into your uterus, you'd find an overlarge head and dark spots where your baby's eyes and nostrils are starting to form. His emerging ears are marked by small depressions on the sides of his head, and his arms and legs by protruding buds. His heart is beating about 100 to 160 times a minute—almost twice as fast as yours—and blood is beginning to course through his body. His intestines are developing, and the bud of tissue that

BabyCenter Buzz

What Other Women Say at 6 Weeks

"My husband thinks I'm totally nuts. *I* think I'm totally nuts. I've never been so bitchy in my life. It's horrible!"   —*Cindy*

"Everything bothers me about a hundred times more than it should. When I lose my cool around my partner, I always have to remind him that I can't help it!"   —*Amy*

"My acne's really flared up."   —*Lisa*

"Week 6 hit, and with it came morning sickness. Healthy eating went out the window. I've been eating a lot of carbohydrates and mozzarella cheese and drinking a lot of milk. I'm definitely getting enough calcium, but my vitamins are coming from a pill."   —*Anonymous*

"Grilled cheese sandwiches are all I can stomach, and I know that can't be good." —*Vicki*

will give rise to his lungs has appeared. His pituitary gland is forming, as are the rest of his brain, muscles, and bones. Right now, your baby is a quarter-inch long and about the size of a lentil.

Your Pregnancy: 7 Weeks
Your Changing Body

Your uterus has almost doubled in size in the last five weeks, and keeping food down may be next to impossible, thanks to morning sickness. (If you're feeling fine, don't worry—you're lucky!) You probably need to use the bathroom a lot more than usual, too, thanks to your increased blood volume and the extra fluid being processed through your kidneys. (By the end of your pregnancy, you'll have 40 to 45 percent more blood running through your veins to meet the demands of your growing baby.)

HOT TOPICS

- Shortness of breath (page 50)
- Why pregnancy can make headaches flare up (page 52)
- What to do if you notice spotting (page 57)
- Miscarriage warning signs (page 58)
- How to deal with a junk-food jones (page 196)
- Which household chores to avoid (page 559)

BabyCenter Buzz

What Other Women Say at 7 Weeks

"Almost every three hours, I'm starving to death. And I don't mean the 'Mmm, I could use a carrot' hungry—I mean the 'Get out of my way and show me some real food!' hungry." —*Anonymous*

"I'm exhausted all the time. All I want to do is sleep, which is hard because I work full-time." —*Carrie*

"I noticed some light pink spotting this weekend and freaked out. We had an ultrasound yesterday, and everything's fine. Whew!" —*Anonymous*

"I wish someone had told me that you can have *no* problems: no morning sickness, no extreme fatigue, no aches and pains, no weird cravings—and still have a healthy baby! When I went to the doctor, I was terrified that she'd tell me I wasn't actually pregnant or that something was wrong with the baby because I had no symptoms." —*Tricia*

While your nausea may diminish during your second trimester (in about seven weeks), get used to making a beeline for the bathroom. Many women report that the need to pee is a constant part of pregnancy.

Your Growing Baby

The big news this week: Hands and feet are emerging from developing arms and legs—though they look more like paddles at this point than the tiny, pudgy extremities you're daydreaming about holding and tickling. Technically, your baby is still considered an embryo and has something of a small tail, which is actually an extension of her tailbone. The tail will disappear within a few weeks, but that's the *only* thing getting smaller. Your baby has doubled in size since last week and now measures half an inch long, about the size of a raspberry. If you could see inside your womb, you'd spot eyelid folds partially covering her peepers—which already have some color—as well as the tip of her nose and tiny veins beneath parchment-thin skin. Right now both hemispheres of your baby's brain are growing, and her liver is churning out red blood cells until her bone marrow forms and takes over this role. She also has an appendix and a pancreas, which will eventually produce the hormone insulin to aid in digestion. A loop in your baby's growing intestines is bulging into her umbilical cord, which now has distinct blood vessels to carry oxygen and nutrients to and from her tiny body.

Your Pregnancy: 8 Weeks

Your Changing Body

Though you haven't gained much weight yet, parts of you are certainly growing—like your breasts. In fact, many women go up a cup size or more during pregnancy (the result of all the new milk-making machinery under construction as your body gears up to feed a hungry newborn), and much of this growth happens in the first trimester. Time to invest in a new bra! Some of the other changes you may be noticing now: Bone-deep fatigue as your body works overtime to create a new human being; gas as your digestion slows to a crawl under the influence of progesterone; and aversions to certain foods and pungent smells as your nose and taste buds go on high alert for potential toxins.

Your Growing Baby

New this week: Webbed fingers and toes are poking out from your baby's hands and feet, his eyelids practically cover his eyes, breathing tubes extend from his throat to the branches of his developing lungs, and his "tail" is just about gone. In his brain, nerve cells are branching out to connect with one another, forming primitive neural pathways.

HOT TOPICS

• Your first prenatal checkup (page 30)

• First-trimester blood tests (page 31)

• Should your mate come to prenatal appointments? (page 35)

• What to do when you can't stomach your prenatal vitamin (page 66)

• From oral sex to anal sex— what's safe and what's not (page 100)

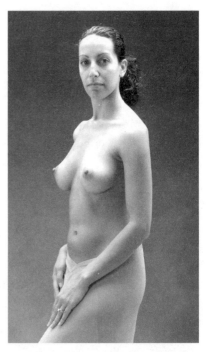

Your belly may no longer be as flat as it once was—though slowed digestion and bloating take most of the blame for making your pants feel snug.

BabyCenter Buzz

What Other Women Say at 8 Weeks

"From morning to night, I feel like gagging. I don't throw up, but I have a queasy stomach. I'd much rather hurl and get it over with." —*Stephanie*

"I crush my prenatal vitamin and mix it with yogurt. So far, that's been the only way for me to keep it down." —*Anonymous*

"I have tingling nipples, and it's driving me crazy!" —*Steph*

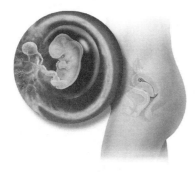

With the beginnings of facial features and fingers and toes, your baby is taking on a more human form now.

Though you may be daydreaming about your baby as one sex or the other, the external genitals still haven't developed enough to reveal whether you're having a boy or a girl. Either way, your baby—about the size of a kidney bean—is constantly moving and shifting, though you still can't feel him.

Your Pregnancy: 9 Weeks
Your Changing Body

You still may not look pregnant (unless this pregnancy isn't your first), even if your waist is thickening a bit. You probably *feel* pregnant, though. Not only are morning sickness and other physical symptoms out in full force for most women, but you may feel like an emotional pinball as well. Mood swings are common now; it's perfectly normal to be ripping into your mate for leaving the toilet seat up one

HOT TOPICS

- Genetic counseling (page 40)
- Chorionic villus sampling (page 43)
- Common sleep problems (page 59)
- Prenatal exercise (page 78)
- Why you're so moody now (page 90)

BabyCenter Buzz

What Other Women Say at 9 Weeks

"I'm so congested that I sound like I've got a whopper of a cold. I have to keep a humidifier going in my room at night and sleep propped up." —*Penny*

"I just had an ultrasound, and there were not one but *two* babies! What am I going do with *two*?" —*Anonymous*

"I'm always hot. I sleep naked, with a fan going and our window open. My husband is freezing!" —*Amy*

"'Morning sickness' is a farce—it's 'all-day sickness' for me. I wish someone had hit me in the head when I told them I'd love every minute of pregnancy. That's a farce, too!" —*Anonymous*

minute and weeping over a sentimental commercial the next. Try to cut yourself (and him!) some slack—it'll be good practice for the months to come. Emotional flip-flopping can persist throughout your pregnancy and well after your baby is born. On the physical front, you may find yourself sweating while others around you are shivering (yet another side effect of all the extra blood pumping through your veins). Some women also notice that they salivate much more than normal now, though the cause is a bit of a mystery.

Your Growing Baby

This week's big news: Your baby—just under an inch long and about the size of a grape—looks practically human for the first time! All of the standard body parts are accounted for—though they'll go through plenty of fine-tuning in the coming months. Other changes abound: Your baby's heart finishes dividing into four chambers, and the valves start to form—as do her tiny teeth. The embryonic "tail" is completely gone. All of your baby's organs, muscles, and nerves are kicking into gear. The external sex organs are there but won't be distinguishable as male or female for another few weeks. Her eyes are fully formed, but her eyelids are fused shut and won't open until week 27. She has tiny earlobes, and her mouth, nose, and nostrils are more distinct. The placenta is developed enough now to take over most of the critical job of producing hormones. Though your baby still weighs just a fraction of an ounce, she's poised for rapid weight gain now that her basic biology is in place.

Your Pregnancy: 10 Weeks

Your Changing Body

HOT TOPICS

• Buying a maternity bra (page 47)

• Excessive saliva (page 51)

• How many calories you need now (page 81)

• Dressing for early pregnancy (page 95)

• Depression during pregnancy (page 210)

Before you got pregnant, your uterus was the size of a small pear. By this week, it's as big as a grapefruit. Though you're probably not yet ready for maternity wear, you may find that your regular clothes are becoming uncomfortably tight. That's because your midsection is thickening (still due to slight weight gain and bloating) and your blossoming breasts are straining the seams of your bra. In these transitional weeks between regular and maternity clothes, pants and skirts with forgiving elastic waists (or low-rise waistlines that sit below your belly) will provide some much-needed comfort.

Your Growing Baby

Major news this week: If you have a prenatal visit scheduled, you should be able to hear your baby's heartbeat during your appointment. The moment can be very dramatic, as the room fills with the sound of a galloping horse. It's confirmation of the power of the new life you've helped create, and for many parents it's an incredibly moving experience.

Other happenings: Your tiny baby, just the size of a walnut, is officially a fetus—meaning that most of his critical development is complete! He's swallowing, moving (thanks to newly functional joints), and kicking up a storm. Vital organs—including his kidneys, intestines, brain, lungs, and liver (now making red blood cells in place of the disappearing yolk sac)—are in place and starting to function, though they'll continue to develop throughout your pregnancy.

If you could take a peek inside your womb, you'd spot minute details, like tiny nails forming on perfect fingers and toes (no more webbing!) and peach-fuzz hair beginning to grow on tender skin.

In other developments: Your baby's limbs can bend now, and his hands are flexed at the wrist and meet over his heart, and his feet may be long enough to meet in front of his body. The outline of his spine is

BabyCenter Buzz

What Other Women Say at 10 Weeks

"I haven't had any cravings until now. Out of the blue, I want olives."   —*Crissy*

"I cry at everything. I just cried watching *Oprah* when she talked about John Steinbeck's death. He died in 1968—and I already knew that! My husband said no more kids for me because this pregnancy stuff is too hard. He was joking, but of course I started to cry."   —*Brenda*

"I have a saliva problem. I keep a washcloth next to me at work and spit out the extra saliva. Gross, I know, but it keeps the trips to the bathroom to a minimum."
—*Anonymous*

clearly visible through translucent skin, and spinal nerves are beginning to stretch out from his spinal cord. Your baby's forehead temporarily bulges with his developing brain and sits very high on his head, which measures half the length of his body. From crown to rump, he's about 1¼ inches long. In the coming three weeks, your baby will again double in size—to nearly 3 inches.

Your Pregnancy: 11 Weeks

Your Changing Body

If you're like many women, you're feeling a bit more energetic now and your nausea may be starting to wane. Unfortunately, you may also be suffering from constipation (caused by pregnancy hormones, which can slow digestion and lead to a bit of "clogging up") and heartburn (pregnancy hormones yet again—this time they're relaxing the valve separating your esophagus from your stomach). Just remember, all this suffering is for a good cause—you're having a baby!

HOT TOPICS

- Hearing the heartbeat (page 15)
- The latest prenatal screening tests (page 31)
- Cures for constipation (page 50)
- Getting your partner involved (page 97)
- Help for heartburn (page 172)

BabyCenter Buzz

What Other Women Say at 11 Weeks

"I'm starting to feel some improvement with the morning sickness and the exhaustion. Granted, I generally go to bed at 7:30 and fall asleep around 8:30!"
—*Staci*

"I was so tired about a month ago, but then it stopped. For the past few days, though, I've been tired again. All I want to do is sleep." —*Heather*

"I've had two miscarriages, and yesterday we heard the heartbeat during our prenatal visit. I feel as though I'm experiencing a miracle." —*Amy*

Your Growing Baby

Your baby, just over 1½ inches long and about the size of a fig, is now almost fully formed. Her fingers and toes have separated, her hands will soon open and close into fists, tiny tooth buds are beginning to appear under her gums, and some of her bones are beginning to harden. As her body grows and becomes functional, she'll start twisting, turning, kicking, and stretching as though she's doing water ballet—cushioned and protected all the while by your amniotic fluid. You won't feel your baby's acrobatics for another month or two—nor will you notice the hiccuping that she may be doing now that her diaphragm is forming.

Your Pregnancy: 12 Weeks

Your Changing Body

By this point, your uterus is almost big enough to fill your pelvis. You might even be able to feel the top of your womb—called the fundus—above the middle of your pubic bone. (*Hint:* It's around the top of your pubic hair.)

HOT TOPICS

- The best position for pregnancy sleep (page 59)
- Travel tips (page 114)
- When morning sickness persists past 12 weeks (page 174)
- Pregnancy-induced forgetfulness (page 326)
- Should you take out your belly button ring? (page 575)

Luckily, your body is beginning to adjust to your changing hormone levels, and for even more women, morning sickness is finally becoming a thing of the past. (Queasiness can return periodically throughout pregnancy, though, and some unlucky mothers-to-be *never* get a break from it.)

Your Growing Baby

The most dramatic development this week: Reflexes. Your baby's fingers will soon begin to open and close, his toes will curl, his eye muscles will clench, and his mouth will make sucking movements. In fact, if you prod your abdomen, your baby will squirm in response (though you won't be able to feel it). His intestines, which have grown so fast that they protrude into the umbilical cord, will start to move into his abdominal cavity about now, and his kidneys will begin excreting urine into his bladder. Meanwhile, nerve cells are multiplying rapidly, and in your baby's brain, synapses are forming furiously. His face also looks unquestionably human: His eyes have moved from the sides to the front of his head, and his ears are right where they should be. From crown to rump, your baby-to-be is 2⅛ inches long (about the size of a lime) and weighs half an ounce.

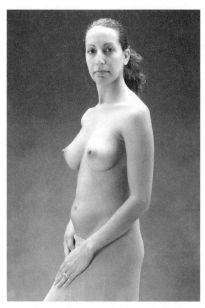

Finally, the beginning of a real "baby belly" as your uterus outgrows the confines of your pelvis and rises into your abdominal cavity. Maternity clothes, here you come!

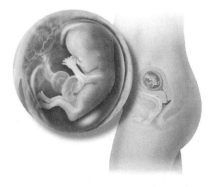

At barely 2 inches long, your baby's head is disproportionately large compared with his body; his forehead bulges with his developing brain, and his eyes are sealed shut. Still, there's no question that his appearance is now distinctly human.

BabyCenter Buzz

What Other Women Say at 12 Weeks

"I feel anything but sexy. My face looks like a pizza. I don't dress up anymore, don't wear makeup, and my hair stays in a ponytail." —*Toya*

"I'm suffering from pregnancy brain. I was getting dressed and put a bra on top of the one I already had on!" —*Susan*

"I had my first baby dream: It was a girl. I've heard that dreams are telling, but who knows?" —*Anonymous*

Your Pregnancy: 13 Weeks

Your Changing Body

Hooray! You're at the end of your first trimester, and not only are your early-pregnancy complaints likely easing, but your long-lost energy and sex drive may finally be staging a comeback. Though birth is still months away, your breasts may have already started making colostrum, the antibody—and nutrient-rich fluid that feeds your baby for the first few days after birth, before your mature milk comes in. What's more, your belly may soon be big enough to announce to the world that you're expecting.

HOT TOPICS

- Handling headaches (page 52)
- Telling your firstborn about the baby (page 105)
- Breaking the news at work (page 107)
- All about linea nigra, that line down your belly (page 123)
- Why you may feel faint (page 168)

Your Growing Baby

This week's big news: Your chance of miscarriage has dropped dramatically, now that your baby's critical development is nearly complete. Go ahead and breathe a sigh of relief.

In other developments: Fingerprints have formed on your baby's tiny fingertips, her veins and organs are clearly visible through her still-thin

BabyCenter Buzz

What Other Women Say at 13 Weeks

"Side sleeping has taken some getting used to. I've found that it's easier to sleep in that position when I hug a pillow and wrap my legs around it." —Clara

"I'm so sick of hearing 'How are you feeling?' I know most people are genuinely concerned, but man, I'm repeating myself over and over." —Sara

"Yesterday I decided it was okay to finally blab our pregnancy news. What a great feeling. My husband and I have been keeping this secret for two months!"
—Anonymous

skin, and her body is starting to catch up with her head—which makes up just a third of her body size now. If you're having a girl, she now has more than 2 million eggs in her ovaries. Your baby is almost 3 inches long (the size of a jumbo shrimp) and weighs nearly an ounce.

Symptoms You Should Never Ignore in the First Trimester

Fortunately, most women get through their first trimester with only run-of-the-mill aches, pains, and other problems. But just to be safe, don't hesitate to call your caregiver if you have any of these symptoms:

- Severe or persistent abdominal pain or cramping
- Vaginal bleeding or spotting (*Note:* If you're bleeding or have severe pain of any kind and can't reach your practitioner, head straight for the emergency room. And if you are soaking through several sanitary pads in an hour, in excruciating pain, having trouble breathing, or feeling "shocky" or like you might pass out, dial 911 right away.)
- Leaking fluid or watery, mucousy, or bloody vaginal discharge
- Discharge that's foul-smelling, frothy, or yellow, green, or gray
- Itching, burning, or other discomfort in the vagina or surrounding area
- Little or no urination
- A painful or burning sensation when you urinate
- Severe or persistent vomiting or vomiting accompanied by pain or fever
- Chills or fever of 101°F or higher
- Coughing up blood
- Persistent, severe leg cramps or calf pain that doesn't ease up when you flex your ankle and point your toes toward your nose
- Trauma to your abdomen from a fall, blunt-force impact like a car crash, or physical abuse
- Sudden, "explosive" headaches, a headache that doesn't go away, or any headache accompanied by blurred vision, slurred speech, or numbness
- Fainting, dizziness, heart palpitations, or a racing or pounding heart
- Breathlessness that comes on suddenly or is severe and accompanied by other symptoms (including worsening asthma, rapid breathing or pulse, pain, pallor, a bad or persistent cough, or a sense of apprehension)
- Severe constipation accompanied by abdominal pain, or severe diarrhea that lasts more than 24 hours
- Any health problem that you'd ordinarily call your practitioner about—even if it's not pregnancy-related (like a cold that gets worse rather than better)

YOUR HEALTH: WHAT TO DO NOW

Your body's just begun an amazing transformation, an exciting—and sometimes scary—process that will continue until the moment you give birth and beyond. It's normal to feel overwhelmed by the changes you're going through—and to have lots of questions about what's going on. In this chapter, you'll learn the best ways to take care of yourself and your growing baby, including what to expect at prenatal checkups, which tests and procedures are right for you, what's safe and what's not, and how to tell the difference between normal pregnancy aches and pains and those that require special attention.

Prenatal Care

Regular checkups are an essential part of a healthy pregnancy and can reduce your risk for problems. Choose a caregiver you like and respect from the get-go. The more confidence you have in her, the less anxious you'll be during the next nine months.

Which Type of Doctor or Midwife Is Best for You?

When it comes to choosing a prenatal care provider, you have four options: an obstetrician, a family physician, a certified nurse-midwife, or a direct-entry midwife. Who you settle on will depend on what kind of prenatal care you envision, the sort of birth experience you want, where you plan to deliver your baby, whether your pregnancy is normal or high risk, and what your insurance will pay for. Use the following guide to sort through the pros and cons of each option.

Obstetrician-Gynecologist

An ob-gyn (or OB) is a physician who specializes in women's reproductive health. She can handle all types of pregnancies, including those that develop complications, and she can perform cesarean sections. OBs who receive further training in high-risk pregnancies are called perinatologists or maternal-fetal medicine specialists. Not all gynecologists treat pregnant women. Before booking an appointment, be sure to ask if the doctor's practice includes obstetric care.

AN OB MAY BE FOR YOU IF . . .

- You're happy with your current ob-gyn and don't want or need to change.
- You have a chronic medical condition—such as high blood pressure, epilepsy, heart disease, diabetes, or certain other health problems—that puts your pregnancy in the high-risk category. (In that case, you may even need to see a perinatologist.)
- You discover that you're having twins or multiples (in which case you may need to see a perinatologist).
- Problems develop during your pregnancy (again, you may need to see a perinatologist).
- You know that you definitely want a hospital birth and you just feel more comfortable with a doctor.

POSSIBLE DRAWBACKS

- Your doctor may not have much time to spend with you at your prenatal appointments.
- Doctors may be more inclined to suggest routine interventions.

HOW TO DECIDE

- Interview several physicians before making your final choice.
- Make sure that you and your chosen doctor see eye-to-eye on labor and delivery issues. Find someone who will respect your wishes and will touch base with you before making decisions on your behalf.
- Ask which labor procedures—such as IVs or continuous electronic fetal monitoring—the doctor or hospital routinely requires.
- Find out under which circumstances she'll induce labor, how often and under what circumstances she does episiotomies, and when she thinks c-sections are warranted and how often she performs them. You can't pre-

BabyCenter Buzz

Why I Chose an OB

"I loved my ob-gyn (he actually delivered *me* 23 years ago!) and couldn't imagine going to anyone else for my first pregnancy." —*Laura*

"We couldn't afford any out-of-pocket costs, so we had to find someone covered by our insurance. For us, that meant choosing an OB. She was kind and reassuring when we went through a couple of unexpected complications." —*Beryl*

"Knowing that my OB could handle an emergency c-section if something went wrong was a big factor in my decision." —*Nicole*

"I knew for sure that I wanted an epidural and didn't really want or need someone to stay with me for my entire labor. I really liked my ob-gyn and didn't see any reason to go doctor shopping." —*Cara*

dict what your individual pregnancy or delivery will require, but you'll get an idea of the doctor's approach.

• See our physician interview worksheet (page 32) for a complete list of questions to ask.

Family Physician (FP)

An FP is a doctor who's qualified to care for patients of all ages. Family practice physicians are trained in obstetrics and gynecology in addition to pediatrics and primary care (though most don't continue to practice obstetrics after their training).

AN FP MAY BE FOR YOU IF . . .

• You like the family doctor you've been seeing for routine health care.

• Your FP has a lot of obstetric experience and routinely delivers babies.

• Your caregiver is well-versed in your medical and personal history and takes the time to answer your questions.

• You want someone who can continue to care for your whole family after you've given birth.

BabyCenter Buzz

Why I Chose a Family Practitioner

"We live in a rural area, and our family practitioner was our only choice. He's delivered just about every baby around here for 20 years, so I felt perfectly comfortable with him." —S

"Our family doctor knows us well. She cares for my husband, my 2-year-old, and me. It didn't make sense to find someone else to deliver our second child." —Jane

POSSIBLE DRAWBACKS

• Even if you already have a family practitioner you know and like, she may not be willing or able to care for you during your pregnancy. Not all FPs practice obstetrics; it's more common in rural areas.

• Not all FPs are trained to care for women with complicated pregnancies, and only a very small percentage can do c-sections. So if problems arise, you may need to be transferred to an OB.

HOW TO DECIDE

• Ask any FP you're considering if she has a backup obstetrician for consultation or referral in case pregnancy complications arise. Also, ask what she'll do if you need a c-section or if there are labor complications or other problems.

• Find out how much obstetrical training and experience she has.

• Make sure that you and your chosen doctor see eye to eye on labor-and-delivery issues. Discuss your preferences and see how she responds.

• Ask which labor procedures—such as IVs or continuous electronic fetal monitoring—the doctor or hospital routinely requires.

• Find out under which circumstances she'll induce labor, how often and under what circumstances she does episiotomies, and when she thinks c-sections are warranted and what percentage of patients in her care get them.

BY THE NUMBERS

Doctor Deliveries

Physician-attended births in 1975: **99%**

Physician-attended births in 2002: **91%**

Source: *Centers for Disease Control and Prevention*

BabyCenter Buzz

Why I Chose a Nurse-Midwife

"I didn't set out to choose a nurse-midwife, but my OB practice had one in their group, and she wound up being the one I saw most—and the one who spent the longest with me, who answered my questions the most thoroughly, who asked *me* questions about what was going on in my head and in my life, and who I just really connected with. Under her care, giving birth to my son was everything I'd hoped it would be. When I became pregnant with my second child, we'd moved 3,000 miles away—but I didn't blink before signing on with a nurse-midwife again." —*Leah*

"A friend who'd used a CNM raved about the care she got, so I decided to give it a try. Now I can't imagine going any other route, since my midwife was with me through my entire labor and birth." —*Georgia*

"I didn't want any pressure to have drugs or other interventions. I thought a midwife would be more likely to help me have the kind of natural birth I wanted." —*Cory*

Certified Nurse-Midwife (CNM)

A CNM is a professional educated in both nursing and midwifery who is certified by the American College of Nurse-Midwives (ACNM). All CNMs have completed an accredited midwifery program and passed a national certifying exam. They provide prenatal care and attend births primarily in hospitals, but also in birth centers and private homes. CNMs have safety records equal to those of physicians. They also provide routine gynecological care (such as performing Pap smears and prescribing birth control) and can continue to care for you after your pregnancy. About 7.6 percent of all births in the United States are attended by CNMs.

A CNM May Be for You If...

• You've been seeing a CNM for routine well-woman care and feel comfortable with her.

• You're in good health and at low risk for pregnancy complications. (If a problem does crop up, a CNM has a backup OB to call on.)

• You're looking for a practitioner who'll have more time to answer your questions than most physicians would.

• You want someone who's more likely to take a holistic approach to health care.

• You want a practitioner who is less likely to recommend routine labor interventions and who will treat you as an active participant in your own care.

• You want to give birth in a hospital but be attended by a midwife rather than a physician.

• You have your heart set on a natural birth in a comfortable setting, such as a birth center (page 369) or your home, with family and friends around. (In some communities, in-hospital birth centers are an option, too.)

• You want someone who'll support your desire for an unmedicated labor (but who can also arrange for an epidural if you give birth in a hospital).

POSSIBLE DRAWBACKS

• Some insurance plans don't cover CNMs. (In more than half the states, though, insurers and HMOs are required to cover CNM care and Medicaid coverage is mandatory in all 50 states.)

• If you develop complications during your pregnancy or labor, you may need to switch to an OB or a perinatologist.

HOW TO DECIDE

• Start by asking for recommendations from friends, neighbors, and coworkers who've used nurse-midwives. Childbirth educators can usually help you find a CNM in your community, too.

• If you want to deliver at a specific hospital or birth center, ask which nurse-midwives practice there.

• Interview several CNMs before making your choice.

• Make sure that you and your chosen CNM see eye-to-eye on labor and birth issues.

• Ask who her backup obstetrician is (you may want to meet her as well).

• Ask how she handles emergencies; if you're considering a home birth or a birth center, find out how far away the hospital is and whether she has privileges there in case you need to be transferred.

• See our midwife interview worksheet (page 36) for a complete list of questions.

BabyCenter Buzz 🧸

Why I Chose a Direct-Entry Midwife

"I wanted a home birth, and that's exactly what direct-entry midwives are trained to do." —*Mary*

A Direct-Entry Midwife

This type of midwife typically delivers babies at home, though some work in birth centers. She may have learned her skills through self-study, through apprenticeship, or at an independent midwifery school or college. Those who've met the standards for certification set by the North American Registry of Midwives (NARM) are called certified professional midwives (CPMs). A few direct-entry midwives are certified according to the requirements of the American College of Nurse-Midwives and are called certified midwives (CMs). Midwives who aren't certified or licensed are known as "lay" or "traditional" midwives. The practice of midwifery by direct-entry midwives (even CPMs) isn't legal in every state. Fewer than 0.5 percent of all births are attended by a direct-entry midwife.

Other Factors to Consider—No Matter Which Type of Caregiver You Choose

Depending on where you live and what type of health coverage you have, you may not be able to decide who'll deliver your baby. But if you do have a choice, keep in mind that the doctor or midwife your best friend raves about isn't necessarily the best match for *you*. In choosing a provider, you're also choosing the place where you'll give birth (page 369)—so when you look for a caregiver, you also need to think about whether you want to deliver in a hospital, in a birth center, or at home. Other things to keep in mind before making your decision:

Bedside manner: Does the doctor or midwife explain things clearly and seem up-to-date in her thinking? (Ask her opinion of a recent pregnancy-related issue you've read about in the news to gauge how well she keeps up on things.) Does she seem interested in you personally, or does she rarely look up from her charts or seem preoccupied?

Accessibility: Some practitioners return routine calls at a certain time each day, while others reserve a special line for messages or have nurses answer routine questions and act as a go-between for other information. Find out how easy it is to speak directly to the doctor or midwife if you have any important questions or are concerned that something is wrong. If it's an emergency or if you're in labor, find out how you'll get in touch with your practitioner at any time, day or night.

Practice size and type: Many group practices rotate on-call duty, so the likelihood that your regular doctor or midwife will be on call the day you go into labor may depend on how many caregivers there are in the practice. Also, some group practices have both doctors and midwives—so if you have a preference, find out if you can be assured you'll get the type of provider you want, even if you can't be promised a particular person. To minimize conflicts with another practitioner and increase your comfort level, try to meet all the partners in the practice and briefly communicate your needs and wishes to them. (When the time comes, a printed birth plan—page 378—is helpful in this regard.) If it's important for you to have your main caregiver deliver your baby, you may be happier with someone in a smaller practice, but even that doesn't guarantee she'll be there on labor day. No one person can be available 24 hours a day, 365 days a year.

Hospital: Before making your final decision, check out the hospital where the doctor or midwife has privileges so you're familiar with its requirements. Ask about policies on things that are important to you, such as the number of support people you can have with you during labor, 24-hour "rooming in" with your baby, securing a private room (if you don't want to share your space), accommodations for your partner, sibling policies, and visiting hours. Find out if the hospital has an anesthesiologist or anesthetist in-house, around the clock (if it doesn't, getting that epidural you have your heart set on may be easier said than done). Ideally, you should be comfortable with the hospital as well as with the practitioner, and both should be within a reasonable distance of home.

Birth center: If you're thinking of going this route, arrange a visit to the birth center. Most offer some kind of tour so you can see the center, meet some of the staff, and learn about their philosophy of care. Look for a birth center that's accredited by the National Association of Childbearing Centers (NACC).

Fees and insurance: Get a breakdown of your practitioner's and the hospital or birth center's fees, and find out what—and who—is covered by your health insurance plan.

Attitude: Consider what kind of labor and postpartum experience you'd like to have and then find out what the practitioner's perspective is on key issues. Things to consider: breastfeeding, pain relief during labor, interventions (like episiotomies, routine IVs, and continuous fetal monitoring), and the presence of fathers, partners, or coaches in labor.

Your First Prenatal Checkup

At your first prenatal visit—usually when you're around week 8—your doctor or midwife will ask about your medical history as well as any concerns you may have, so come prepared. At this appointment, your caregiver will:

Take your health history. She'll want to know when your last period started so she can determine your due date, any symptoms or problems you've had since then, whether your menstrual cycles are regular and how long they usually last, and details about any gynecological problems (including sexually transmitted infections) you have now or had in the past. She'll also want to know all the details of any prior pregnancies. She'll review other medical history—such as drug allergies, psychiatric problems, and any past surgeries or hospitalizations—and ask you about lifestyle issues, such as smoking or drinking, that may affect your pregnancy.

Take your family health history. Your doctor or midwife will ask if any of your relatives or your baby's father or his relatives have any chronic or serious diseases. Many health problems are hereditary, so knowing your family's medical history will help your provider stay on the lookout for potential problems.

Do a genetic and birth defect screening. She'll want to know if you, your baby's father, or anyone else in either family has a chromosomal or genetic disorder or was born with another birth defect. She'll want to know, too, about all the medications and nutritional supplements you've taken since your last period, any potential toxic exposures you've had, and whether you've recently had any rashes or viruses or other infections. If you're going to be 35 or older on your due date or you have any other risk factors for genetic problems, your provider will talk to you about genetic counseling and genetic testing.

Check you out and run some tests. Your practitioner will give you a thorough physical, including a pelvic exam. And unless you've recently had one, she'll take a Pap smear to test for abnormal cells and cervical cancer. She might also do a culture to check for chlamydia and gonorrhea. Next, she'll order routine blood tests to identify your blood type and Rh factor and to check for anemia. She'll also have the lab test your blood for syphilis, for hepatitis B, and for immunity to German measles (rubella), and offer to test for HIV. If your caregiver doesn't offer you an HIV test and you want one, ask for it. Being treated for HIV during pregnancy can dramatically reduce your chances of passing the infection to your baby. Depending on your ethnic background and medical history, you may also be tested for sickle-cell disease, Tay-Sachs disease, cystic fibrosis, and thalassemia. If you're at high risk for gestational diabetes, you might have a glucose challenge test done at the first visit. In some cases, your provider may also do a skin test to see if you've been exposed to tuberculosis. Finally, she'll ask for a urine sample to check for signs of kidney problems, urinary tract infections, and other conditions.

Counsel you and let you know what's coming. Before you leave, your caregiver should give you advice about eating right and gaining weight, describe the common discomforts of early pregnancy, talk about the benefits of getting a flu shot and warn you about symptoms that require immediate attention. She'll also talk to you about the dangers of smoking, drinking alcohol, using drugs, or taking certain medications. She should also highlight the do's and don'ts of exercise, travel, and sex during pregnancy and discuss environmental and occupational hazards that may affect your baby (including how to avoid toxoplasmosis). She should ask you about domestic violence—if you have ever been or are currently a victim of abuse. Finally, she'll let you know about prenatal tests that you may want to consider.

First-Trimester Prenatal Tests

Here's a look at the routine lab tests you can expect to be offered in early pregnancy and the other first-trimester tests you may need.

Blood Tests

Your practitioner can find out a lot about your health by analyzing a sample of your blood. You can expect the following blood tests at your first prenatal visit:

(continued on page 34)

INTERVIEWING THE DOCTOR

Use this list to help you choose an obstetrician or family physician. Most doctors limit consultation to 15 minutes, so ask your most important questions first and save fee and insurance issues for the office manager or the billing department. If you go over 15 minutes, the doctor may charge a fee.

THE BASICS

How long have you been practicing obstetrics?

How many babies have you delivered?

How much time do you allow for each prenatal visit?

How long is the average wait in your office?

What percentage of your own patients do you deliver in a month? _____%

How can I reach you in an emergency?

Are you in a solo or group practice? solo/group

If you're solo, who covers for you when you're not available?

If you're in a group practice, how often will I see other doctors?

Where do you have admitting privileges?

PRENATAL CARE

What prenatal tests do you routinely recommend?

What if I have a concern about a specific test?

How much experience do you have with high-risk pregnancies?

If my pregnancy becomes high-risk, what changes might I expect in my prenatal care?

LABOR AND DELIVERY

What kind of childbirth classes do you recommend?

Will you help me develop a birth plan?

At what point in my labor do you come to the hospital, and who will be in charge of my care until then?

What do you suggest to help me deal with labor pain?

What procedures do you routinely employ during labor and delivery (that is, enemas, continuous fetal monitoring, IVs, episiotomies, and so on)?

What if I don't want them?

What percentage of your patients have forceps- or vacuum-assisted deliveries? _____%

What percentage of your patients have episiotomies? _____%

What percentage of your patients end up with c-sections? _____%

Do you encourage vaginal birth after cesarean (VBAC)?

What percentage of your patients who've had prior C-sections attempt VBAC? _____%

What's your rate of success with VBAC? (Sixty to 80 percent is the norm.) _____%

Is an anesthesiologist (or anesthetist) available in the hospital around the clock if I want an epidural, attempt a VBAC, or need an emergency c-section?

FOR OBSTETRICIANS

Are you a board-certified ob-gyn?

If you're seeing a perinatologist: Are you board-certified in maternal-fetal medicine?

FOR FAMILY PHYSICIANS

Have you had extra training in obstetrics beyond your family medicine residency?

If I have complications you don't handle, who's your backup obstetrician?

Do you perform c-sections?

If you don't do c-sections yourself, is there an obstetrician available in the hospital around the clock should I need an emergency c-section?

POSTPARTUM

Will I be separated from my baby after birth?

If so, when and for how long?

Can my baby room in with me if I choose this option?

Do you or someone on the staff assist with breastfeeding questions or problems?

If I deliver a boy whom I want to have circumcised, will you perform the procedure?

QUESTIONS TO ASK YOURSELF

Did you feel comfortable with the doctor?

Why or why not?

If you attended the interview with your partner, did the doctor make an effort to include both of you in the conversation?

Is the office conveniently located?

How long were you kept waiting? _____ minutes

How helpful were the nurses and support staff at the office?

QUICK TIP

Minimize Your Time in the Waiting Room

Most pregnancy practitioners' offices are incredibly busy, and waits of up to an hour for scheduled appointments aren't unheard of. You'll get in to see your caregiver sooner if you schedule your appointments for first thing in the morning or right after lunch— that way, there's no backlog of patients still waiting to be seen. If that's not possible, call your doctor or midwife's office before you leave to see if they're running on schedule.

BLOOD TYPE AND RH FACTOR AND ANTIBODY SCREENING

In addition to checking your blood type (A, B, AB, or O), your practitioner will also want to know if your blood is Rh negative. If you're Rh negative, you'll get a shot of Rh immune globulin at least once in your pregnancy, and after delivery if your baby turns out to be Rh positive. This will protect you from developing antibodies that could be dangerous during this or later pregnancies. (*Note:* If your baby's father is also Rh negative, then Rh immune globulin won't be necessary.)

BLOOD COUNT

A complete blood count will tell your practitioner if you have too little hemoglobin in your red blood cells (a sign of anemia) and, if so, whether it's likely due to iron deficiency. If you're iron deficient, she may recommend iron supplements and iron-rich foods, such as lean meat. The test also checks your white blood cell and platelet counts.

GERMAN MEASLES (RUBELLA) IMMUNITY

This test looks for antibodies (and thus immunity) to the rubella virus. Luckily, the vast majority of women are immune because they either were vaccinated or had the disease as a child. If you're *not* immune and contract rubella during pregnancy, it can lead to miscarriage, stillbirth, or serious birth defects.

CHICKEN POX IMMUNITY

If you haven't been vaccinated against it or aren't sure if you've ever had chicken pox, some providers will also test you for immunity to the disease, which can cause complications during pregnancy.

HEPATITIS B TESTING

Many women with this chronic liver disease have no symptoms and can unknowingly pass it along to their babies. If you're a carrier, your caregiver will protect your baby by giving him injections of hepatitis B immunoglobulin as well as the standard hep B vaccine right after birth.

Just for Dad

Should You Go to Prenatal Checkups?

Yes—as often as you can. Being by your partner's side during these appointments is a great way to show her your support and to learn about pregnancy, birth, and your developing baby. At the very least, be there for important milestones and tests, like the first appointment (when you'll be asked about your family health history), hearing the baby's heartbeat (around week 11), and the ultrasound or amniocentesis.

How Often Dads Attend Prenatal Appointments

37%   attend every one
21%   go most of the time
15%   come along sometimes
21%   rarely show up
 6%   never attend prenatal appointments with their partners

Source: A BabyCenter.com poll of more than 7,600 pregnant women

HIV Testing

Counseling and testing for the human immunodeficiency virus is recommended for all pregnant women. If you test positive, you can get treatment that greatly reduces the chance that you'll pass the disease on to your baby.

Syphilis Screening

This sexually transmitted infection is rare, but if you have syphilis and don't treat it, both you and your baby can develop serious problems. In the unlikely event that you test positive, you'll be given antibiotics to treat the infection.

Urine Tests

At your first prenatal visit, you'll be asked to wipe carefully with an antiseptic pad and pee into a sterile cup. Your urine will then be checked for bacteria and other abnormalities, even if you don't feel like you have a bladder infection. About 10 percent of women have bladder or urinary tract infections with no symptoms. It's important to identify and treat these infections when you're pregnant.

At the rest of your prenatal visits, your caregiver or her assistant (or

(continued on page 38)

INTERVIEWING THE MIDWIFE

Use this list to help you choose a midwife. Many midwives limit consultations to 15 minutes, so bring up your most important concerns first and save insurance and fee questions for the office manager or the billing department. If your conversation takes longer than 15 minutes, she may charge a fee. Also, if you have a health condition or other potential complication, tell the midwife before you make an appointment. If you're interested in an out-of-hospital birth, find out in advance whether she attends them.

THE BASICS

How long have you been practicing, and in what settings?

How many babies have you delivered?

How many babies do you deliver in a month?

Did you graduate from a nationally accredited midwifery education program? Which one?

Are you certified by the American College of Nurse-Midwives?

Are you licensed by the state?

How much time do you allow for each prenatal visit?

How long is the average wait in your office?

How can I reach you in an emergency?

Who's your backup obstetrician?

Are you in a solo or group practice?

If you're solo, who covers for you when you're not available?

If you're in a group practice, how often will I see other practitioners?

Do you have hospital admitting privileges? If so, where?

Do you do birth center deliveries? Is the center accredited by the NACC?

Do you attend home births?

PRENATAL CARE

What prenatal tests do you routinely recommend?

What if I have a concern about a specific test?

Can you give me some examples of when you might manage my care jointly with a physician or transfer me to a doctor?

LABOR AND DELIVERY

What kind of childbirth classes do you recommend?

Will you help me develop a birth plan?

Will you meet me at the hospital when I'm first admitted? If not, who will be in charge of my care until then?

Do you stay with me throughout labor?

What labor-pain options will be available to me?

Do you (or any hospital policies) require that I have continuous fetal monitoring, IVs, or other interventions?

What percentage of your patients have episiotomies? _____%

What percentage of your patients end up having forceps- or vacuum- assisted deliveries? _____% c-sections? _____%

If I have complications or need a c-section, who's your backup OB?

Are there an anesthesiologist and an obstetrician in the hospital around the clock should I need an emergency c-section?

If I needed a c-section, would you stay with me during the procedure?

Do you encourage vaginal birth after cesarean (VBAC)?

What percentage of your patients who've had prior c-sections attempt VBAC? _____%

What's your rate of success with VBAC? (60 to 80 percent is the norm.) _____%

For birth centers and home birth midwives: Do you have admitting privileges at the backup hospital so you can take care of me if I need to be transferred?

If not, are you allowed to accompany me if I need to be transferred?

POSTPARTUM

Will I be separated from my baby after birth?

If so, when, why, and for how long?

Can my baby room in with me if I choose this option?

Will you, or someone on your staff, teach me how to breastfeed?

If I deliver a boy whom I want to have circumcised, will you perform the procedure?

QUESTIONS TO ASK YOURSELF

Did you feel comfortable with the midwife?

If you attended the interview with your partner, did the midwife make an effort to include both of you in the conversation?

Is the office conveniently located?

How long were you kept waiting? _____ minutes

How helpful was the support staff at the office?

perhaps even you!) will do a series of quick dipstick tests to check for a variety of conditions. Here's what your practitioner's looking for:

SUGAR

Although an occasional slight increase in the amount of sugar in your urine isn't unusual during pregnancy, a urine sugar level that's high and *stays* high could be a red flag for gestational diabetes.

PROTEIN

Excess protein in your urine can signal a urinary tract infection. Later in pregnancy, protein in your urine—along with high blood pressure—is a sign of preeclampsia.

KETONES

Ketones are produced when your body starts breaking down stored fat for energy. If you're having severe nausea and vomiting or if you've lost weight since you got pregnant, your practitioner may check your urine for ketones. If the ketone reading is high and you can't keep any food or liquid down, you'll need intravenous fluids and medications. Ketones in combination with sugar can signal diabetes.

BLOOD CELLS OR BACTERIA

Blood cells or nitrites (produced by certain bacteria) in your urine can signal a urinary tract infection. In that case, you'll need a urine culture to check for infection and to pinpoint the best type of antibiotics to treat it.

BabyCenter Buzz

How I Cope with My Needle Phobia

"Ask for a butterfly needle (it's smaller and less painful than the regular kind). Lie down and prop your feet up. Ask someone to come along and distract you."
—*Jenny*

"Request the most experienced nurse or lab technician, and remember the spot where she finds the best vein so there will be no need for future 'searches.'"
—*Andrea*

Ultrasound

WHAT: An ultrasound (sometimes called a sonogram) is a noninvasive diagnostic test that your practitioner will use to see your baby and gather valuable information about his health.

WHO: Women who aren't sure exactly when they conceived or whose practitioners have questions or concerns about the pregnancy or the developing baby.

WHEN: Most women have a routine ultrasound between 18 and 20 weeks—but you can have one at any time, depending on the particulars of your situation.

WHY: Your practitioner may recommend a first-trimester ultrasound to:

Date your pregnancy. If you have irregular cycles or if you're not sure when your last period started, an early ultrasound will reveal how far along you really are. Taking certain measurements can help your doctor or midwife pinpoint the baby's gestational age (and thus your due date) within three or four days.

Check for more than one baby. If you got pregnant with the help of fertility treatments, or if you're simply measuring large for your stage, there's a chance you're carrying twins or more. An ultrasound will let your practitioner know for sure.

Confirm or rule out miscarriage or ectopic pregnancy. If you have vaginal bleeding or severe abdominal pain or cramping, your practitioner may be concerned about miscarriage (page 543) or ectopic pregnancy (page 546) and will schedule an ultrasound to check on you and your baby.

To assist with other tests. If you choose to have a test called the nuchal fold scan or a diagnostic test called chorionic villus sampling (CVS), an ultrasound will help your practitioner collect the information she needs.

HOW: A trained sonographer will place a handheld device on your belly (or, more likely in early pregnancy, in your vagina). The device sends out sound waves, which bounce off solid masses within your body to form a picture of your baby, uterus, and surrounding organs. That picture can be seen on a nearby computer monitor.

Genetic Tests

Depending on your personal or family health history (or, for certain tests, on your race or ethnicity), your doctor or midwife may offer you one or more of the following genetic tests.

Just the Facts

Genetic Counseling

A genetic counselor is a medical professional who can help you sort through complex information about your chances of having a child with a genetic disorder or birth defect, as well as help you navigate the testing, treatment, and other options available to you. Your pregnancy caregiver may refer you to a genetic counselor if you'll be 35 or older when your baby is due or if you have other risk factors for giving birth to a child with chromosomal abnormalities or other problems. Though being referred for genetic counseling is understandably nerve-racking, many couples find that the information they get from a genetic counselor is reassuring rather than alarming.

Screening tests help determine your potential risk for carrying a baby with genetic problems such as Down syndrome or inherited genetic disorders. *Diagnostic* tests help confirm—or rule out—suspected genetic problems.

Blood Tests for Specific Genetic Disorders

If you fall into a high-risk category for certain genetic disorders, your practitioner should recommend that you be screened for them as early as possible in your pregnancy. This will give you time to talk to a genetic counselor and figure out if you want to go forward with diagnostic testing like CVS or amniocentesis.

CYSTIC FIBROSIS SCREENING

Your practitioner may offer to screen you and your mate for the genetic mutations that cause cystic fibrosis (CF). CF is a very serious (and frequently fatal) disease of the mucus and sweat glands that makes breathing and digestion difficult. Until recently, CF screening was offered only to couples with a family history of the disease, but experts now recommend that all Caucasian parents-to-be (who are at higher risk of the disease than other groups) be offered screening, too—as should other couples who request it. (Whether or not you take the test is a personal choice.) If you *and* your partner carry the gene for this disease, you may decide to undergo a diagnostic test such as CVS or amniocentesis to find out if your baby is affected.

SICKLE-CELL SCREENING

You may be offered a blood test to screen for the gene that causes sickle-cell disease, a debilitating red blood cell disorder—particularly if you're of African, Caribbean, South or Central American, Mediterranean, Indian, or Arabian descent. If you're a carrier (in other words, if you have sickle-cell trait), your partner will be tested as well. If you *and* your partner are carriers (or your partner is a carrier of a related blood disorder), your practitioner will suggest further testing to find out if your baby will be affected.

TAY-SACHS SCREENING

If you're a descendant of Central or Eastern European (Ashkenazi) Jews or of French Canadian, Cajun, or perhaps Irish ancestry, your practitioner will recommend screening for the gene that causes Tay-Sachs, a fatal disease of the central nervous system. (Ashkenazi Jews are also at risk for carrying the gene that causes another severe central nervous system disorder called Canavan disease and can be screened for that as well.) If you *and* your partner carry the gene, your caregiver will recommend further testing to find out if your baby is affected.

THALASSEMIA SCREENING

Thalassemia encompasses a varied group of inherited blood disorders that affect people of Italian, Greek, Turkish, Middle Eastern, Southeast Asian, Southern Asian, Chinese, Indian, and African ancestry. If you have a family history of this disease, your practitioner will screen you for the gene that causes it. People who have the thalassemia trait may have a mild form of anemia called thalassemia minor. If your initial blood count shows that your red blood cells are small (but your iron status is normal), a special test will be done to check for the thalassemia trait. If you have it, your partner should be tested as well. If you and your partner are carriers (or if your partner is a carrier for another red blood cell disorder, such

---

BY THE NUMBERS

Cystic Fibrosis Stats
Chance that your baby will develop CF if you *and* your partner are carriers: **1 in 4**

Sickle-Cell Stats
Chance that your baby will develop sickle-cell disease if you *and* your partner are carriers: **1 in 4**

Tay-Sachs Stats
Chance that your baby will develop Tay-Sachs if you *and* your partner are carriers: **1 in 4**

Sources: *March of Dimes; National Institutes of Health; March of Dimes, National Tay-Sachs and Allied Diseases Association*

Just the Facts

First trimester combined screening

Another test, called first trimester combined screening (sometimes called the ultra-screen), combines the nuchal fold measurement with two blood tests, thereby assessing the risk for Down syndrome more accurately than other available screening tests. (But it's still an *estimate* of risk and not a definitive diagnosis.) As with nuchal fold screening, the combined screening isn't yet available everywhere.

as sickle-cell disease), your practitioner will advise further testing to see if your baby is affected.

Screening Tests for Chromosomal Abnormalities

In addition to screening for genetic disorders, which tend to be inherited, you may also be offered screening for certain chromosomal problems, which involve abnormalities in the number or structure of your baby's chromosomes. These types of disorders include "trisomies" (three chromosomes instead of the normal two at a certain point in the DNA chain that forms your baby's physiological blueprint) such as Down syndrome (trisomy 21) and Edward's syndrome (trisomy 18).

NUCHAL FOLD SCAN

WHAT: Also known as the nuchal translucency screening test ("nuchal" refers to the neck), this test measures the clear space in the "nuchal fold" at the back of your developing baby's neck. Babies with Down syndrome and some other chromosomal abnormalities tend to have more fluid in this spot during the first trimester, causing the clear space to be larger. The nuchal fold test can be combined with a blood test to increase its detection role for chromosomal anomalies.

WHO: This noninvasive screening test may be offered to women of all ages, but it's not yet available everywhere.

WHEN: Once, between 11 and 14 weeks.

WHY: Like any screening test, this one won't give you a definite diagnosis, but it can help you decide whether to undergo further testing. And unlike diagnostic tests such as CVS, it's painless and noninvasive.

HOW: Done during an ultrasound, this test simply involves taking one extra measurement of your developing baby.

Diagnostic Tests for Chromosomal and Genetic Abnormalities
CHORIONIC VILLUS SAMPLING (CVS)

WHAT: This test examines fetal cells collected from the tiny fingerlike projections (called chorionic villi) on your placenta to detect chromosomal abnormalities and some genetic disorders. One advantage of CVS is that it can be done several weeks before amniocentesis (page 154), a more commonly used technique that's performed in the second trimester.

WHO: Your practitioner may offer CVS if you're going to be 35 or older on your due date, if you've previously conceived a baby with a chromosomal problem or other birth defect, if an earlier screening test indicate an increased risk of a genetic problem, or if you or your partner has a family history of inherited genetic disorders.

WHEN: Generally at 10 to 12 weeks (though it's occasionally done as late as 13 weeks).

WHY: CVS can detect hundreds of genetic disorders and chromosomal abnormalities. There are certain disorders that everyone gets tested for, such as Down syndrome, and others—such as Tay-Sachs, cystic fibrosis, and sickle-cell disease—that your practitioner will look for only if your ethnic background, family history, or prior screening tests warrants it. That said, CVS isn't for everyone. Some women at risk for having a baby with genetic problems opt instead for amniocentesis in the second trimester, and others choose to bypass invasive testing altogether. Meeting with a genetic counselor will help you sort through your options.

HOW: First, you'll get an ultrasound to confirm how far along you are and to make sure that collecting a good sample is possible. Then, depending on where the placenta is attached to your uterus, the doctor doing the procedure will use either a thin catheter to withdraw chorionic villus cells through your cervix or a needle to collect the sample through your abdomen.

For the more common cervical pro-

BY THE NUMBERS

CVS Stats

Risk of miscarriage from CVS:	**1 to 2%**
Accuracy of CVS:	**more than 99%**
Wait for results:	**7 to 10 days**

Source: *March of Dimes*

QUICK TIP

How to Minimize the Risks of CVS

Make sure the doctor performing the test is experienced. Your best bet is to find someone who does at least 50 CVS procedures a year and is expert at both the transcervical and transabdominal procedures so she can choose the route that's safest for you. Ask your practitioner or a genetic counselor for a recommendation. Finally, make sure that an experienced registered diagnostic medical sonographer provides continuous ultrasound guidance during the procedure. This greatly increases the odds that the doctor will be able to collect enough sample tissue on the first try, so you won't have to repeat the procedure.

cedure, she'll swab your vagina and cervix with antiseptic (to prevent bacteria from being carried by the catheter into your uterus, where it could cause an infection). Next, she'll thread the catheter through your cervix, then use gentle suction to collect a sample from your placenta (many women say this feels similar to getting a Pap smear). For the abdominal procedure, the doctor will numb a spot on your belly with local anesthetic. Then she'll insert a long needle through your skin, muscle, and uterine wall to extract the sample.

Either way, the amniotic sac where your baby is growing won't be disturbed. When the doctor's done, she'll check your baby's heartbeat via sonogram. Though CVS might hurt a little, it's over relatively quickly, taking no longer than a half-hour from start to finish, with the extraction itself running only a few minutes.

You'll need to take it easy immediately after the test, so arrange for someone to drive you home. Then rest for the remainder of the day and abstain from strenuous physical activity, sex, and exercise for three days. You may have some cramping and light bleeding, which is normal, but report it to your caregiver anyway.

Common Symptoms and Complaints

There's no getting around it: Pregnancy brings about dramatic changes, and your body will most likely behave in a series of bewildering new ways over the course of the next nine months. Some of these changes are obvious (your growing belly and baby), while others are invisible (rising levels of pregnancy hormones). But both types of changes can lead to a host of *other* symptoms. Some—such as filling out your bra like you never have before—

are a pleasant surprise, while others—like headaches and vomiting—can be downright annoying or sometimes even signal more serious problems. A guide to common early pregnancy complaints—and tips for making them more bearable:

Surprising Ways Pregnancy Affects Your Body

You can't expect to grow a new human being without a little collateral damage to yourself! Here's a look at three physical changes caused by pregnancy and the unexpected symptoms they cause.:

• **Pregnancy hormones surge.** Your hormone levels are rising dramatically. The combined effect is that you really *aren't* yourself, at least hormonally speaking. Estrogen, for instance, helps maintain your pregnancy and triggers fetal maturation—but it's also to blame for breasts so tender they feel like they've been punched every time your arm brushes against them and for your sudden aversion to the smell of your partner's deodorant. Progesterone wards off contractions—but it makes things sluggish elsewhere in your body, too. And relaxin helps loosen the connective tissue in your pelvis so your baby will have room to pass through—but it may also loosen other joints, making you feel more like Jim Carrey than Nicole Kidman, and leaving you more vulnerable to injury.

• **Your heart rate increases, and your circulatory system expands.** The amount of blood circulating through your body rises by as much as 45 percent during pregnancy (all the better to deliver nutrients and oxygen to your developing baby, and to make up for the blood you'll lose on delivery day). But these changes can also play a role in some of the symptoms you may experience during your pregnancy, from nosebleeds to swelling ankles.

• **Your uterus expands.** As your pregnancy progresses and your womb grows up and out of your pelvis, it will push, pull, and weigh on other organs in your abdomen and groin—leading to abdominal aches, pains, and other strange sensations.

Early-Pregnancy Symptoms and How to Cope

Bleeding Gums

When you're pregnant, increased progesterone and estrogen levels and changes in your blood vessels can make your gums extra-sensitive to the

QUICK TIP

Rh Alert

If your blood is Rh negative (page 34), you'll need a shot of Rh immunoglobulin after having CVS because a tiny bit of your baby's blood may have mixed with yours during the procedure, possibly triggering an immune system response.

bacteria in plaque—resulting in swollen, tender gums that may bleed when you brush or floss. This problem, known as "pregnancy gingivitis," affects half of all pregnant women.

If pregnancy gingivitis persists and isn't treated by a dentist, it can sometimes progress to a more serious condition called periodontitis, in which the infection spreads into the bone and other tissue that support your teeth. Research has found that pregnant women with periodontal disease are seven times more likely to have a premature baby (page 440). If you do develop periodontitis, getting treated can significantly reduce your risk. Pregnant periodontitis sufferers who are treated with a plaque-and-tartar-removal procedure known as "scaling and root planing" have far fewer preterm babies than untreated women. What's more, other research has shown a link between periodontitis and preeclampsia (page 531), though it's unclear whether the gum disease *causes* the preeclampsia or if there's another factor to blame for both conditions.

In rare cases, you may develop a nodule on your gums during pregnancy that bleeds when you brush. These "pregnancy tumors," or "pyogenic granulomas," can grow up to three-quarters of an inch in size. The nodule is generally painless and harmless and usually disappears after delivery. But if it causes you discomfort, interferes with chewing or brushing, or starts to bleed excessively, you can have it removed. (If you notice a lump or bump on your gums, no matter how painless, point it out to your dentist.)

To care for your teeth during pregnancy:

• Gently brush at least twice a day (after every meal, if possible), for five minutes at a time, using a soft-bristled brush and fluoride toothpaste.

• Floss daily and rinse your mouth well with water or an antimicrobial rinse after flossing.

• Get regular dental care. Your dentist or periodontist can remove plaque and tartar that brushing can't get to. If you haven't seen your dentist recently, schedule a visit now for a thorough cleaning and checkup. Let her know that you're pregnant and how far along you are. She'll likely want to see you once more during your pregnancy (or even more frequently if you already have gum disease, because pregnancy is likely to exacerbate the problem).

• Schedule a dental appointment right away if you have a toothache or if your gums are bleeding frequently and causing you pain. Also call if you have any other signs of gum disease, such as swollen, tender, or receding gums; persistent bad breath; or loosening teeth. If you notice a growth in your mouth, don't wait to have it checked out.

Bloating, Gassiness, and Indigestion

Don't be surprised if you find yourself belching like a champion beer guzzler or having to unbutton your pants many weeks before you're actually showing. Your symptoms are caused mainly by increases in progesterone, a hormone that relaxes the smooth muscles throughout your body—including those in your gastrointestinal tract. This slows digestion, in turn causing gas, bloating, burping, flatulence, and generally miserable sensations in your gut, especially after a big meal.

To help prevent gas, have four or five small meals a day, instead of three large ones, and eat them slowly. Drink lots of water between, not during, meals. Exercise to help keep your digestive tract moving. Try to avoid gulping air. Eat plenty of foods rich in fiber, like wheat bran. (Be careful, though: Some high-fiber foods, like oat bran, can actually *cause* gas.). If you're really uncomfortable, ask your caregiver about trying an over-the-counter, simethicone-based gas-relief remedy, like Gas-X or GasAid.

When a gas attack strikes, get moving. Many women find that some form of exercise or stretching helps release the gas from their bodies. Try getting on your hands and knees and arching and flexing your back. If that doesn't work, wiggle or dance around.

Breast Tenderness, Growth, and Other Changes

Breast tenderness is one of the earliest hallmarks of pregnancy, usually starting around four to six weeks and lasting through the first trimester or beyond. Your breasts may feel swollen, sore, tingly, and unusually sensitive to touch—similar to how they feel before your period, but much more in-

Just the Facts

Gassy Foods

Avoiding foods that cause gas seems like a no-brainer, but the list of gas producers is so long that if you eliminated every one of them, you'd put your diet in jeopardy. And every body is different. What causes your gas might be completely different from what causes another woman's. Here's a list of some of the most common culprits. To get to the bottom of your gas problem, eliminate one group of food at a time. If you feel better, add items back in one at a time until you isolate your personal offenders.

- Asparagus, beans, brussels sprouts, broccoli, cabbage, cauliflower
- Candy or gum sweetened with sorbitol
- Milk and dairy products, especially if you're lactose intolerant. You'll need to substitute other calcium- and protein-rich fare, if you eliminate this group from your diet.
- High-fiber foods like oat bran (wheat bran is okay)
- Artichokes, onions, and some fruits, like pears
- Certain starches, like pasta and potatoes (rice is okay)
- Carbonated drinks and fruit drinks sweetened with fructose

tense. This is probably due to increased blood flow as well as tissue changes—spurred by rising hormone levels—that help prepare your breasts for making milk.

You may be expecting your breasts to get bigger during pregnancy, but many women are surprised by how early they start seeing their chests grow. Breast blossoming usually begins in the first trimester, sometimes even within the first weeks of pregnancy. How much bigger will you get? Most women go up at least one cup size during the course of their pregnancy. (On the other hand, don't worry if your breasts don't seem to be growing much— that's normal, too, and has no bearing on your ability to breastfeed.)

Bigger breasts mean you'll likely need new bras. You may also experience these changes: itching and possibly stretch marks as a result of skin stretching, more visible veins, bigger and darker nipples and areolas (the pigmented skin around your nipples), and more pronounced bumps on your areolas (oil-producing glands called Montgomery's tubercles).

BabyCenter Buzz

"The Boom–Bust Cycle"

"Believe it or not, I actually wore my most comfortable bra to *bed*. I found that any sort of jiggling movement caused incredible discomfort during those early weeks—so the bra stayed on 24/7." —*Leanne*

"I went from a small B to a C cup during my first pregnancy, then went back to normal after weaning. My breasts stayed small when I was pregnant with my second, though, which worried me until my daughter was born. They may not have grown much, but they made plenty of milk!" —*Marie*

If your newly voluptuous form requires a new bra, keep these tips in mind:

• Try a variety of maternity bras, which offer the extra support you need and are specially designed for your pregnant body.

• Pass up bras with underwires, which may be too binding now.

• Think carefully before buying a front-clasp or O-ring bra. It may feel fine now, but as your abdomen expands, you'll likely find the clasp or ring digging into your rib cage.

• Cotton bras are more comfortable and breathable than synthetic ones. To prevent chafing, look for soft, smooth material with no seams near the nipple to prevent chafing.

• For nighttime, try a pregnancy sleep bra—a soft, nonrestrictive cotton bra that provides gentle support.

• When you work out, you'll need a snug exercise bra to provide additional support and minimize painful bouncing.

• Check your size. Just because you were a 34B six months ago doesn't mean you're one now. (Plus, pregnant or not, most women wear the wrong bra size to begin with.) To pinpoint your true size: Measure around your chest, just under your breasts; then add 5 inches. This is your band size. (For example, 31 inches plus 5 inches equals 36.) Next, measure around the fullest part of your breasts. Now subtract your chest measurement from this number. If there's a 1-inch difference, you're an A cup; 2 inches is a B, 3 inches is a C, 4 inches is a D, 5 inches is a DD, and so on. (So if your chest measurement is 31 and your breast measurement is 34, you're a 36C.)

• Buy bras with a bit of room to grow, since your breasts will continue to swell, and your rib cage will expand throughout pregnancy. If you can, buy the cup a little on the big side, though not so much so that the material creases or puckers when it should lie flat. Although it's still a bit early, you could pick up a nursing bra with several different hook closures for the cup, which you can adjust as you need. For the band size, buy bras that fit when the clasp is on the tightest setting, so you have room to let them out.

Breathlessness

Right now, you may be feeling as if you can't get enough air. This sensation of breathlessness probably comes from your need to breathe rather than from your actually being out of breath. Rising hormone levels, particularly progesterone, affect your lungs directly and also stimulate the respiratory center in your brain. The number of *breaths* you take each minute has actually changed very little—but the amount of air you take in with each breath increases significantly as your pregnancy progresses.

Constipation

If it's any consolation, constipation is par for the course during pregnancy—at least half of all pregnant women report bouts of it. In your first trimester, the main culprit is rising levels of progesterone, which makes your digestion sluggish. Later in pregnancy, the pressure of your growing uterus on your intestines and rectum, along with extra iron you may need to take for anemia (page 163), can also make you feel stopped up.

To help you stay "regular":

• Eat high-fiber foods such as cereals, whole-grain breads, and fresh fruits and vegetables every day. Add a couple of tablespoons of unprocessed wheat bran (available at health food stores) to your cereal in the morning and follow it with a glass of water.

• Drink eight 8-ounce glasses of water a day. Fruit juice, especially prune juice, can also help.

• Exercise regularly. Walking, swimming, stationary cycling, and yoga can all help ease constipation.

• Never "hold it"—doing so can cause your bowels to get backed up.

• Try a warm beverage when you first get up in the morning—it might stimulate your bowels.

Enjoy a **FREE** Subscription to BabyCenter's magazine

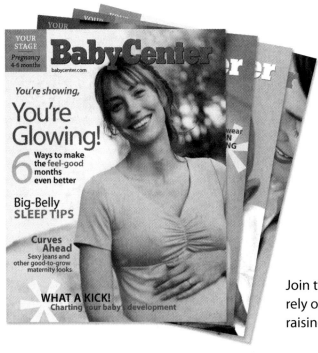

Get our magazine and enjoy:

- **Timely and relevant articles** for exactly where you are in your pregnancy
- **Features of real moms** sharing their stories, tips and insights
- **Multiple expert opinions** on various topics, so you can choose what works for you
- A new issue delivered to your home **every three months**
- Content from the award-winning editors at BabyCenter.com

Join the millions of parents who rely on BabyCenter for guidance raising healthy, happy families.

>> **Subscribing is easy!**
Go to **www.babycenter.com** or mail in the card below

Sign me up for a FREE Subscription to BabyCenter's magazine!

Name

Address 1

Address 2

City   State

Zip Code

Due Date

or Baby's birth date

E-mail address

• Try an over-the-counter psyllium-fiber supplement, or ask your provider to recommend a bulk-forming supplement or a stool softener.

Cramps

You may feel a faint crampy or "stretching" sensation early in your pregnancy, or you may notice a bit of brief cramping during or right after orgasm. As long as it's mild and short-lived, this cramping is perfectly normal and nothing to be alarmed about. It's usually caused by your growing uterus and the stretching of abdominal ligaments to accommodate it. Call your caregiver if you have persistent severe cramps or abdominal pain with or without accompanying symptoms.

Excessive Saliva

If you feel like your mouth is a never-ending fluid factory right now, you're not alone. No one knows for sure what causes excess salivation during pregnancy (also known as ptyalism or sialorrhea), but hormonal changes may be the root of the problem. It's also possible that nausea is making you avoid swallowing, and that's causing saliva to pool in your mouth. Or, if you've been throwing up a lot or have heartburn, your salivary glands may crank up their output to help buffer the digestive acids backing up into your esophagus. In rare cases, the saliva may be so excessive that you need to spit constantly into a tissue or cup. The good news is, excess salivation usually wanes around the end of your first trimester.

Fatigue

Growing a new human being can make you feel bone tired, and even avowed night owls may find themselves nodding off by 9 P.M. now. Rising progesterone levels are behind that sluggishness, but late-night trips to the bathroom and frequent nausea and vomiting certainly deplete your energy reserves, too. No wonder you feel as if you've run a marathon at the end of the day! Some women continue to feel tired for the whole nine months, but most notice that their energy returns as the first trimester winds to a close.

QUICK TIPS

Staunching the Spit Flow

• Brush your teeth gently and use mouthwash several times a day.

• Eat frequent, small meals.

• Drink more water. Keep a water bottle with you and take frequent small sips.

• Suck on a hard candy or chew sugarless gum (but avoid sour candies and gum, which *stimulate* saliva production).

Some quick tips to fight fatigue:

• Go to bed early. Try to get nine or ten hours of sleep a night if you can manage it. Nap whenever you have the chance.

• If you can, cut back on your commitments at work or arrange to take work home over the weekend so you can cut out early or come in late once in a while. Or take an occasional midweek vacation or sick day and use the time off to power nap.

• Don't rely on quick pick-me-ups like caffeine or sweets—they may give you a temporary energy boost, but you'll crash quickly and hard. Instead, drink plenty of water to stay hydrated, and snack on healthy foods, like fruit and yogurt, that will give you energy without making you feel sluggish.

• Get a little exercise every day. Even a short walk around the block can make you feel better, and the fresh air will help keep fatigue at bay. Take frequent breaks throughout your day to stretch and breathe deeply.

• Let the housework go—no one will blame you if you turn a blind eye to the dust bunnies for now.

Frequent Urination

You may find yourself running for the bathroom with alarming frequency these days. In fact, an increased urge to pee is one of the most common early pregnancy symptoms, starting around week 6. Why do you suddenly need to go all the time? Mainly because your blood volume is increasing dramatically, which leads to a lot of extra fluid getting processed through your kidneys and ending up in your bladder.

Headaches

It's not unusual to get tension headaches in your first trimester—especially if you've always been susceptible to them. The hormonal free-for-all happening in your body is probably to blame, though going cold turkey on caffeine can also make your head pound. Other potential perpetrators include fatigue, sinus congestion, allergies, eyestrain, depression, stress, hunger, and dehydration. If you're like most women, pregnancy headaches will diminish and finally disappear during your second trimester, when your body gets used to its altered chemistry. (Migraine headaches are a different story. See page 492 for coping tips.)

To ease tension headaches, try to:

- Get some fresh air.

- Apply a warm compress around your eyes and nose for sinus headaches or a cool or warm compress at the base of your neck for tension headaches. Or try a warm bath or shower.

- Get a massage. This works especially well for headaches caused by tension that builds in your neck, shoulder, and back muscles.

- Eat smaller, more frequent meals to stave off hunger—which can lead to headaches for some women. If you're on the go, keep snacks like crackers, nuts, or fruit in your bag.

- Have your vision checked if you feel eyestrain or notice that reading or looking at a computer screen seems to trigger your headaches.

- Use relaxation techniques such as meditation, yoga, or biofeedback.

- Take acetaminophen. Though most headache medications, such as aspirin and ibuprofen, are off-limits during pregnancy, acetaminophen (page 551) is considered safe when taken as directed.

> **QUICK TIPS**
>
> **Cutting Down on Bathroom Trips**
>
> To reduce the number of times you need to visit the loo:
>
> - Cut down on coffee and tea which can have diuretic effects.
> - Drink plenty of fluids during the day, but taper off several hours before bedtime to limit sleep interruptions.
> - When you pee, lean forward to help completely empty your bladder.

Morning Sickness

Three out of four pregnant women suffer from nausea—and sometimes vomiting, too, especially in their first trimester. For many, symptoms are worst in the morning, hence the name "morning sickness." For others, stomach churning lasts morning, noon, and night. Queasiness usually begins at around week 6 (but can come on as early as week 4), and about half of morning sickness sufferers get complete relief by week 14. For most of the rest, nausea gradually tapers off during the second trimester—although some unlucky women feel sick to their stomach until their babies are born.

No one knows exactly what causes morning sickness. But as with so many pregnancy symptoms, it's likely triggered by increasing levels of pregnancy hormones, which can result in an enhanced sense of smell and sensitivity to noxious odors, as well as a more sensitive stomach. You're more likely to suffer from morning sickness if you have a history of nausea or vomiting from taking birth control pills, if you're susceptible to motion sickness or migraine headaches, if you're carrying twins or multiples, or if your mother or sisters had morning sickness.

If you're one of the few who *don't* get sick, consider yourself lucky. It doesn't mean that your body isn't producing enough hormones, as many believe; it's just that everyone reacts differently to pregnancy. While it's true that women who end up miscarrying or whose pregnancies aren't viable are less likely to feel nauseated, a lack of nausea does *not* mean that there's anything wrong with your pregnancy. Most women with "symptom-free" pregnancies go on to give birth to perfectly healthy babies.

QUELLING THE QUEASIES

Do your best to avoid foods and smells that make your gorge rise. If that list includes just about everything, rest assured that it's okay to eat only the things that *do* appeal to you right now, even if they don't add up to a totally balanced diet. Better to eat something and keep it down than eat perfectly and lose your lunch.

Try eating foods that are cold or at room temperature. They'll give off less intense odors than hot foods.

Keep simple snacks, such as crackers, by your bedside. When you first wake up, nibble a few crackers, and then rest for 20 to 30 minutes before getting out of bed. Snacking on crackers may also help if you wake up feeling nauseated in the middle of the night.

Eat small meals or snacks throughout the day so your stomach is never empty (a surefire invitation for nausea). Aim for bland foods that are high in protein, since it may help fight nausea. (But in a pinch, go for whatever appeals to you.)

Avoid fatty foods, which take longer to digest. Also avoid rich, spicy, acidic, and fried foods, which can irritate your already traumatized digestive system.

Sip, don't chug. Though it's important to stay hydrated, you don't want to drink so much at once that your stomach feels full, since that'll leave less room for nausea-fighting food. If you've been vomiting a lot, try a sports drink that contains glucose, salt, and potassium to replace lost electrolytes.

Rather than popping your prenatal vitamin on an empty stomach first thing in the morning, try taking it with food or just before bed. You might

Ask the Experts

Are there safe medications for morning sickness?

Gerald Briggs, pharmacist clinical specialist: It's best to avoid exposing your developing baby to any kind of medication when you can make do without. However, nausea and vomiting that's severe (but falls short of hyperemesis gravidarum, below) can be treated with a variety of drugs, though not all of them work for all women. Vomiting suppressants such as trimethobenzamide hydrochloride (Tigan) and prochlorperazine (Compazine), either alone or combined with an antihistamine like Benadryl, work well in some cases. Sometimes, a different antihistamine like Phenergan (promethazine) is used alone. One drug, ondansetron (Zofran), which was designed to control nausea in chemotherapy patients, is effective for some women, but it's very expensive. Sometimes over-the-counter (OTC) antireflux medications such as ranitidine (Zantac) and famotidine (Pepcid) work for expectant mothers whose nausea and vomiting is triggered by gastrointestinal distress. A dextrose-levulose-phosphoric acid combo (Emetrol) is another OTC drug that may soothe your stomach and minimize morning sickness symptoms—plus, it's one of only two nausea medications currently approved by the Food and Drug Administration (FDA) for use in pregnancy.

Bendectin, an antihistamine-and-vitamin-B_6 combo, was once widely used to treat morning sickness. But controversy over its safety during pregnancy—despite there being no evidence that it was harmful—forced the drug's manufacturer to pull it from the market. Interestingly, the FDA has since classified the combination of ingredients in Bendectin (doxylamine and B_6, both available over-the-counter) as "safe and effective for nausea and vomiting in pregnancy."

If your morning sickness is really intolerable and other coping strategies aren't working, ask your caregiver if any of these treatments might work for you and, if so, what dose to take. Remember, though: Never take *any* medications—prescription or OTC—during pregnancy without first getting your practitioner's okay.

also want to ask your practitioner if you can temporarily switch to a prenatal supplement with less iron, because this mineral can be hard on your delicate digestive system.

Try ginger, an alternative remedy that research has shown to settle the stomach. Look for ginger ale made with real ginger (most common sodas aren't). Or grate some fresh ginger into hot water for ginger tea. Ginger lozenges and candied ginger are also worth a try. (Ask your healthcare provider before taking ginger supplements because—as with many other things that are helpful in small amounts—the effects of megadoses are unknown.)

BabyCenter Buzz

How I Cope with the Queasies

"If you've got a kitchen sink with a garbage disposal and a spray nozzle attachment, it's easier and more comfortable to vomit in there than in the bathroom or in a trash can." —*Super KK*

"Peppermint oil really helps me. When I feel nauseated, I just hold it to my nose." —*SVDUB*

"If I don't get enough sleep, I feel horrible the whole next day. When I do sleep, my morning sickness is more manageable." —*Karen*

"Lemon ices really seem to help. Friends who've been truly ill have even tried sucking on a lemon itself." —*Wendy*

"Sucking on peppermint candy helps a ton. I carry them with me all the time, and I constantly have one in my mouth." —*Amanda*

Consider wearing an acupressure band. These soft cotton wristbands, available at drugstores, are designed to ward off seasickness but can also keep morning sickness at bay. The bands strap on so that an attached plastic button puts gentle pressure on a specific acupressure point on the underside of your wrist, which is thought to affect the nausea center in your brain. You can also ask your practitioner about an electronic wrist device that stimulates the same point with a mild electric current. It's available by prescription only but it's safe and research suggests it works well for some women.

Try hypnosis. There's no scientific evidence that hypnosis combats nausea, but some mothers-to-be have used hypnotherapy to help them deal with severe morning sickness. Learning (with the help of audio- or videotapes, classes, workshops, or private training) to get into this relaxed state may help your mind tune out the unpleasant sensations emanating from your belly.

Ask your practitioner about taking vitamin B6, which some women find helpful, though, no one knows exactly why. The recommended daily allowance for B_6 is 1.9 milligrams (mg), but your doctor or midwife may give you the go-ahead to take 10 to 25 milligrams three times a day to battle

When Morning Sickness Is Unmanageable

Though morning sickness is normally a relatively minor and short-lived complaint, some women get such a severe case that keeping anything down becomes an incredible challenge and simple treatments aren't enough to solve the problem. You may be suffering from this condition, called *hyperemesis gravidarum* (literally "excessive vomiting in pregnancy") or HG, if your vomiting is so frequent, prolonged, and severe that you're losing weight and you can't keep *anything* (including water, juice, liquids, food, prenatal vitamins, and medication) down for 24 hours. If you suspect you have HG, call your health-care provider right away; if you don't yet have one, go to the emergency room. HG causes dehydration and malnutrition, leading to weight loss and metabolic imbalances that could harm you and your baby. Women who suffer from it often require hospitalization for treatment and to rule out other disorders that may be causing the symptoms.

• •

severe queasiness. Don't take this or any supplement without your caregiver's okay, though.

If nothing else eases your misery, ask your caregiver about taking antinausea medications that are considered safe during pregnancy.

Vaginal Spotting

Very light vaginal bleeding or spotting, similar to what you might see at the beginning or end of your period, can vary in color from pink to red to brown. Spotting doesn't necessarily mean that your pregnancy is at risk, but to be on the safe side, call your practitioner right away, even if the bleeding seems to have stopped. You'll probably need an exam to rule out any complications and to see how your baby is doing. Spotting may be brought on by:

• **Conditions unrelated to your pregnancy.** A vaginal yeast infection (page 181) or bacterial vaginosis (page 497), or a sexually transmitted infection (page 503), such as trichomoniasis, gonorrhea, chlamydia, or herpes, can cause cervical irritation or inflammation, which in turn can

Ask the Experts

How Is HG Treated?

Gerald Briggs, pharmacist clinical specialist: If you have hyperemesis gravidarum, or HG, your practitioner will most likely want to treat you with intravenous fluids and medications in the hospital. Many drugs have been used to help women with HG, but the most effective and powerful is droperidol. Droperidol will rapidly curb your nausea and vomiting and allow you to resume eating and drinking within a day or two. Once your HG is under control, you can go home with oral antinausea medications and a special diet designed to make morning sickness more manageable. A small percentage of women may need to be hospitalized more than once for treatment.

bring on light bleeding after sex or a vaginal exam. You might also spot or bleed after sex or an internal exam if you have a benign growth called a cervical polyp.

• **Implantation bleeding.** This might happen a few days before your period is due, as the fertilized egg burrows into the lining of your uterus. Your practitioner might make this diagnosis after ruling out other causes—though there's no way to confirm it.

• **Miscarriage or ectopic pregnancy.** Spotting—especially spotting accompanied by abdominal pain or cramping—warrants an immediate call to your caregiver.

Vaginal Discharge

Mild-smelling or odorless, milky discharge called leukorrhea is common in your first trimester—and there's a lot more of it than there was before you got pregnant, partly due to increased estrogen levels and greater blood flow to your vagina. This discharge is made up of vaginal and cervical secretions, old cells shed from your vaginal walls, and normal vaginal flora (fungus and bacteria).

Don't douche during preganancy. It can introduce an air bubble into your circulatory system through your more-engorged-

BY THE NUMBERS

Spotting Stats

Women who experience some spotting or bleeding during their pregnancy: **1 in 4**

than-normal vagina, which in turn could lead to rare but potentially fatal complications, such as stroke. More likely, though, you'll upset the normal balance of vaginal flora and increase your risk of yeast and other infections—a good reason to skip douching even when you're *not* pregnant.

Getting Enough Sleep
Sleep Problems—and Solutions

Pregnancy symptoms that plague you throughout the day can make for an uncomfortable night, too. A look at some typical first-trimester troublemakers, plus tips for getting the sleep you need:

> ### QUICK TIPS
> **Dealing with Discharge**
>
> - Use panty liners—not tampons—to absorb it.
> - Wash your genital area with warm water and a gentle cleanser once or twice a day.
> - To avoid vaginal irritation (which causes even more discharge), always wipe from front to back to avoid introducing anal bacteria into your vagina; wear breathable cotton underwear; and avoid tight pants, nylon fabrics, bubble bath, feminine hygiene sprays, scented pads or toilet paper, and scented or deodorant soaps.

Frequent Urination
They don't call them the wee hours for nothing! You can reduce the number of trips you take to the bathroom by limiting how much you drink before bed. While it's important to drink plenty of fluids, you can make up for it by drinking more during the day.

Nausea
To help keep nausea at bay while you're trying to settle down to sleep—and when you wake up in the middle of the night—keep some simple snacks, such as crackers, on your bedside table. At dinnertime, avoid fatty foods, which take longer to digest. Steer clear of rich, spicy, acidic, and fried foods, too, which can irritate your stomach and digestive system and make nausea worse. (For more on coping with a queasy stomach, see page 54.)

A Need to Nap
Early in your pregnancy, you may start feeling sleepy during the day. This sudden craving for naps may be caused by increasing levels of progesterone, a pregnancy hormone that has a sedative effect. Unfortunately, there's no way around this problem other than to rest as much as you can and grab a

Just for Dad

"Sympathy" Symptoms

It's not a myth: Many dads-to-be have symptoms similar to their pregnant mate's, including weight gain, indigestion, fatigue, and changes in sexual appetite—to name just a few. Though the phenomenon, known as couvade syndrome (from the French word *couver*, meaning "to hatch"), is well-documented, no one knows exactly what lies behind these "sympathetic" pregnancy symptoms. Interestingly, the response appears to be universal, affecting expectant fathers of different ethnicities and cultures around the world. The symptoms typically start around the third 3rd month of pregnancy and end when the baby's born. Researchers cite a wide range of possible causes, including stress or anxiety about becoming a father, close emotional attachment to an expectant mother, and possibly even hormonal changes. It's a harmless and relatively common condition, so don't worry too much if it suddenly seems like there are two pregnant people in your house.

quick catnap whenever possible. Keep in mind, though, that napping *too* late in the day (or for more than 30 to 60 minutes) can disrupt a good night's sleep.

Evening Drowsiness

Even if you're an avowed night owl, you may suddenly find it impossible to keep your eyes open after 9 P.M. Don't fight it—your body is sending you the message that you (and your baby) need more sleep. It's better to turn in earlier than you're accustomed to than to doze off on the couch. That way, you're more likely to get a longer stretch of uninterrupted sleep—instead of waking up hours later and having to turn out the lights and drag yourself to bed, where you may find yourself staring at the ceiling and trying to will yourself back to sleep.

Trouble Getting Comfortable

Trying to sleep on breasts so tender that they feel like hot rocks are buried within them can make it hard to find a comfortable sleeping position, especially if you're used to sleeping on your stomach. Some women find it helpful to wear a soft bra at night (try a sports bra, a seamless cotton bra, or even a snug tank top made with supportive spandex). Or start training yourself to sleep on your side, which you'll need to do later in pregnancy to improve the flow of blood and nutrients to your baby. It's fine to sleep on your back now if that's how you're most comfortable, but the sooner you get used to side sleeping, the better you'll be able to rest when your belly is bulging.

Though pregnancy itself can bring on many sleep disturbances, these problems are often aggravated by bad sleeping habits that took hold *before* you got pregnant. Here are some sleep strategies to help you get a better night's sleep—in pregnancy and beyond.

• Regulate your sleep-wake schedule by going to bed and getting up at the same time every day, even on weekends.

• Establish a regular bedtime routine. Have dinner at a leisurely pace; afterward, do something quiet, such as reading or taking a bath.

• Say no to smoking and alcohol. Not only can nicotine and alcohol harm your developing baby, but both can make it difficult to get to sleep.

• Limit caffeinated foods (such as tea, coffee, and soda), too much of which aren't good for your baby, anyway, and avoid them entirely in the afternoon and evening.

• Don't exercise right before bedtime. Exercise is great for your mental and physical health and can help combat insomnia, but drifting off can be difficult if your body doesn't have two to three hours to unwind after a workout.

• Make your bedroom a sleep sanctuary. Because you may feel warmer than usual when you're pregnant, keep your room on the cool side. Block out light and noise, too—they can rouse you from a light sleep. If you live in a noisy city, try using a fan or a white-noise machine to cover the din.

• If you're in the habit of paying bills or watching TV in bed, stop. Reserve your bed for enjoyable activities, like sleep, sex, and maybe a little light reading.

BY THE NUMBERS:

Men with "Sympathy Symptoms"

26%	of dads-to-be said they were gaining more weight than their partner was
25%	felt better than ever
23%	had a variety of sympathetic pregnancy symptoms
17%	said they're moodier than normal
10%	felt a little queasy

Source: *A BabyCenter.com poll of more than 3,000 men*

BabyCenter Buzz

How I Cope with Drowsiness at Work

"Getting as much rest as I can prior to a big day of meetings helps me cope with those midday yawns." —Hopamommy

"Here's what works for me: I 'disappear' into an unused conference room, then lay my head down on the table and take a quick catnap. One of my coworkers keeps an eye on the clock and comes to wake me after 15 or 20 minutes. Of course, you have to have both sympathetic friends and an accommodating work environment to pull this off!" —Holly

"If you have a safe parking spot, take a nap in your car during your lunch break. Just make sure someone knows where you are and can wake you up when you need to get back!"   —Amanda

• Experiment with relaxation techniques. Sleep-promoting practices such as guided imagery, deep breathing, and progressive muscle relaxation can help you nod off. Try this: Close your eyes and imagine all of the stress and tension you're holding in each part of your body seeping out of your pores and dissipating into the air. Start at your toes, then move on to your feet, your ankles, your calves, and so on—all the way up to the top of your head. Chances are, you'll be snoozing before you get to your shoulders.

• Write down tomorrow's to-do list and anything else that's worrying you (along with possible solutions) before you turn in.

• Ask your partner for a back rub or foot massage.

• If you're still awake 20 to 30 minutes after turning in, get up and go into another room. Listen to soothing music or read a magazine. When you feel drowsy, go back to bed.

Worry

It's normal to spend an occasional night tossing and turning while you worry about whether your baby's developing properly, how you'll survive labor, and the parental responsibilities that loom ahead of you, but if anxiety is becoming all-consuming or regularly disrupts your slumber, it's time to find a better way to deal with it.

Just for Dad

What *You* May be Dreaming About

Just as with your mate, your own feelings of excitement, anticipation, anxiety, and worry will probably open a floodgate of imagery, according to dream expert Patricia Garfield. During the first few months of your partner's pregnancy, you may have more sex-filled dreams than usual. These dreams often involve having sex with your partner, with other women, with prostitutes, or even with other men. Sexual and other macho dreams (such as triumphing on the football field) may express a need to be more "masculine" at a time when you're feeling protective of your partner and unborn child. In fact, another common dad-to-be dream theme during early pregnancy is of protecting and caring for your partner. The frequency of your sexual dreams will likely subside once your mate enters her second trimester, Garfield says.

To start, share your fears with your partner; chances are he's harboring similar concerns. Communicating openly about your anxiety can help you both feel—and sleep—better. Turn to friends and family members for support, too. Other moms-to-be offer a crucial support network, since they're likely experiencing the same worries you are. If anxiety still plagues you, you may want to seek professional counseling to help you rest easy.

YOUR NUTRITION
AND FITNESS

Eating Well

We know how hard it can be to eat a well-balanced diet, especially if you're battling waves of nausea one minute and answering the siren song of the doughnut the next. Don't beat yourself up if you can't stomach the sight of vegetables right now—but make an effort to sneak in healthy foods and snacks as often as you can. And if you're feeling overwhelmed by the constant barrage of nutrition advice and cautions, consider these healthy yet realistic guidelines.

Prenatal Vitamins: A Nutritional Insurance Policy

If you're very tuned in to nutrition and regularly eat a broad range of foods (including meat, dairy products, fruits, vegetables, grains, and legumes), your

---

Just the Facts

Why Folic Acid Is So Important

Getting the recommended daily amount of folic acid—starting a month before you become pregnant and continuing through your first trimester—can reduce your baby's risk of neural tube defects (such as spina bifida) by up to 70 percent. There's also research suggesting that folic acid decreases the risk of other birth defects and possibly the risk of repeated early miscarriages. So how much is enough? At least 400 micrograms (mcg) a day before you become pregnant and at least 600 mcg a day once your pregnancy is confirmed. You can get folate (the natural form of folic acid) from food, but because your body doesn't absorb much from natural sources, you still need to take a daily folic acid supplement or a multivitamin with folic acid.

diet will provide almost all the nutrients you and your baby need. Realistically, though, most women—especially those in the throes of morning sickness—can benefit from taking an all-in-one prenatal vitamin-and-mineral supplement.

In general, prenatal supplements contain more of certain nutrients (such as folic acid and iron) that are hard to get enough of from food alone. Find one that includes no more than the recommended amounts of other nutrients (particularly vitamin A, and possibly vitamins D, E, and K as well) that in very large amounts can be harmful to your baby. Your practitioner may give you a prescription for a prenatal vitamin or just suggest that you buy a particular over-the-counter brand. Whichever type you take, be careful not to take additional nutritional supplements without running them by your practitioner first.

Making the Food Groups Work for You

As long as you eat a wide variety of foods from the major food groups, you'll get most of the vitamins (except for folic acid), minerals (except for possibly iron), and fiber you need. While few women are able to eat a perfectly balanced diet—at least in early pregnancy—here's what to strive for and why.

QUICK TIPS

Coping with Lactose Intolerance

- Most women who have trouble digesting lactose (the sugar in milk) can tolerate at least 1 cup of regular milk with meals. (Don't worry if you're not one of them—you can get your calcium from other sources.)

- Drinking lactose-reduced milk is another option-as is adding over-the-counter lactase (the enzyme needed to help you digest lactose) drops to your milk to break down the lactose or taking enzyme supplements to help you digest lactose.

- Choose low-fat or hard, aged cheeses, which have the lowest lactose content and may be easier to digest.

- Eat yogurt, which contains beneficial bacteria that may produce lactase.

- Opt for calcium-fortified soy milk or orange juice.

Dairy Products

Dairy products, such as milk, cheese, and yogurt, are excellent sources of calcium, protein, vitamin D, and phosphorus—nutrients important for your baby's developing bones, teeth, muscles, heart, and nerves, as well as for blood clotting.

You need about 1,000 mg of calcium a day, so aim to eat three to four servings of calcium-rich foods. (A serving usually equals about 1 cup,

What to Do If Prenatal Vitamins Upset Your Stomach

In your first trimester, when your digestive tract is roiled enough as it is, forcing yourself to choke down a giant horse pill of a prenatal vitamin can send you running for the nearest bathroom. Strategies for keeping your supplement down when your stomach is acting up:

- Don't swallow your pill on an empty stomach. Instead, take it with meals.

- If your stomach is particularly upset in the morning, wait until bedtime to take your supplement.

- Try breaking your pill in half, then taking the halves several hours apart.

- If *swallowing* the pill seems to trigger your gag reflex, try a chewable vitamin, or ask your doctor about a liquid formulation (available in many health food stores) that you can mix into your morning juice.

- If all else fails, ask your caregiver if you can stop taking an all-in-one supplement for a while. In the meantime, take an individual supplement of folic acid and any other nutrient your practitioner recommends.

or 1 ounce of cheese.) Unless you're having trouble putting on weight, choose low-fat or fat-free dairy products whenever possible—you'll get all the nutrients without the added fat.

Fruits and Vegetables

Packed with essential nutrients and full of fiber, fruits and vegetables are absolutely vital when you're pregnant. Aim for about two to four servings of fruit and three to five servings of lightly steamed or raw vegetables a day (a serving is one piece of fruit or ½ cup of vegetables). A good rule of thumb for getting a variety of nutrients is to vary the colors of the fruit and vegetables you eat.

Grains

Grains (whole wheat, oats, barley, corn, and rice, to name a few) are packed with nutrients, especially the B vitamins (including B_1, B_2, folate, and niacin) that your growing baby needs to develop just about every part of his body. Most grains have plenty of fiber, too-and you need 20 to 35 grams of fiber a day to help prevent constipation and hemorrhoids. And be sure to look for "whole grains"—whole wheat bread, for instance, or brown rice—over their "refined" counterparts.

Try to eat 6 to 11 servings of grains a day. That may sound like a lot, but a serving of grains equals just ½ cup of cereal, cooked rice, 3 tablespoons of wheat germ or noodles, or one slice of bread.

Just the Facts

Vitamin A Is Dangerous in Large Doses

Vitamin A, a fat-soluble nutrient stored in your liver, is important for your health and for your baby's development. But this is *not* a case of "more is better." Getting very high doses (more than 3,000 micrograms RAE or 10,000 IU) of so-called preformed vitamin A from supplements, animal sources, and fortified foods can cause serious birth defects. This is one reason that you should never double up on prenatal vitamins or take additional supplements that your practitioner hasn't recommended. Most prenatal formulations contain at least part of their vitamin A in the form of beta-carotene, but some over-the-counter brands—and other multivitamins—may have excessive amounts of preformed vitamin A. So before you try a new supplement, check the label carefully—or, better yet, show it to your practitioner. Also check the labels of fortified foods—such as energy bars—that you tend to eat a lot of, since they may contain a lot of vitamin A. (*Note:* This caution doesn't apply to beta-carotene, which is found in some fruits and vegetables; it is converted into vitamin A by your body only as needed, so you can consume as much of that as you want.) One last thing: Avoid eating liver while you're pregnant because it contains an enormous amount of vitamin A. One 3-ounce serving of beef liver, for instance, can contain more than *eight times* the recommended daily allowance of vitamin A.

Meat, Fish, Poultry, and Beans

Beans are a great source of protein, as are lean meats, poultry, fish and shellfish, eggs, milk, cheese, tofu, and yogurt. Aim for 60 grams of protein a day (the equivalent of a glass of milk, a serving of chicken, and a bowl of yogurt, for example). Most women in the United States regularly eat more protein than they need, so you probably won't have any trouble meeting your quota. If you don't eat meat, you'll need to get your protein from other sources, such as dairy, beans, or soy products. Eat three to four servings of protein a day. One serving equals about 3 ounces of lean meat, poultry, or fish, or one egg. A half cup equals one serving of beans.

QUICK TIPS

Getting Enough H_2O

- If you don't like the taste of plain water, try adding a wedge of lemon or lime or a splash of juice for flavor. Carbonated water-flavored or unflavored-is perfectly okay, too.

- If you're not sure how much water you actually drink each day, fill a 64-ounce container in the morning and try to finish it by bedtime—but if frequent urination is keeping you up at night, do the lion's share of your guzzling by late afternoon.

Water

Water plays many vital roles in your body. In fact, none of your organs could function without it. Your body uses even more water during pregnancy; among other things, it's needed to make the plasma essential for your expanding blood volume and to form the amniotic fluid that bathes and cushions your baby. You also need water to help flush out waste, and getting enough can help prevent the bladder infections that dog many mothers-to-be. If you drink plenty of H_2O, your urine will stay diluted and you'll urinate more often—thus lessening the chance that bacteria will hang around in your bladder and multiply. What's more, water can ward off constipation and help prevent hemorrhoids. And though it may seem counterintuitive, the more water you drink during pregnancy, the *less* water your body will retain (and the less likely you are to be plagued by pudgy fingers and swelling feet as your pregnancy moves on).

You need eight 8-ounce glasses of water a day (a total of 64 fluid ounces), plus an extra 8 ounces for each hour of light activity you do. Juice contributes to your fluid intake, but keep in mind that it can also pack in a lot of extra calories. Caffeinated beverages, such as coffee, cola, and tea, don't count as part of your fluid intake because they're diuretics—in other words, they make you urinate more, so you actually *lose* water.

Nutrition Advice for Vegetarians

If you're a pregnant vegetarian—especially a vegan who doesn't eat *any* animal products, including dairy—you may worry that you're not getting enough protein. Rest assured, it's pretty easy to

---

QUICK TIPS

When You Can't Stomach Vegetables

If the mere *idea* of a salad or whiff of cooked broccoli sends you running for the nearest barf bin:

- Try *drinking* your vegetables in the form of tomato or carrot juice (or whatever veggie juice strikes your fancy). Many supermarkets and health food stores sell fruit-and-vegetable juice blends—carrot and orange juice, for instance—in which the vegetable juice is disguised by the more dominant (and palatable) flavor of the fruit juice.

- Eat more fruits, since many contain some of the same vitamins and minerals found in vegetables.

- If all else fails, be sure to take your prenatal vitamin every day—and try greens again in a few weeks, when your stomach settles down a bit.

meet your protein needs just by drinking soy milk and eating beans, rice, tofu, and nuts. Instead, what you may need to focus on is getting enough omega-3 fatty acids, zinc, iron, vitamin B_{12}, vitamin D, folic acid, and calcium. With a little menu planning, though, most of these essentials are easy enough to get from foods that even strict vegans can eat. (The exceptions are the omega-3s—because they're found mainly in fatty fish like salmon—and folic acid. You can get your omega-3s by eating flaxseed and walnuts, and you can take folic acid in pill form.) You should also take a prenatal vitamin-and-mineral supplement to make sure you're getting all of the nutrients you need.

To be on the safe side, review your eating habits with a nutritionist, who can point out where you're falling short and help you come up with a healthy eating plan. Ask your pregnancy-care provider for a referral.

The Lowdown on Alcohol
Nobody knows exactly how much—or how little—alcohol can harm a developing baby, so experts recommend that mothers-to-be play it safe by avoiding alcohol entirely. (If you had a drink or two before your period was due, don't panic. The most important thing to focus on is staying healthy from now on—and that includes swearing off alcohol for the rest of your pregnancy.)

You don't have to be a heavy drinker to endanger your baby. One

> **QUICK TIPS**
>
> **Balanced Eating for Pregnant Vegetarians**
>
> • Aim for four servings a day of cooked dried beans and peas—they're full of folate, magnesium, iron, protein, and other important nutrients. Throw in a few nuts and seeds, too.
>
> • You need four daily servings of calcium- and vitamin D-rich foods, including fat-free or low-fat milk (if you consume dairy products) or calcium- and vitamin D-fortified soy milk.
>
> • Work in eight to ten servings of fruits and vegetables—they're packed with fiber, vitamins, and other important nutrients.
>
> • Eat six to 11 servings of whole grains—including foods such as brown rice, oatmeal, and whole wheat bread-to provide the energy and B vitamins that you and your baby need.
>
> • Have one or more servings of vitamin B_{12}-rich food-milk and egg yolks (if you eat them), as well as fortified soy milk and fermented soy foods, like miso and tempeh, are all good candidates.

Ask the Experts

Are Low-Carb Eating Plans Safe during Pregnancy?

Bridget Swinney, registered dietitian: If you mean the very low carbohydrate diets that've taken the country by storm—then the answer is an emphatic *no!* That's because there are major questions surrounding the safety of restricting carbohydrates during pregnancy.

For one thing, a very low-carb diet kicks your body into an altered metabolic state called ketosis, in which it relies on stored body fat for energy. Problem is, without carbs, the fat is incompletely broken down, causing the production of ketones. An abnormal buildup of ketones, the products of this breakdown, signals a starvation-like state. And according to the National Women's Health Information Center, constant exposure to ketones in the womb can increase your baby's risk of mental retardation.

What's more, research looking at high-protein, low-carb diets in late pregnancy found that they may raise levels of the stress hormone cortisol. The thinking is that exposure to increased cortisol might "program" your baby to produce too much cortisol during his own lifetime, which could in turn lead to high blood pressure. Another study found that a low-carb diet during late pregnancy may alter a newborn's insulin production—thus putting him at greater risk for diabetes.

Despite current eating fads, there are lots of reasons to keep carbs on your maternity menu:

• Carbohydrates aren't the dietary villains they've been made out to be. The fruits, vegetables, and whole grains that make up this food category provide vitamins that play a vital role in your pregnancy. For instance, folic acid—the B vitamin found in many grain products—is responsible for proper neural tube development. So following a low-carb eating plan—and thus skimping on folic acid—before you get pregnant and in early pregnancy could put your baby at risk for a neural tube defect.

• Well-chosen carbs contain plenty of fiber, a necessity for your prenatal diet—as you may know all too well if you have problems with constipation or hemorrhoids. Try to eat 25 to 35 grams of fiber a day now.

• Your baby's healthy growth and development requires a proper balance of nutrients—about 50 percent carbs, 30 percent fat, and 20 percent protein.

That said, there are benefits to being carbohydrate *aware*. If you know the carbohydrate content of juices, sodas, and other simple-carb (that is, low-nutrient) fare, for instance, it's easier to eat them in moderation. Instead, choose complex carbs, such as whole grain breads, cereals, and pasta; raw fruits and vegetables; legumes; and brown rice.

Just the Facts

Eating Peanuts May Increase Your Baby's Allergy Risk

Peanuts are a good source of protein (2 ounces provide a quarter of your daily quota), but if severe allergies run in your family, you may want to cool it on the nuts. The reason: Research suggests that consuming peanut products (peanuts, peanut butter, and peanut oil) during pregnancy may expose your developing baby to peanut allergens. For the vast majority of babies, this isn't a problem—but for the one in 100 who is genetically predisposed to peanut allergies, this in-utero sensitization can up the odds that a potentially severe allergy might form later in life. (What's more, if you plan to breastfeed and you have a personal or family history of nut allergies, hold the peanuts until you wean your baby.) As for other common food allergens—including milk, fish, and eggs—feel free to indulge (unless you're allergic to them yourself, of course). Research has found no benefit in avoiding these foods during pregnancy.

drink a day during pregnancy can increase the odds of miscarriage, preterm labor, and low birthweight, as well as raise your child's risk for learning, speech, attention, language, and hyperactivity problems. Some research has even shown that pregnant women who have as little as one drink a week are more likely than nondrinkers to have children who later exhibit aggressive and delinquent behavior.

If you have a drinking habit—even a moderate one—it's vital to get

Just the Facts

"Nonalcoholic" Wine and Beer

The term "nonalcoholic" is a bit of a misnomer when it comes to the supposedly sin-free versions of beer and wine. In fact, all "nonalcoholic" beers and many "nonalcoholic" wines *do* contain some alcohol—typically less than 0.5 percent. While few would say that the trace amount of alcohol in an occasional glass of "nonalcoholic" beer is going to do your baby harm, it's something to be aware of—especially if you imbibe often or in large amounts. So before you drink up, read labels carefully, and remember that "nonalcoholic" and "alcohol-free" aren't interchangeable: Drinks labeled "nonalcoholic" can contain trace alcohol, while those labeled "alcohol-free" cannot.

QUICK TIPS

Delicious "Virgin" Drinks

If you're hankering for a cocktail or a celebratory sip, whip up one of these alcohol-free classics:

Virgin Strawberry Daiquiri: The perfect drink for a hot summer day, this fruity blend is tangy and thirst-quenching. To make it, fill a blender with cracked ice. Add 1 ounce of lime juice, 3 ounces of fresh or frozen strawberries, and 1 teaspoon sugar. Blend until smooth, and then pour into a chilled glass. Garnish with an extra strawberry or an orange slice. Makes one serving.

White Sangria: Mix a batch of this refreshing drink to have on hand whenever you need a bubbly beverage break. In a large pitcher, combine 4 cups of white grape juice, 1 cup of pink grapefruit juice, and 1 tablespoon of lime juice. Refrigerate. Just before serving, add a 750-milliliter bottle of soda water and grapefruit slices. Makes 12 servings.

Sin-Free Champagne: This concoction is ideal for an elegant baby shower—or any festive occasion. Combine ⅔ cup of sugar and ⅔ cup of water in a saucepan over low heat, stirring until the sugar is dissolved. Bring to a boil and reduce for 10 minutes, then cool. Add the resulting sugar syrup to 1 cup of grapefruit juice and ½ cup of orange juice. Chill thoroughly. Stir in 3 tablespoons of grenadine and 28 ounces of ginger ale just before serving. Makes 1 quart.

help giving up alcohol as soon as possible. Talk to your provider about counseling or treatment options.

Caffeine Cautions

First, the good news: You can still enjoy your favorite caffeinated drinks—as long as you don't overdo it. After years of controversy over the issue, researchers now believe that moderate amounts of caffeine (approximately 300 mg, about what you'd get from three 8-ounce cups of coffee) won't harm your baby. Even so, most mothers-to-be limit their intake even further or cut out caffeine completely.

When it comes to heavy caffeine consumption—more than three cups of coffee a day—the science isn't quite so clear-cut. Some studies have found that this raises the risk of miscarriage. One study even suggested that high caffeine consumption during pregnancy might influence a baby's sleep patterns in the womb, and another found that the babies of big caffeine consumers exhibited withdrawal symptoms soon after birth. Though the research isn't conclusive, it makes sense to cut back if you're downing more than three cups of java a day (or more than 300 mg a day from all sources—sodas, tea, coffee, and chocolate—combined).

Avoiding the Most Common Foodborne Illnesses

When you're not pregnant, eating something a little "off" can mean spending the

Just the Facts

Four Reasons to Cut Down on Caffeine

1. Caffeine is a nutritional loser, containing absolutely no vitamins or minerals.
2. It's a stimulant, increasing your heart rate and metabolism, and it can cause insomnia, nervousness, and headaches.
3. Caffeine stimulates the secretion of stomach acids and can contribute to heartburn.
4. It's a diuretic, causing you to lose fluids and calcium—both of which you need to maintain a healthy pregnancy.

night hung over the toilet seat—unpleasant, but usually not serious. During pregnancy, foodborne illnesses, like salmonella, listeriosis, and toxoplasmosis are much more dangerous to you and your baby. Fortunately, there are easy ways to protect yourself.

Caffeine in Common Foods and Beverages

To help you limit your caffeine consumption to no more than 300 milligrams a day, here's a list of caffeine counts in common foods and beverages.

Item	Amount	Caffeine (in milligrams)
Coffee, brewed, drip method	5 oz	60–180
Coffee, brewed, percolator	5 oz	40–170
Instant coffee	5 oz	30–120
Espresso	Single	100
Cappuccino	Single	100
Decaffeinated coffee	5 oz	1–5
Brewed black tea	5 oz	20–110
Green tea	5 oz	8–36
Instant tea	5 oz	25–50
Soft drinks	12 oz	40–59
Milk chocolate	1 oz	1–15
Dark chocolate, semisweet	1 oz	5–35
Baker's chocolate	1 oz	26
Hot cocoa	8 oz	7

Key Pregnancy Nutrients and How They Help Your Baby Grow

Nutrient	How Much You Need Each Day	What It Does	Where to Get It
Calcium	1,000 mg (1,300 mg for women under age 19)	Grows strong bones and teeth, healthy nerves, heart, and muscles; develops heart rhythm and blood clotting	8 oz skim milk: 302 mg 8 oz calcium-fortified orange juice: 300 mg 3 corn tortillas: 150 mg
Chromium	30 mcg	Regulates blood sugar levels; stimulates protein synthesis in developing tissues	1 Tbsp peanut butter: 41 mcg 3 oz broiled skinless chicken: 22 mcg 1 slice whole grain bread: 16 mcg
Fluoride	Up to 3 mg	Needed when teeth begin to form at 10 weeks; later, in the second and third trimesters, needed to develop primary incisors, molars, and permanent teeth	Fluoride-fortified water: varies 1 cup cooked kale: 0.21 mg 1 medium apple: 0.01 mg
Folic Acid	600 mcg	Helps form spinal fluid, close the tube housing the central nervous system, synthesize DNA, and normalize brain function	1/2 cup lentils: 179 mcg 1/2 cup cereal (fortified): 146–179 mcg 4 spears steamed or boiled asparagus: 88 mcg
Iron	27 mg	Makes red blood cells, supplies oxygen to cells for energy and growth, and builds bones and teeth	Combine heme (in animal sources) and nonheme iron (in plants) 3 oz beef sirloin: 2 mg ½ cup lentils: 3 mg ½ cup boiled spinach: 3 mg ¾ cup iron-fortified cereal: 2 mg
Magnesium	350–360 mg	Helps build strong bones and teeth; regulates insulin and blood sugar levels; builds and repairs tissue	1 oz dried pumpkin seeds: 152 mg 3 oz halibut: 91 mg 1 cup spinach spaghetti: 87 mg
Manganese	2 mg	Aids bone and pancreas development and synthesis of fats and carbohydrates	1 cup cooked brown rice: 7 mg 1 cup cooked whole-oat oatmeal: 1 mg 1 cup cooked black beans: 1 mg
Pantothenic Acid	Up to 6 mg	Regulates adrenal activity, antibody production, growth and metabolism of protein and fat	1 medium hard-boiled egg: 1 mg ½ medium avocado: 1 mg 1 cup fat-free milk: 1 mg

Nutrient	How Much You Need Each Day	What It Does	Where to Get It
Phosphorus	700 mg	Builds strong bones and teeth; develops blood clotting and normal heart rhythm	1 cup cooked pinto beans: 273 mg 1 cup fat-free milk: 247 mg 1 cup cooked black beans: 241 mg
Potassium	Up to 2,000 mg	Aids muscle activity and contractions, energy metabolism, and nerve function	1 medium baked potato: 844 mg 1 medium banana: 806 mg 8 oz prune juice: 707 mg 1 cup cubed melon: 404 mg
Riboflavin	1.4 mg	Promotes growth, good vision, and healthy skin; essential for bone, muscle, and nerve development	1 cup fat-free yogurt: 0.5 mg ½ cup boiled mushrooms: 0.2 mg ½ cup part-skim ricotta cheese: 0.2 mg
Thiamin	1.4 mg	Converts carbohydrates into energy; essential for brain development; aids heart and nervous system growth	3 oz pork tenderloin: 0.8 mg 1 cup enriched spinach noodles: 0.4 mg 1 cup split peas: 0.4 mg 1 cup enriched cereal: 0.35 mg
Vitamin A	770 mcg RAE (retinol activity equivalents) or 2,565 IU	Important for cell growth, eye development, healthy skin and mucous membranes, infection resistance, bone growth, and fat metabolism	1 baked sweet potato: 1,403 mcg 1 cup boiled spinach: 1,146 mcg 1 raw carrot: 433 mcg
Vitamin B_6	1.9 mg	Aids metabolism of protein, fats, and carbohydrates; helps form new red blood cells and develop the brain and nervous system	1 medium banana: 0.7 mg 1 medium baked potato: 0.7 mg 1 cup chickpeas: 0.6 mg 3 oz chicken breast: 0.5 mg
Vitamin C	85 mg	Essential for tissue repair and collagen production; aids proper growth and strengthens bones and teeth	8 oz orange juice: 124 mg 1 cup strawberries: 85 mg 1 kiwi: 84 mg ½ cup boiled broccoli: 58 mg 1 mango: 57 mg ¼ cup raw bell pepper: 30 mg 1 tomato: 24 mg
Vitamin D	5 mcg	Helps build bones and teeth	3 oz herring: 35 mcg 1 cup milk: 2 mcg
Zinc	11 mg	Helps form organs, skeleton, nerves, and circulatory system	3 oz beef blade roast: 9 mg 3 oz Alaskan king crab: 7 mg ⅓ cup toasted wheat germ: 5 mg

Healthy Weight Gain

Weight gain during pregnancy can be one of the greatest struggles for expectant moms. Many fear that if they gain too much, too fast, they'll never get it off, while others, too sick to keep anything down, worry that slow weight gain could harm their babies.

Your caregiver will help you determine how many pounds you should put on over the next nine months, based on your height, how much you weighed before you conceived, and whether you're carrying a single baby or multiples, but here are some general recommendations from the *Journal of Midwifery and Women's Health* American College of Nurse-Midwives.

If you've struggled with your weight or body image in the past, you may have a hard time accepting that it's okay to gain weight now. It's normal to feel anxious as the numbers on the scale creep up, but the weight you gain during pregnancy is vital to your baby's health. In fact, *not* gaining enough weight increases the odds that your developing baby won't gain weight properly and could be born prematurely.

On the other hand, while pregnancy may seem like a good excuse to throw caution—and calorie counting—to the wind, it's important not to gain too *much* weight now because excess pounds can lead to complications that could affect the health of you and your baby. In general, you need to put on only about 2 to 5 pounds in the first trimester.

Another consideration: Extra weight you gain during pregnancy may stick with you after your baby's born.

If You Started Your Pregnancy Underweight

If you're very thin, you may be starting pregnancy with a nutritional disadvantage, since you likely have inadequate stores of fat. Some studies have

Herbal Teas Not Always Healthy for Pregnant Women

Despite claims that herbal teas are "all natural" and "good for you," that isn't always the case—especially if you drink too much or drink the wrong kind. High doses of certain herbs can bring on diarrhea, vomiting, and heart palpitations, and some have even been known to cause miscarriage. The FDA doesn't regulate herbal products as it does traditional drugs—which means you can't know for sure what's in that tea bag you're steeping.

The same cautions apply to teas touted as beneficial to pregnant women. While the makers of some of these "pregnancy teas" promote their products as all-around aids and tonics for expectant moms, their claims often lack scientific support. Granted, many of the pregnancy teas sold in health food stores and supermarkets are made with benign ingredients such as alfalfa, lemongrass, lemon verbena, nettle, and strawberry leaf. But if you have any doubts about a particular herbal tea, bring the box to your next prenatal checkup and get an okay from your provider.

∙∙∙

even linked being underweight at conception to an increased risk for preterm birth and low birthweight. Luckily, other studies show that there is no added risk if you gain enough weight over the course of your pregnancy. So work closely with your caregiver to map out a healthy weight-gain and eating plan—especially if your morning sickness is so severe you can't keep anything down. You may also want to seek the advice of a nutritionist.

It's particularly important to get help with your pregnancy weight and nutrition goals if you have an eating disorder. Not only are you and your baby at greater risk for pregnancy complications, but you may also need assistance to break unhealthy eating patterns that may have been a part of your life for years.

If You Started Your Pregnancy Overweight

If you've struggled with your weight all your life or recently gained a few too many, you may be fearful that the extra pounds will be burden on your baby's health. The truth is many overweight women have normal pregnan-

QUICK TIPS

Reducing Your Risk of Food Poisoning

- Cook your meat well. Use a food thermometer to test the internal temperature of meat; most meat should be cooked to a temperature of 160°F (180°F in the thigh for whole poultry). If you can't actually measure the temperature of the meat, cook it until it's no longer pink.

- Wash or peel fruits and vegetables before eating.

- Keep uncooked meats separate from produce, cooked foods, and ready-to-eat foods.

- Don't eat raw eggs or drink unpasteurized milk.

- Don't touch your mouth, nose, or eyes while preparing food.

- Wash your hands well before eating and after handling raw meat, soil, sand, or cats (all of which can harbor the parasite that causes toxoplasmosis) and other pets (reptiles can harbor salmonella).

- Wash your counters, cutting boards, and utensils with hot, soapy water after preparing food, and toss your dish sponge in the dishwasher or microwave every few days (one minute on high) to kill lurking germs.

- Drink only bottled water when you're camping or traveling to developing countries.

cies and healthy babies, but being overweight does put you at greater risk for complications such as preeclampsia and diabetes. And the risks increase, especially if you were more than 20 percent over a healthy weight when you conceived. Being overweight also increases your odds of having a larger-than-normal baby, which in turn boosts your chances of having a c-section. (This risk is increased even further if you gain too much weight during pregnancy.)

Though you'll probably need to gain less weight during your pregnancy than the average mom-to-be, you should still aim to put on at least 15 pounds. But don't attempt to control your weight on your own. It can be tough to do if you feel ravenous, as many pregnant women do, and dieting is risky for your baby. Work closely with your healthcare provider to put on pounds at a healthy pace. If you need more assistance or you can't seem to control your urge to overeat, ask your doctor or midwife to recommend a nutritionist who can help you work up a detailed eating plan that's both satisfying and sensible.

Staying Fit

You may not feel like doing much besides napping these days, but there are compelling reasons to stick with—or get started on—a regular exercise program (working your way up to 30 minutes or more of moderate exercise a day).

Can't live without your weekly work-outs? Have no fear—you don't have to. You may need to alter your routine or skip a few sports that could be risky as your pregnancy progresses (talk to your healthcare provider), but staying active will pay huge dividends during your pregnancy and after your baby's born.

Eight Reasons to Get Moving Now

• **Exercise will give you an energy boost.** Pregnancy can be draining, but regular exercise actually increases your energy level. Not only does it immediately perk you up by getting your blood pumping, but over the long run, aerobic exercise helps your body better utilize food and oxygen and strengthens your cardiovascular system so you don't tire as easily. So when you're fit, you need less effort to engage in *any* activity, be it grocery shopping or sitting through meetings at the office.

• **It will prepare you for the rigors of childbirth.** Giving birth is akin to running a marathon—it requires stamina, determination, and focus. The better shape you're in, the stronger you'll be come delivery day.

• **Working out will help ease and prevent pregnancy aches and pains.** Stretching and strengthening your muscles can help your body cope better with the myriad aches and pains of pregnancy. Walking, for instance, improves circulation—and may help ward off constipation, leg cramps, varicose veins, and swelling.

• **You'll sleep better.** Later, when you're carrying an extra 25 pounds in front of you, getting comfortable enough to sleep at night can be a real challenge, and anxiety may cause you to toss and turn. Exercise helps decrease stress and burn off excess energy, lulling you into a deeper, more restful slumber.

• **Exercise helps reduce stress and lifts your spirits.** Pregnancy is a big deal. Having a child is a life-changing, momentous decision that can leave

---

BY THE NUMBERS

Pregnancy Pounds

Women who gain 15 pounds or less during pregnancy:	**12%**
Women who gain 16 to 25 pounds:	**25%**
Women who gain 26 to 35 pounds:	**32%**
Women who gain 36 to 45 pounds:	**19%**
Women who gain 46 pounds or more:	**12%**
Average weight gain for all pregnant women:	**30.5 lbs.**

Source: *National Center for Health Statistics*

you feeling ecstatic yet overwhelmed and anxious at the same time. Some research suggests that exercise boosts levels of certain body chemicals like serotonin (which is linked to mood) and endorphins (which relieve pain). But what's known for sure is that exercise has a positive effect on your overall sense of health and well-being.

• **Your self-image will soar.** Watching the scale inch its way up to numbers you've never seen before can be disheartening. Staying active will make you feel good about yourself and make you less likely to put on more weight than you should.

Just the Facts

Where the Weight Goes

If the average newborn weighs just 7.5 pounds, and the average woman is advised to gain 30 pounds during pregnancy, where do those other pounds go? Here's a look.

Uterine growth, placenta, and amniotic fluid: 5.5 pounds

Breast growth: 2 pounds

Extra blood and body fluids: 8 pounds

Fat stores: 7 pounds

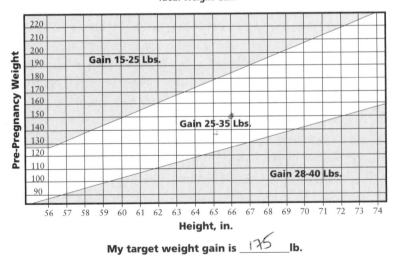

Ideal Weight Gain

My target weight gain is ____175____ lb.

Ask the Experts

Can I Diet during Pregnancy?

Dr. Thomas Bader, obstetrician: Pregnancy is *not* the time to diet. On average, you should be getting about 2,500 calories a day now (up from about 2,200 before you got pregnant). Even if you're overweight, you *need* those calories and nutrients, and your baby does, too. Not only is there a likelihood of poor fetal growth if you're not nourished well, but you increase your odds of having a preterm birth. Research also suggests that dieting early in pregnancy may raise your risk of delivering a baby with a neural tube defect such as spina bifida. My approach is to think of these nine months as part of a larger piece. Any weight you feel you need to lose, you probably put on during the years before you got pregnant. So instead of trying to lose that weight now, use this time to develop the good eating habits that will carry you through the rest of your life.

• **You'll get your body back faster after giving birth.** This alone is reason enough for many women to embark on a pregnancy exercise regimen. If you manage to maintain (or even build) your strength and muscle tone during your pregnancy, you won't be starting from square one when you try to get back into your old jeans after the baby arrives.

• **Exercise may reduce your risk for some pregnancy complications.** Researchers think that exercise decreases your odds of developing pregnancy-induced high blood pressure or gestational diabetes, as well as helping to maintain normal blood-sugar levels if you *do* get gestational diabetes. Some studies also show that exercise in early pregnancy helps your placenta grow and function properly.

Prenatal Exercise Guidelines

Your cardiovascular system changes when you're pregnant—something you need to take into account as you're planning (or modifying) an exercise program. Among other things, your resting heart rate rises by ten to 15 beats a minute, and your blood volume increases between 40 and 50 percent by your third trimester. Working out spurs your heart to beat even faster (and your breathing to become more rapid) so that your body can deliver more oxygen to your muscles. If you've been exercising regularly and you're in good health, your body can meet the dual demands of moderate exercise and pregnancy, but if you're just starting out, you'll

QUICK TIPS

Calorie Boosters

For some women, being thin comes naturally. If you have trouble eating enough and keeping weight on, try these tips.

- Eat breakfast every day. For an extra protein boost, try some peanut butter or a slice of cheese on your morning toast.

- Add a couple of slices of avocado and a handful of nuts or seeds to your salads for extra protein and (good) fat.

- Snack often—and wisely—between meals. Choose foods like yogurt or cheese (for protein and calcium), dried fruits (for vitamins, minerals, and fiber), or a fruit-and-yogurt smoothie (for protein, calcium, vitamins, and minerals).

- Carry cashews or other nuts to nibble on throughout the day. Nuts are packed with calories and protein.

- Drink a milk shake when you crave something sweet. The milk and ice cream combination will give you the calcium and calories your body needs.

need to begin slowly. A few things to keep in mind:

- A "moderate" level of activity depends on what kind of shape you're in, but whether you're fit as a fiddle or a newly reformed couch potato, don't exercise to exhaustion or so hard that you get out of breath. You should be able to carry on a conversation while you're exercising. If you can't, then you need to slow down until you can.

- Your risk for injury may also rise because pregnancy hormones cause your ligaments and joints to become looser than normal. This will allow your baby to descend more easily through your pelvis at birth, but it may also make exercise-related strains, tears, and sprains more likely. That's why it's a good idea to avoid any activity that includes jumping, jarring motions, quick changes in direction, or heavy weights.

- Don't start exercising when you're wiped out, and stop exercising if you start to feel fatigued.

- Forget "going for the burn"—stop *before* your muscles start to hurt.

- Allow at least five to ten minutes to warm up before you exercise and another five to ten minutes to cool down and gently stretch afterward.

- Have a healthy snack of complex carbs after you cool down, to replace the energy you've used exercising.

- Be careful not to get overheated or dehydrated. Dress in layers, and drink plenty of water before, during, and after exercising—even if you don't feel thirsty. Avoid exercising outdoors when it's hot and humid. Instead, get out in the morning or in the evening, or exercise indoors in an air-conditioned space.

• Wear shoes that provide good support and cushioning, and a well-fitting, supportive bra.

• The higher up you go, the less oxygen is in the air, so if you're working out at a high altitude, you'll need to ease in to exercise carefully. You'll likely do fine at altitudes up to 6,000 feet (some experts even say up to 8,000 feet), but above that level, exercise could be risky.

• If you're an elite or competitive athlete who wants to continue strenuous activity, work closely with your doctor or midwife to make any modifications necessary to protect the health of your baby and yourself.

The Best Exercises for Early Pregnancy (and Beyond)

At your first prenatal appointment, be sure to go over your exercise regimen with your health-care provider. Aerobic exercise (that is, activities that increase your respiration and heart rate) strengthens your heart and lungs and helps maintain your muscle tone. Other forms of exercise, such as yoga and weight lifting, are good for toning and strengthening your body. Most women with normal pregnancies can safely take part in any of the following activities.

Low-Impact Aerobics

BENEFITS: You can work out at home with the help of an exercise video or get on the stairclimber at your local gym,

---

QUICK TIPS

Managing Your Weight Gain

If you're overweight, you'll need to take a careful look at your eating habits and make sure you're not gaining too much, too fast. Some strategies for staving off hunger and upping the nutrition quotient of meals and snacks:

• Eat breakfast, lunch, and dinner, plus two healthy snacks—one at midmorning and one in the afternoon—to avoid excessive hunger and overeating.

• Choose high-fiber foods such as whole grain breads and cereals, whole fruit, and legumes. They tend to fill you up, they're packed with nutrients, and they help stave off constipation, a common pregnancy complaint.

• Savor a cup of hot chocolate with skim milk to satisfy a sweet tooth and get a serving of calcium at the same time. Low-fat chocolate pudding is another good choice.

• Include some vegetables in every meal. Mix a handful of chopped veggies into your morning eggs, stack some sliced tomatoes and cucumbers on your turkey sandwich at lunch, and add a handful of your favorites to your dinner salad. Carrot sticks dipped in salsa or hummus make a quick, nutritious snack.

BabyCenter Buzz

How I Find Time to Exercise

"I walk to work. It takes less than an hour, saves on commuting costs, and helps me clear my head." —Belinda

"I found a lunchtime workout partner. I don't have to get up early, and it gives me energy to get through the rest of the day. I have a snack about an hour before I exercise, then eat lunch afterwards at my desk." —Anonymous

"I schedule exercise into my calendar. I called my mom and promised to go to the gym with her, called a friend to see if she could go for a regular evening walk, and signed up for a once-a-week prenatal aerobics class. Making exercise 'appointments' has really helped me get off my butt." —Anonymous

"I walk with a friend at the mall. We have company, air-conditioning, and easy access to drinking fountains and bathrooms." —Anonymous

but an aerobics class designed specifically for expectant moms may be your best bet. Not only will you enjoy the company of other pregnant women, but you'll also benefit from the expertise of an instructor who understands how to keep you and your baby safe. Many community recreation centers offer prenatal aerobics classes.

CAUTIONS: As long as you choose a low-impact aerobic program (meaning it involves no high kicks or leaps) and you have one foot on the ground at all times to minimize stress on your joints and decrease your risk of falling—you should be able to continue your routine throughout most of your pregnancy. If you're already signed up for a regular aerobics class and want to stick with it, let your instructor know that you're pregnant so she can suggest ways to modify any movements that may be too strenuous for you.

Stationary Bicycling

BENEFITS: While it's usually safe to continue riding a bicycle during pregnancy, riding a stationary bike is a great way to get an excellent cardiovascular and lower-body workout—without the risk of falls.

CAUTIONS: If you're plagued by lower-back pain, use a model with upright handlebars or consider a recumbent bike. With a cushioned, chair-like seat and with pedals in front, a recumbent model offers better support for your lower back than a regular bike.

Swimming

BENEFITS: Swimming is one of the best forms of exercise for pregnant women. Not only does it work your large muscle groups (like your arms and legs), but it also provides good cardiovascular benefits and allows you to feel weightless while you're in the water (which will become increasingly important as your girth expands). It's also very safe, with a low risk of injury and little chance of your becoming overheated (unless the water is too warm—over 85°F). (And don't worry: Chlorinated water won't hurt you or your baby.)

CAUTIONS: If you enjoyed swimming regularly before you got pregnant, you should be able to continue now without too much modification. If you didn't exercise at all, you should still be able to start swimming—check in with your practitioner first. You'll need to start slowly, stretch well before and after you get into the pool, warm up and cool down gradually, and be careful not to overexert yourself.

Walking

BENEFITS: One of the best cardiovascular exercises for pregnant women, brisk walking keeps you fit without jarring your knees and ankles too much. It's also safe to do right up to delivery day, and it's one of the easiest ways to start exercising if you haven't been very active in the past.

CAUTIONS: If you're already a regular walker, keep it up. If you haven't been out for a stroll longer than the one from the door to your car in a while,

QUICK TIPS

Walk This Way

- Make sure you have proper walking shoes so your feet get the support they need. Look for shoes that are well-cushioned, to lessen the impact on your joints.

- During warm weather, wear a sun hat and carry a bottle of water to keep yourself cool and hydrated. Dehydration can bring on contractions and raise your body temperature to dangerous levels. And always protect your skin with sunscreen.

- If it's very hot and humid outside, avoid overheating by going for a walk in an air-conditioned mall or on a treadmill at the gym or at home.

start with a slow walk a few times a week and build yourself up to brisk daily 20- to 30-minute jaunts. As with all exercise, start with a five- to ten-minute warm-up (slow walking in this case) and slow down for the last five minutes of your walk;, followed by five minutes of gentle stretching.

Weight Training

BENEFITS: Weight training strengthens and tones your muscles and helps build stamina, which you'll need in spades during labor and delivery (and beyond).

CAUTIONS: Whether you use the free weights and resistance-training machines at your local gym or do simple weight-training exercises at home—such as lifting hand and ankle weights, start with short sets (five to ten repetitions) with lighter weights (2 or 3 pounds each) and gradually work up to more repetitions and slightly heavier weights.

Yoga

BENEFITS: Prenatal yoga, combined with cardiovascular exercise such as brisk walking, is an ideal way to stay fit when you're pregnant. When you stretch or do yoga, you're toning your muscles, improving your balance and circulation, and limbering up with little, if any, impact on your joints.

Yoga is also beneficial because it teaches you to relax and breathe deeply, which in turn helps you prepare for the physical demands of pregnancy, labor, birth—and yes, motherhood. Learning how to take deep breaths, for instance, teaches you to stay calm when you need it

---

QUICK TIPS

Weight-Training Moves to Avoid

- Never use quick, jerking movements, which can injure your looser-than-normal joints. Slow, controlled movements will prevent injury.

- Work with much lighter weights than you normally would; you can compensate for the lower weight by doing more repetitions (but stop *before* your muscles get too fatigued).

- If you're doing arm exercises that require you to stand still, move around between sets to keep blood from pooling in your legs.

- Avoid moves such as the Valsalva maneuver (bearing down like you do when you have a bowel movement) which can cause dizziness, and walking lunges, which can strain your ligaments.

Exercise Alerts

Use your common sense and listen to your body—if it hurts, don't do it! And stop before you feel sore or get too tired. Also stop exercising immediately and contact your healthcare provider if you notice any of the following symptoms when you're working out at any time during your pregnancy:

- Difficulty walking, calf pain, or swelling
- Dizziness, light-headedness, or nausea that persists
- Shortness of breath
- Increased heart rate that doesn't return to normal after several minutes of rest
- Chest pain, palpitations, or an irregular heartbeat
- Headache
- Pain—especially in your back, abdomen, or pelvis
- Uterine contractions
- Vaginal bleeding
- Fluid gushing or leaking from your vagina
- Decreased fetal movement once you've been feeling your baby move regularly

most. When you're afraid—during labor, say—your body produces increased amounts of adrenaline, which can decrease your contractions and slow your labor. Yoga training helps you resist the urge to tighten up during contractions and shows you how to breathe instead.

The benefits of yoga aren't all physical, either: Taking a prenatal yoga class (or any prenatal exercise class) is also a great way to meet other expectant mothers. Being in a positive, supportive environment with your fellow moms-to-be will give you a regular emotional boost—and motivate you to keep coming back.

CAUTIONS: Seek out an instructor who's been trained in prenatal yoga. If you don't want to drop out of your regular class, tell your instructor that you're expecting—and ask her to help you safely modify your regular routine. If you do Bikram yoga, though, you'll need to drop the class

Buying Guide

Prenatal Exercise Videos

Overwhelmed by the number of prenatal fitness videos? You might want to check what's available to rent before you invest in a tape or DVD of your own. A few specifics to look for when making your choice:

- An instructor who has plenty of experience with prenatal exercise, who's certified by the American Council on Exercise, and who follows the prenatal exercise guidelines set by the American College of Obstetricians and Gynecologists (ACOG)

- A low-impact routine, especially if you're not used to exercising regularly

- A routine that includes an adequate warm-up and cool-down period (at least five minutes each)

- Instructions on how to modify the routine for each trimester as well as for your fitness level

- A workout that includes abdominal and pelvic-floor exercises but that doesn't have you lying on your back (or suggests alternative positions to use after your first trimester)

- Maneuvers that don't require any sudden moves or quick changes of direction that could cause you to lose your balance

- Bonuses, such as tips or routines for postpartum exercise

- A tape that looks like fun—because if you don't enjoy it, you won't *do* it

until after your baby arrives, since the excessive heat pumped into the room could be dangerous to both of you. Whatever kind of class you take, skip the inversions—head and shoulder stands are *not* for pregnant women. Also avoid positions that stretch your abdominal muscles too much, such as deep forward and backward bends, which can lead to muscle strains and tears and back pain during pregnancy.

When Exercise Is a No-Go

Sometimes exercise during pregnancy is strictly forbidden, to protect the health of you or your baby. Check with your healthcare provider before starting, continuing, or changing an exercise regimen. If you have—or develop—any of following conditions, she'll probably advise you *not* to exercise for the duration of your pregnancy:

• Heart disease
• Lung disease
• Cervical insufficiency or cerclage
• Intrauterine growth restriction
• Persistent vaginal bleeding
• Pregnancy-induced hypertension or preeclampsia
• Preterm labor in this pregnancy
• Placenta previa (after 26 weeks)
• Preterm rupture of the membranes

Your practitioner may also advise you not to exercise if you have certain other medical conditions, such as poorly controlled diabetes, high blood pressure, or severe anemia. If you're a heavy smoker or are obese or extremely thin, aerobic exercise may be out, too. And in certain other circumstances, such as having had preterm labor in a previous pregnancy or having risk factors for preterm labor in this pregnancy (if you're carrying twins or higher-order multiples, for instance), you may be able to exercise in your first trimester but will have to take it easy after that.

YOUR EMOTIONS

Excitement, joy, anticipation—all of these emotions go into high gear once you find out you're pregnant. But so, too, do moodiness, anxiety, and irritability. Repeat this mantra: *I'm not crazy; I'm just pregnant!*

Managing Mood Swings

Are you fine one minute and in tears the next? Snapping more at your partner, friends, or coworkers? Welcome to the club. It's practically expected for you to have major mood swings during pregnancy. Your seesawing emotions may be caused by hormone changes that alter your levels of neurotransmitters (brain chemicals that affect mood), along with the broad range of feelings you may have about the big life changes that becoming a parent bring about. Most women find that moodiness flares up at around six to ten weeks, eases up in the second trimester, and then reappears with a vengeance as their pregnancy winds to a close. Everyone responds differently to these changes—some women experience heightened emotions both good and bad; others feel more depressed or anxious.

While there's no one-size-fits-all approach to moodiness, you can handle the mood monster by finding ways to take care of yourself emotionally.

- If you're feeling frustrated and overwhelmed, take frequent breaks: Put your feet up, get some fresh air, or concentrate on another task for a few minutes. If these feelings are a constant in your life, take steps to reduce your stress load.
- Spend time with your partner and friends, doing things that you find relaxing and enjoyable.
- You're more likely to feel moody when you're not babying your body, so get plenty of sleep and make sure you're eating well.
- When you feel a bad mood coming on, try going for a walk, prac-

BabyCenter Buzz

Dealing with Mixed Emotions

"Even though my pregnancy was very much planned and wanted, my first reaction when the test turned positive was, 'Oh s--t—what've I *done*?' The reality of a human being in the making and the end of childless life as I knew it was just really sobering. I gave myself permission to feel those emotions—panic, fear, even a little regret—and eventually they faded and allowed me to concentrate on my excitement and happiness."   —*Leah*

"Listening to the experiences of other pregnant women helps me. It's reassuring to know that I'm not the only one with ups and downs."   —*Melissa*

"When I have a bad day, I write down all the positive things that are happening in my pregnancy, how excited we are about the little one's arrival, and then I sort of 'talk' to the baby. It gives me a sense of hope and excitement about what's to come."   —*Anonymous*

"My moods and emotions become hard to handle when I haven't had enough rest and I'm eating badly. When I feel down, taking my dog for a walk seems to help."   —*Anonymous*

"I was excited when the pregnancy test was positive, but my husband was so worried about our finances and how our lives were going to change that I wondered if we'd done the right thing. Talking each other through the emotional ups and downs—we never seem to hit them at the same time!—helps both of us immensely."   —*Heather*

ticing breathing exercises, popping in a pregnancy yoga video, having a prenatal massage, or even doing meditation.

• Air out your less positive feelings with friends and family or, if you prefer, with your healthcare provider or a therapist.

Worry: A Mother-to-Be's Constant Companion

Pregnancy brings out the worrywart in all of us. And for good reason: You're growing a *life* inside of you. It's natural to fret about what you eat, drink, think, feel, and do. It's also perfectly normal—provided you don't obsess about it— to worry about whether your baby is healthy, how this new person will change your life and relationships, and whether you're truly up to the task of parenthood. But if your anxiety is becoming all-consuming and regularly interferes with your day-to-day functioning, it's time to find a better way to deal with it.

BabyCenter Buzz

What I Worry About

"I wish I'd known how *much* I would worry—about how the baby is doing, how he or she is growing, and every little twinge I feel. There are just so many unknowns." —*Julie*

"What an overwhelming feeling it is to know that you and you alone are solely responsible for the life and well-being of this unborn miracle! I worry about every 'bad' thing I've ever done to my body over the last 28 years!" —*Amie*

"I worry that I may neglect my four-year-old daughter. She's been my whole world." —*Jennifer*

"I fret about the money situation. Both my husband and I work, but I have a firm belief that children do better with a parent at home." —*Anonymous*

To start, gently share your fears with your partner—even if they're about *him*; chances are he's harboring concerns of his own. Communicating openly about your anxiety can help you both feel better. Turn to friends or family members for support, too. Other moms-to-be are another source of comfort, as they're likely experiencing the same worries you are. If you're extremely anxious or have a specific reason to be concerned about your baby's health, share your concerns with your caregiver. If, after you've aired your worries and checked in on your baby's well-being, anxiety *still* plagues you, professional counseling can help you get to the bottom of your troubles.

Managing Stress: How to Relax and Reduce Anxiety

If you're used to caring for others or giving 110 percent at work, making *yourself* a priority may seem unnatural or even selfish. But taking care of yourself is an essential part of taking care of your baby. Cutting down on or learning how to manage stress makes for a healthier pregnancy. While everyday pressure is a part of modern life, a high level of chronic stress can boost your odds of preterm labor or of delivering a low-birthweight baby—all the more reason to get it under control now.

Just for Dad

What *You* May Be Worried About

Security fears. The biggest fear men face is the one most deeply ingrained in our culture: Will I be able to protect and provide for my family? When a baby arrives, there's often a sudden—if temporary—shift from two incomes for two people to one income for three. And that's a tough burden to carry. Plus, you have to be strong in ways you hadn't counted on before. You have to provide support not just financially but also emotionally. Your partner will need your help; she'll be undergoing dramatic emotional shifts, and you have to be ready for her to lean on you.

Paternity fears. You won't find many expectant dads fessing up to it, but it's common to question—ever so fleetingly—how this baby can really be *yours*. It's not that you mistrust your partner's fidelity; it's just that you're momentarily overwhelmed by the idea that you had a hand in creating something as miraculous as a child.

Mortality fears. When you're a part of the beginning of a new life, you can't avoid thinking about the *end* of life. Thoughts about your own mortality can loom large: You're not the young buck anymore, the next generation is in the works, and if everything turns out the way it's supposed to, you'll die before your child does. For a lot of young men who go around thinking they're immortal or invincible, that's a lot to absorb.

Here are some simple ways to keep stress at bay.

• Vent your frustrations with friends and family. Keeping your feelings bottled up inside will only add to your stress.

• Join (or create!) a support group. If you're coping with a difficult situation, spending time with others in the same boat can help ease your burden. (Many women create support networks online; visit http://bbs.babycenter.com/boards/bbs-preg to connect with other moms-to-be grappling with similar issues.)

• Cut back on chores—and use that time to put your feet up, nap, or read a book.

• Make time for the things you love doing. Any activity that you can lose yourself in—listening to or playing music, painting, knitting, cooking, even dinner with a girlfriend—are great ways to distract yourself from worry and recharge.

• Use some vacation days whenever possible. Spending a day—or even an afternoon—resting at home will help you get through a tough week. And, if you're not feeling well, take a sick day.

• Try deep-breathing exercises, yoga, or stretching, and get regular physical activity such as swimming or walking.

• Do your best to eat a healthy, well-balanced diet so you have the physical and emotional energy you need.

• Go to bed early. Your body is working overtime to nourish your growing baby and needs all the sleep it can get.

• Limit "information overload." Reading books and magazines, surfing pregnancy Web sites, and listening to your friends' pregnancy stories is great—but don't delve into all the scary things that *might* (but probably won't) happen during your pregnancy. Focus instead on how you're feeling and what's happening to you *now*.

• Practice saying "no." Now is as good time to disabuse yourself of the notion that you can do it all. You can't, so learn to let your superwoman ideals go. Make slowing down a priority, and get used to the idea of asking your friends and loved ones for help.

• If you're under unusual stress, feel like you're at your breaking point, or think you may be depressed (page 210), ask your practitioner to refer you to a therapist.

THE REST OF YOUR LIFE

Though you look pretty much the same as you normally do, you may wonder what to wear before it's time for true maternity clothes. You may also be concerned about whether various aspects of your normal beauty regimen are safe to continue now that a baby's on board.

How Your Appearance Will Change

Other than a green tinge around your gills from morning sickness, some bleariness from fatigue, a bit of thickening around your middle from bloating and gas, and perhaps a little twinkle in your eye from your happy secret, you may look much the same as you did before you became pregnant.

Dressing for Early Pregnancy

If you can't resist trendy new maternity clothes now available everywhere, feel free to indulge. But if your clothes are feeling a little tight and you aren't ready to come out of the pregnancy closet by sporting maternity wear, try these time-tested ideas.

 Scour your closet—and your man's. What woman *doesn't* have some things to wear when she's a few pounds heavier than usual? Loose tops, pants or skirts with elastic or drawstring waistbands, and just about anything made out of stretchy fabric are terrific for getting you through the first

QUICK TIP

Adapting Nonmaternity Pants and Skirts

To get a few weeks' extra wear out of your regular pants and skirts, try this trick: Loop a rubber band or ponytail holder through the buttonhole and then wrap it around the button to provide that crucial extra inch or two of breathing room.

95

few months. You can also wear a favorite cardigan—just leave it unbuttoned—or a much-loved T-shirt under a partly buttoned blouse or blazer. A-line shifts, Empire-waist dresses and tops, and pencil skirts paired with swingy shirts work like a charm. For a sporty, hip look, pair low-rise pants with a fitted tee. Don't forget menswear, either: A man's oxford shirt worn unbuttoned over a formfitting tee or tank is a classic look.

Buy several "transitional" pieces. Pick up a couple of pairs of inexpensive nonmaternity pants and tops a size or two larger than you normally wear; some women have great success finding transitional clothes in boutiques and departments that specialize in "plus sizes"—they tend to be less expensive than maternity retailers, too. An added bonus: You'll be able to wear these transitional clothes during the awkward months *after* you deliver, as well.

Your Relationships and Sex Life

Getting pregnant changes forever your relationship with your partner, your friends, and your family—sometimes in unexpected ways.

BabyCenter Buzz

How I Shared the Big News with My Mate

"We went out to a Chinese restaurant, and I had the waiter put 'Michelle is having a baby' in his fortune cookie. It was a hit!"   —*Michelle*

"My husband was with me when I took the test. We left the room for the requisite five minutes—which seemed more like five *hours*—then nervously held hands as we climbed the stairs to learn our fate."   —*Julia*

"I bought a book for expectant *fathers* and put it in a gift bag, along with the pregnancy test I'd taken. His reaction was priceless."   —*Sue*

"I gave my partner the children's book *Heather Has Two Mommies*. She knew right away what it meant—we'd been trying artificial insemination for months—and she laughed and then burst into tears!"   —*Anonymous*

"I gave my husband a birthday party invitation. On the front it read: 'There's a party and you're invited!' I filled out the information blanks inside with the baby's information: 'Guest of honor: Our son or daughter; Date: On or around September 17; Time: To be announced; Location: Memorial Hospital.' He was thrilled."   —*Barbara*

$$BabyCenter\ Buzz$$

My Partner's Not Excited about Our Pregnancy

"Men are confusing: They send mixed signals and aren't always good about expressing their feelings. He may be overjoyed about the new baby, but he may also be afraid of what's to come." —*Carolyn*

"It's likely your husband has deep worries about your health, how your relationship is going to change, and general worries about the future. Talk to him about your feelings and ask about his. Don't condemn him for seeming unexcited at this point." —*Terry*

"Don't let your partner's lack of enthusiasm dampen your spirits. Happiness is contagious. Find support from other family members and girlfriends until he comes around." —*Jeannie*

You and Your Partner

While it's true that you're the one undergoing massive physical and emotional changes, your partner's changing, too. You're in this together! That can make your pregnancy a time of great joy and increasing closeness or a time of incredible turmoil and stress. More than likely, you'll experience your share of both. Most couples do. Becoming parents is probably the biggest life change you'll ever face together. Open communication is the key to keeping your bond strong, and if you can set the groundwork now for that, you'll be in prime position to tackle the even greater challenge of raising a child. When times get tough, look to—not away from—each other, and remember to involve your partner, have some fun, and celebrate the good times.

You're Thrilled, He's Not (or Vice Versa): When You and Your Partner Have Different Reactions to Your Pregnancy

When it comes to having a baby, men and women don't always work off the same sheet music. While you may be jumping for joy, your partner's reaction may be much more subdued. If that's the case, cut him some slack. It sometimes takes a few months for men to get used to the idea of becoming a father. He can't yet see or feel the tremendous changes that are front and center in your mind—so until you start to show or he can actually feel the baby kick when he puts his hand on your belly, your pregnancy may seem purely theoretical to him. He may also be worried about how your relationship (sexual and otherwise) is going to change and whether he'll be a good father. Finally, impending fatherhood often goes hand in hand with increased pressure for men to boost their earning power, to get on the fast track at work, and to shoulder more responsibility in their daily lives. No wonder he's a little freaked!

Of course, women aren't immune to this phenomenon, either. Your partner may be over the moon about becoming a father, but you may not feel emotionally ready to be a mother or may already be stretched to your limits by other children or other commitments in your life—especially if this pregnancy wasn't planned. On the other hand, perhaps you *thought* a baby was

Just the Facts

Domestic Violence during Pregnancy

One final thought on your relationship with your mate now that you're expecting a baby. Though many women mistakenly believe that pregnancy will reform an abusive partner, it won't. Sadly, pregnancy itself is a common *trigger* for domestic violence. If you need help getting out of an abusive relationship, call the 24-hour National Domestic Violence Hotline at (800) 799-7233 for confidential crisis intervention and counseling. If you ever fear that your partner is about to hurt you, call 911 or your local police department immediately. Consider these sobering stats:

- One in six abused women reports that her partner first abused her when she was pregnant.

- Nearly one in ten pregnant women reports suffering from domestic violence during pregnancy.

- Staying in an abusive relationship comes at a high cost: Partner violence puts not only you at risk but your baby as well. Domestic abuse is associated with miscarriage, low birthweight, and fetal injury or even death.

- Abuse isn't limited to physical violence. Name-calling, humiliation, constant criticism, attempts to isolate you from friends or family, extreme jealousy, restriction of personal freedom, tight control of family finances, and threats of physical harm are all hallmarks of an abusive relationship.

- Abuse doesn't have to happen every day or even every week for it to be classified as domestic violence.

- Women of all ages, races, religions, nationalities, educational backgrounds, sexual orientations, and socioeconomic levels are victims of abuse.

Just for Dad

What Your Partner *Really* Wants from You

- Be a sympathetic listener, especially when she's feeling lousy.
- Give her foot or back massages to ease pregnancy aches and pains.
- Clean the bathroom (without being asked). If she has to throw up, don't let it be in a dirty toilet.
- Be sensitive to her food aversions and bionic nose. If red meat turns her stomach, don't suggest a night out at the local steak house. If the smell of brewing coffee sends her running for the bathroom, pick up your java on the way to work instead.

everything you wanted, but now, faced with the reality of your situation, you're not so sure. If your career is taking off, for instance, you may be worried about how having a baby will affect your ability to stay focused. Or maybe you're simply so sick and tired from morning sickness and other early-pregnancy symptoms that you're having a hard time feeling excited about anything.

Having out-of-sync reactions to your pregnancy doesn't spell disaster for your relationship, but you and your mate will need to start talking openly and honestly about your feelings in order to avoid having a blowup or letting the pregnancy drive a wedge between you. Have a heart-to-heart talk to keep your feelings from festering. Or, if talking is too stressful, write a letter outlining your concerns. If the pregnancy seems to be coming between you or if things weren't so great to begin with, you may want to seek the help of a couples counselor or a family therapist. Pregnancy can bring deeper relationship problems to the forefront that may be better tackled on neutral ground. Ask your caregiver for a recommendation.

Pregnancy Without a Partner

Whether by choice or circumstance, more women than ever are going through pregnancy without a committed partner by their side. So if you're doing this alone—well, you're *not* alone. In fact, more than 10 million American women are raising children without a mate at home. And as you've

BabyCenter Buzz

I'm Pregnant—and on My Own

"I'm 22 and pregnant. My boyfriend split, and I don't think he's coming back. It hurts me a lot knowing that he won't be there when the baby is born. I can't afford to pay all the bills by myself, so I'll be moving back home with my mom. I never thought I'd be a single parent." —Anonymous

"I just found out that I'm pregnant—after six months of attempting artificial insemination on my own. I know that it will mean I'll need to make more sacrifices for my child than a married parent. I'm over 40 now, and I haven't yet met Mr. Right, but I want the experience of motherhood—morning sickness and all." —Linda

"I'm single and expecting my first child. I've found unexpected support and have been pleased by how open my friends and family have been. I know that some people will have issues with my decision, but it's my life and my responsibility. I have no room for small-minded negativity." —Michele

"Early in my pregnancy, I found out that my boyfriend was cheating, and he left me shortly thereafter. It's hard being pregnant by myself, but you have to play the cards you're dealt. I do believe that it's better for him not to be in my baby's life than for him to be a source of negativity and pain. It's a wonderful thing for a child to have a loving and responsible father—but if that's not possible, a single mother can raise a well-adjusted child." —Anonymous

surely discovered by now, single moms experience many of the same pregnancy highs and lows as their married and partnered counterparts: elated expectation, profound fear—and, yes, morning sickness.

But as a single person, you may be grappling with other issues as well: unique legal or financial concerns, judgmental friends and family, difficulties with an ex or with a partner who comes and goes, or even dating. You may also need to secure a birth partner in the short run and a support network in the long run. Above all, figure out how to take good care of *yourself*—and then you can take good care of your baby.

Sex in the First Trimester

Sex is, in all likelihood, how you found yourself in this situation in the first place, whether you and your mate indulged often in your quest to make a baby—whether it was a happy (or unhappy) accident. But now that your pregnancy test is positive, you may be plagued by questions and worries about having sex. Is it safe? Will it be different? Will my partner still want to make love to me? The short answer to all is almost certainly yes. But the longer answer is: While sex during pregnancy is almost always safe—actually *wanting* to do it may be the furthest thing from your mind right now.

The big physical and emotional changes you're undergoing are bound to change your sex life, too. Many women are just too tired or nauseated to make love during the first trimester. Don't beat yourself up about it—you can hardly expect to feel like a tigress in the bedroom when your main goals are keeping your dinner down and your eyes open. But do your best not to turn your back on your mate—intimacy is important, but it doesn't have to include sex. Give him lots of hugs, kisses, and other displays of affection; gently explain why you're just not up to making love right now (he's not a mind reader); ask him to be patient and help him understand that your lack of interest doesn't mean that you love him any less than before. You both should be reassured to know that your desire will likely return when you're feeling better. In fact, you may find that making love in the second trimester (page 000) is better than ever.

When you *are* up to making love again, you'll notice that the sensations of sex also change when you're pregnant—mostly for the better, but occasionally for the worse. You may find that, finally free from worries about getting (or not getting) pregnant, you enjoy sex more than ever. Increased vaginal moistness helps smooth the way, and increased blood flow to your pelvic area causes genital engorgement and heightened pleasure. But the same engorgement can also give you an uncomfortable feeling of fullness after intercourse ends. What's more, you may have mild and harmless abdominal cramps during or immediately after intercourse, and if your breasts feel swollen and tender, your mate's caresses may actually feel painful.

BY THE NUMBERS

How Orgasm Changes When You're Pregnant

48% said it felt the same as it always did

36% said the big O was more intense

16% said it was less intense

Source: *A BabyCenter.com poll of more than 17,000 women*

If you're worried that your partner will be turned off by your condition, rest assured that most men find their pregnant mates as attractive as ever—and often even *more* so. The new life growing inside you is, after all, a potent reminder of your bond. Don't be surprised if he loves your bigger breasts and new curves as well.

But your mate's desire may also be dampened by concerns for your health, apprehension about the burdens of parenthood, fear that sex could cause a miscarriage or hurt the baby, or, later, even self-consciousness about making love in the presence of your unborn child. Reassure him (and yourself) that sex is perfectly safe during pregnancy (see opposite page for exceptions) and that your baby, ensconced behind your closed cervix and strong uterine muscles and cushioned by the amniotic fluid, will be blissfully unaware of any action the two of you are getting.

How Pregnancy Changes the Father's Sex Life

For some men, sex during pregnancy is an incredible turn-on—but for others, it's not even on their radar screen. Both are perfectly natural responses. Where you stand on the issue depends on a lot of factors, but one thing is pretty much guaranteed: When your partner is pregnant, your sex life will change.

In truth, you probably won't have sex as often as you did before. One of the most common reasons that expectant couples cut back on lovemaking during the first trimester is fear they'll cause a miscarriage or hurt their baby. If you're concerned about that, you can stop worrying right now. The baby is safely cushioned in your mate's fluid-filled amniotic sac, and unless you're having *very* rough sex, you have almost no chance of injuring anyone.

When Sex May Be a No-Go

As long as your pregnancy is normal, intercourse and orgasm pose no threat to you or your baby. There are some situations, however, in which you may have to forgo sexual pleasure for the time being. If you have any of the following conditions, ask your healthcare provider exactly what you can and can't do, and *when* in pregnancy the rules apply:

• Vaginal spotting or bleeding or unusual discharge
• Abdominal cramping
• Placenta previa or a very low-lying placenta
• Cervical insufficiency
• Preterm birth in a previous pregnancy or a bout of preterm labor in this pregnancy
• Ruptured membranes
• An unhealed genital herpes lesion in either you or your partner, or the presence of any other untreated sexually transmitted infection (if either of you has oral herpes, you'll need to avoid kissing or having oral sex during an outbreak)

If you have to hold off on a roll in the hay, you can still kiss, engage in foreplay (as long as it doesn't lead to orgasm for you), give each other long massages, and share your feelings for each other.

Family and Friendships

At first, if those around you don't know you're pregnant, they may be mystified by changes in your behavior (especially if morning sickness has you in its grip) or puzzled by your moodiness. When you do decide to spill the beans, accept everyone's good wishes, but don't expect them all to feel as excited as you do. Friends or family members struggling with infertility or pregnancy loss may have a hard time at first sharing in your happiness. Others may simply shrug off your good news. Try not to be too hard on them—your pregnancy may just not seem "real" to anyone but you yet.

Just for Dad

The Difference Is in Desire

Changes in sexual desire—for you and for her—are common during any time of major physical and emotional upheaval. At first, your partner's pregnancy might make you hornier than ever. For some men, pregnancy is an exciting confirmation of their masculinity and virility. In addition, a lot of dads-to-be feel closer to their mates than ever, and that closeness is often expressed erotically.

For other guys, the first trimester (and possibly the entire pregnancy) is a time of decreased desire. Before your partner got pregnant, she was the sexy woman you loved, and her breasts and vagina were all about recreation. But now that she's pregnant, you may find her body less fun and more functional. Even worse, when her pregnancy's over, she's going to be a mother. And mothers aren't always seen as sexy.

As the pregnancy progresses, the differences between the wanna-have-sex's and the don't-wanna-have-sex's continue. Most men, for example, find their partner's growing body to be the essence of femininity and, therefore, quite attractive. Others don't. Their partner's growing abdomen and leaking breasts in late pregnancy may seem more messy than enticing.

Your mate's ideas about sex during pregnancy can also change from week to week or even day to day. She may feel more connected to you than ever and may be much less inhibited now that you don't have to worry about birth control. She may find the idea of having created a life with you to be wildly erotic, and she may be delighted with her blossoming body and newfound curves. On the other hand, she may be spending a lot of her first trimester hunched over the toilet in the grip of morning sickness—hardly an aphrodisiac. She may be thinking that mothers aren't supposed to have sex, worrying about having a miscarriage or hurting the baby, or simply feeling fat as her belly grows.

The solution is to talk about each other's desires and needs. If you're as turned-on by her as ever—or even more so—tell her. She may want you just as much but be feeling insecure about her body right now. You can put that anxiety to rest by being loving with or without sexual intercourse. If she's giving you the cold shoulder, ask her why. Chances are, she's simply too tired or too sick to give sex much thought right now—and may not realize that you're feeling rejected. If penetration is uncomfortable, now may be the perfect time to explore other forms of sexual expression. Think back to the time when you did "everything but" have intercourse. It was exciting then, and it's just as fun now. Mutual masturbation, oral sex, and playing with vibrators and other sex toys can be as enjoyable as intercourse and are practically guaranteed to keep things interesting in the bedroom.

BabyCenter Buzz

My First Reaction to Finding Out That I Was Going to Be a Father

"I've realized that a woman becomes a mother right from conception, but a man really doesn't become a father until the baby is born. I admit that I'm having a hard time dealing with the fact that I'm going to be responsible for another person. When I feel frustrated with the whole pregnancy thing, I remind myself that she's already a mother and that I'm not *quite* a dad yet."   —*Anonymous*

"We've been trying for three years. I'm kind of excited but still in disbelief—I find it sort of unreal. After two miscarriages, my wife is cautious about getting our hopes up, but once she believes we're out of the deep water, reality may set in."   —*H.R.*

"I'm 21 and my fiancée is 18. I felt a lot of anxiety when she told me she was late, and I was shocked when her pregnancy test was positive. I'm excited about the baby now, but also very worried about health complications and financial problems."   —*John*

"I was happy and nervous at the same time. My main worry is that my wife and I will lose the private time we have with each other. We've been together for over ten years, and all that time we've been each other's best friend. I don't want to lose that."   —*Anonymous*

"I was scared but also excited. I feared that I wouldn't know what to do. I feared that I'd need to have a steady income in a very volatile job market. I feared that with a baby, we'd no longer be able to do the things that we enjoyed—eating out, going to movies—on the spur of the moment. But at the same time, the whole prospect of being a dad excited me. The idea of bringing a new life into this world, a little human being—it wasn't just exciting, it was profound. Now when I look at my son, all the worries (which I sometimes still have) just melt away. I know it sounds cliché, but it's true."   —*David*

"For men, finding out that we're going to be a father just scares the crap out of us at first, for a million reasons: money, our feelings, our wife's feelings, etc. But the fact that we worry about it is a good sign—if we're worried, it means we care about doing a good job."   —*AJ*

When and How to Tell Your Child a Sibling's on the Way

You're thrilled that your firstborn is going to be a big sister or brother—but that doesn't mean *he* will be. Though you may want to share the news with your child shortly after you find out yourself, it's often best to wait until the end of your first trimester. That way, your pregnancy will be well-established

BabyCenter Buzz

How We Broke the News to Family and Friends

"I made a sign using crayon and wrote in childish handwriting: 'I'm going to be a big sister.' I took pictures of my daughter holding the sign and e-mailed it to our loved ones." —*Mishalay*

"We bought a few baby items, including a bib that says, 'Grandma loves me,' and wrapped it up for my mother's birthday gift." —*Dianne*

"I mailed out tiny disposable diapers with a note attached that said, 'Arriving in September.' We received many excited phone calls." —*Anonymous*

"I created a 'Vacation Request Form' for my mother that stated she would need time off for the arrival of her grandchild. I faxed it to her work and waited a few minutes to call. She was still screaming when she picked up the phone." —*Sharon*

and you won't have to grapple with explaining a loss to a child who's too young to comprehend it. (Even so, if you're too nauseated or exhausted during your first trimester to interact with your child the way you normally do, an explanation may be in order.)

The best way to break the news about the new baby is briefly and simply, though exactly what you say will depend on your child's age and maturity. You might say something like "You're going to have a new brother or sister. Right now he or she is growing inside Mommy but will be ready to come out after Halloween" (or some other seasonal landmark your child will recognize; "November" probably doesn't mean much to a toddler or preschooler). By not overloading your firstborn with facts, you'll leave him space to absorb this startling revelation at his own speed and to ask questions when he's ready to hear more. If you plan to find out about your baby-to-be's sex, go ahead and tell your child once you know—it'll help make the upcoming arrival more real to him.

Your *Other* "Baby"

Okay, maybe you're not losing sleep over how to break the news to your furry friend. But that tiny baby may mean big changes for your pet.

Your Job and Finances

Most healthy women can work right up until their water breaks. But having a baby—even one whose arrival is nine long months away—usually brings up a slew of work- and money-related issues. How will your pregnancy affect your job duties? When should you share your news with your boss and coworkers? Will you keep your job after your baby arrives? And, speaking of the baby, how are you going to make ends meet when you have another mouth to feed and possibly one fewer paycheck? We'll help you sort through the questions—and find answers that work for you.

Pregnant on the Job

The smell of coffee brewing in the office kitchenette makes you gag, you can't concentrate, and you'd give anything to sneak off for a midday snooze. Sound familiar? Normal early-pregnancy symptoms can wreak havoc on your workplace routine (even more so if you're keeping your condition under wraps). But once you've devised some on-the-job coping strategies, including figuring out when and how to tell your boss that you're expecting, you'll likely feel better (emotionally, at least!).

Taking Care of Yourself at Work

Even if your job requires nothing more strenuous than lifting a telephone, early-pregnancy symptoms can make you so sluggish you can barely move. Some strategies for getting through the day—and babying your body on the job:

Take breaks. Putting your feet up if you've been standing—or walking around every two hours if you've been sitting—should help you feel more comfortable. Try stretching in place, too, if you're starting to feel stiff.

Stay hydrated. Keep a water bottle or a tall glass at your workstation, and refill it often. And don't hold it in: Go to the bathroom as often as you need to—even if it means discreetly leaving meetings.

Eat wisely. Take time to eat a balanced nutritious lunch to keep your energy up and provide the right nutrients for yourself and your growing baby. Also, stock your workstation or office fridge with healthy, handy snacks—such as fresh and dried fruit, nuts, trail mix, yogurt.

Reduce stress. You can't wish away a difficult boss, an annoying coworker, or impossible deadlines, but you can learn to cope with them in a healthy way. Deep-breathing exercises, meditation, yoga, stretching, and simply taking a short walk are proven stress busters.

Get enough sleep at night. If you feel dog tired right after dinner, don't fight it. The extra R & R you get from hitting the sack early will help you get through the next day.

Rest when you can. The more strenuous your job, the more you should take it easy outside of work so you can stay rested and relaxed. If you find yourself feeling especially lousy, take an occasional sick day to rest. Or, if you can, take an hour or two of vacation time here and there to shorten your workdays.

Cut back. Turn down excessive overtime, especially in jobs requiring physical activity (this includes housework, too). Think twice about raising your hand for high-stress or time-consuming new projects. If scaling back to a part-time schedule is a viable option for you, you might want to give that some consideration. And if you're in a position to do so, adopt a new mantra: Delegate, delegate, delegate.

Accept help. If coworkers who are in the know about your pregnancy want to baby you a little, let them. Consider yourself lucky to have the support.

Handling Early-Pregnancy Symptoms at Work

Nausea and crushing fatigue are probably the worst symptoms you'll have to deal with when you're punching the clock, but a constant need to visit the ladies' room can be a distraction, too. Some solutions:

• Keep something handy to nibble on when queasiness strikes. Many women swear by crackers, but one study showed that protein-rich foods, such as cheese or nuts, might provide more relief.

• If you're prone to vomiting, keep plastic bags, a hand towel, and a toothbrush and toothpaste or mouthwash in your bag.

• Map out the quickest route to the bathroom from various points in your workplace.

• If you haven't yet told your boss or coworkers your news, and someone comes in to the bathroom while you're indisposed, simply say you're not feeling well and leave it at that.

• Always visit the restroom before meetings or the start of a shift that's difficult to interrupt.

• If fatigue is making your brain feel fuzzy, try to grab a quick catnap in vacant conference room or office, your car, or other vacant space. A portable alarm clock can help you keep snoozes short enough that no one will notice you're gone—15 to 20 minutes is ideal. Or take a brisk walk around the block to clear your head and get your blood pumping.

When to Break the News

If you're confident that your employer will handle your pregnancy news positively and professionally, you may want to announce it sooner rather than later so you won't have to invent cover stories for prenatal appointments or your frequent sprints to the bathroom. You can also take advantage of employer-provided services designed to make your pregnancy healthier and less stressful. Some of these services (health-mentoring programs, for instance) are most valuable in the early stages of your pregnancy; you could also use similar programs offered by your health insurance company without spilling the beans at work.

Unfortunately, many employers are less than enlightened when it comes to pregnant employees. If you're concerned about your boss's reaction, proceed cautiously and be informed about your legal rights. Consider waiting to share your news until you've made it through your first trimester—and perhaps until your burgeoning belly threatens to make the announcement *for* you. By that point, you will have already demonstrated that pregnancy doesn't hinder your job performance.

You may also want to time your announcement to coincide with the successful completion of a big project. By doing so, you'll send a strong message: I'm a third of the way through my pregnancy, and my productivity is unaffected. Finally, you could wait to break the news to your boss until *after* a salary or performance review to make sure the news doesn't influence how

BY THE NUMBERS

When Women Announce Their Pregnancy at Work

21% spill the beans right away

22% wait a few weeks

3% are outed by morning sickness and other pregnancy symptoms

37% wait until after their first trimester

15% wait until they start to show

77% tell someone *other* than their boss first

Source: *A BabyCenter.com poll of more than 4,300 women*

QUICK TIPS

Maintaining a Professional Image

During your first trimester, fatigue, discomfort, and absent-mindedness don't stay at home when you go to work. Even though these symptoms are normal, carefully consider which coworkers you want to share those feelings with. Someone who's been pregnant before (and whom you can trust) is your best bet.

Even after your pregnancy is public knowledge at work, try not to complain or talk about it too much. Be prudent when you're among your coworkers or with customers or clients.

you're treated. (For pointers on *how* to reveal a baby's on the way, turn to page 109.)

Some key questions to consider as you're determining the timing of your announcement:

Are you having problems with your pregnancy? If you're suffering from severe morning sickness or need to take it especially easy for other reasons, telling your colleagues early in your pregnancy might be a big relief. Even if you're just feeling a bit off your game, knowing about your pregnancy may make others a little more understanding.

What kind of job do you have? For your baby's sake and your own, you'll probably want to come clean early on if you have a strenuous or very stressful job. And if your job exposes you to toxic chemicals or other hazardous agents, it's crucial to get a job reassignment immediately. Making your announcement right away allows you to talk about shifting job responsibilities in a timely manner.

What's the culture of your workplace? If you're the only woman in a macho office, you may have to deal with some unenlightened reactions and a lack of on-site support. In that case, do some research on your rights before making your announcement. Companies with a reputation for being family-friendly are more apt to have policies in place for handling these situations—and tend to be familiar with existing policies and laws regarding pregnant employees.

Dangerous Jobs

You'll need an immediate job reassignment if you work in a field where you're regularly exposed to reproductive hazards, including heavy metals (such as lead and mercury), chemicals (such as pesticides and solvents), biological waste, anesthetic gases, and radiation. These are teratogens—agents that can cause problems such as miscarriage, premature delivery, birth defects, and abnormal fetal and infant development. You may come into contact with these hazards if you work in a computer chip factory, darkroom, manufacturing plant, dry-cleaning operation, rubber factory, operating room, tollbooth, pottery studio, shipbuilding plant, printing shop, or laboratory, for instance.

Ask your employer to provide you with information about any harmful substances you may be exposed to at work. The Occupational Safety and Health Administration (OSHA) requires that chemical manufacturers and importers thoroughly evaluate the chemicals that they produce and to create a material safety data sheet (MSDS) on any potential hazard. Your company should be able to provide you with an MSDS for any chemical you may be in contact with at work. If you're in a union, it will be helpful to talk to a representative on the health and safety committee. If you have concerns about health hazards at your workplace, discuss them with your health-care provider and bring your MSDS (if you have one) to your next prenatal appointment. (Also let your caregiver know if your *partner* is regularly exposed to hazardous substances—there's a chance he could be carrying some of it home on his clothes or equipment.)

Just the Facts

Job Stress

High levels of stress, including work-related stress, have been linked to an increased risk of pregnancy complications, including miscarriage, preeclampsia, premature birth, smaller birthweight, and possibly miscarriage. Still, no one completely understands the role emotional stress plays in prenatal health. Your body's physical response to a stressful situation (releasing stress-related hormones and raising your blood pressure and heart rate) may be to blame, but complications could also be related to lifestyle changes brought on by stress (such as fatigue or lack of sleep, poor eating, and harmful habits like smoking).

What *is* clear is that stress can take a toll on your emotional and physical health. You may get depressed (page 210) or suffer more aches and pains than normal. Healthy coping strategies, such as getting enough rest, cutting back on your to-do list, and getting regular exercise (swimming, walking, or yoga, for instance), can help you feel better about—and be better able to deal with—challenges at work and home. If taking these steps doesn't do the trick, talk to your doctor or midwife. She may recommend counseling or, if job stress seems to be affecting the health of you or your baby, even draft a "doctor's order" to reduce your work hours or otherwise lighten your load.

Certain occupations require modifications when you're pregnant. For instance, expectant mothers who have physically strenuous jobs (including heavy lifting, standing for more than three hours at a time, and physical jobs with long hours) may be somewhat more likely to develop high blood pressure, deliver prematurely, and have smaller babies. If your job is strenuous, you'll have to decide how to safely accommodate your pregnancy. Ideally, it's best to switch to lighter duty for the duration of your pregnancy. If that's not possible, take an occasional sick or vacation day to rest, take breaks as often as you can, or reduce the number of hours you work or the time you spend on your feet during a typical workday.

Above all, be straightforward with your practitioner about what your job entails so she can help you come up with a plan to keep your baby safe while you still fulfill your work duties.

Dollars and Sense: How Having a Baby Will Affect Your Finances

Smart Money Moves to Make Now

Why wait? Start researching important money matters now so you won't be hit with any nasty surprises later.

Check your health coverage. You may not be able to change your insurance coverage now that you're pregnant, but you should find out exactly what your policy will cover so you'll be prepared for out-of-pocket expenses.

Eventually, you'll need to add your baby to your health coverage. Most insurance companies have special rules and policies for babies. Ask your carrier to send you the specifics on which of your baby's medical expenses will be covered and which ones won't.

Look into childcare costs. Childcare can be expensive—anywhere from a few hundred to more than a thousand a month, depending on where you live and what type of care you choose. Research the different types of care now—daycare centers, home providers, and nannies are the big three. In some big metropolitan areas, you may need to put your name on a day care's waiting list *now* to secure a spot for your baby in a year or more. Weigh the financial costs against your daycare needs and child-rearing phi-

BabyCenter Buzz

I'm Worried about Money

"My husband and I don't have health insurance, and I'm worried about covering the medical bills." —*Sarah*

"I'm really worried about how I'm going to afford being on maternity leave. I haven't been at my job long enough to qualify for paid time off." —*Dee*

"How can we cut back to one income and still save to buy a house?" —*Laura*

"I want to stay home with the baby, but I know we can't afford to lose my salary." —*Marilyn*

"I worry about how we'll pay for day care. We don't have a lot of extra money left over *now*, and we haven't even calculated the cost of diapers, formula, and other baby items yet." —*Anonymous*

"As a single mom, I wonder how I'll be able to save for the future. I want to live on my own instead of with my parents, but I'm afraid those dreams will be on hold indefinitely." —*Anonymous*

losophy before deciding whether you can afford a particular type of care. (Keep in mind, too, that there are often childcare subsidies available to low-income parents.)

Open a dependent-care account at work. Many employers allow workers to sock away pretax money in dependent-care savings accounts. Doing this allows you to save taxes on up to $5,000 worth of income that's earmarked for qualifying dependent-care expenses, such as a daycare center, licensed family day care, or an on-the-books nanny. Most plans accept new enrollees only in the fall for the following calendar year, though many make exceptions for "life events"—such as having a baby. In either case, find out from your human resources or union rep when you're eligible to enroll, and then be sure not to miss the boat. Be warned, though: You'll need to carefully estimate your anticipated childcare expenses first because these accounts have a "use it or lose it" policy.

Open a 529 college savings plan—or ask the baby's grandparents-to-be to open one. These investment accounts allow your college savings to

BabyCenter Buzz

Savings Strategies That Work for Us

"We've been putting my husband's check into a savings account to get used to the idea of living on one income, since I'm planning to take several months of unpaid maternity leave."   —A

"We deposit all of our tax refund into savings, and as we pay off long-term debts, we continue to make those payments—right into our savings account." —Leslie

"We cut up all but one of our credit cards and use it for emergencies only. If we can't buy something with cash or a check, then we don't need it."   —Anonymous

"Automatic payments! We have ours set up so that our house, car, and computer payments all come out of my husband's check before he even sees it." —Monica

"We've never subscribed to anything more than basic cable (no HBO or other special channels). After eight years, that's more than $1,500 right there."   —Carolee

grow tax-free, meaning that when you take money out to pay for college (including room and board) 18 years from now, you won't have to pay any taxes on your earnings. Even better, you can start an account with as little as $25.

Travel Plans

If you're thinking about taking a trip, don't let being pregnant stand in your way. As long as you have a clean bill of health, a road trip, airplane flight, train ride, or cruise won't pose any extra risks to you or your developing baby. But consider this: During your first trimester, you may not *feel* much like hitting the road. For most moms-to-be, the second trimester is the ideal time to travel, since that's when energy levels typically rebound and morning sickness subsides. Still, if a business trip, a family visit, or a much-deserved getaway is on the agenda, by all means go for it—bearing in mind the following advice.

Safety First: Precautions for Pregnant Travelers

Before you head out of town, a few safety steps are in order.

Get the go-ahead from your healthcare provider. Ask your doctor or midwife if there are any medical concerns that might impact your plans. While travel *itself* isn't risky for healthy moms-to-be, certain destinations or vacation activities may be off-limits. Also, if you're having prenatal testing done that must be performed at a specific time, plan your trip with that date in mind.

Gather your medical records and vital health information. Ask your practitioner for a copy of your prenatal health record to take on the road, and don't forget to pack your health insurance card. Or see the emergency contact sheet (below) for a complete list of medical information you may need while you're away. Copy it, fill it out, and bring it with you on your trip.

Make sure you have all your meds. Be careful to pack a supply of any prescribed medications, prenatal vitamins, and over-the-counter remedies you may need during your trip, especially if you're going someplace where those items won't be readily available. And bring extra so you'll have enough if any get lost or damaged on the road or your return home is delayed. Be sure to keep prescription medicine in its original container—especially if you are traveling outside the country and will be going through customs.

Check your health insurance policy. Find out if it covers pregnancy complications as well as local emergency medical transportation and evacuation home during travel to your intended destinations (such as foreign countries). If not, you may want to buy additional travel health insurance.

Look into trip-cancellation insurance. If you bail out of a trip you've already booked, it could cost you a bundle. A special travel insurance policy pays for cancellation fees and nonrefundable payments or deposits if you miss all or part of your trip.

Avoid being stranded. Take along the phone numbers for any airlines you'll be flying, in case you need to confirm or reschedule flights while you're on the road. If you will be driving and don't already belong to an auto club that provides emergency road service, join one. Finally, carry a cell phone—especially if you're traveling solo.

Coping with First-Trimester Symptoms and Problems on the Road

Although the first trimester is free of such logistical challenges as squeezing your sizable girth into a tiny airline seat, it has its own share of difficulties, notably morning sickness and fatigue. While you can't escape these two complaints, a few pointers will keep them from ruining your trip.

Eat wisely. Try not to toss restraint out the window just because you're away from home. (On the other hand, don't let a hectic travel schedule get in the way of regular meals and snacks.) Besides doing your developing baby a favor, smart eating will help keep queasiness under control.

Drink up. Staying hydrated is vital for a healthy pregnancy, and it's especially important when you're stuck on a plane (where the air is notoriously dry), outside in warm weather, or spending your day trekking around tourist destinations without a break.

Keep your blood moving. If you're on a long car ride or plane flight, keep your blood circulating by strolling the aisle or getting out of the car every hour. When you're sitting, rotate your ankles and wiggle your toes every half-hour or so, and don't cross your legs or wear constrictive clothing. Also gently flex and point your foot to stretch your calf muscles. Wearing support hose will help the circulation in your legs, something to consider if you're going on a long flight.

Don't overdo it. It's normal to feel pooped when you're pregnant, and

Ask the Experts

Can Altitude or Temperature Changes Make Morning Sickness Worse?

Dr. Jack Schneider, obstetrician: Increases in altitude or temperature can aggravate nausea—especially if you're heading to extremes of height or heat, like a ski resort in the Rockies or a tropical island. If you're having a particularly rough first trimester, consider postponing your trip until you're feeling better. But in other cases, the additional discomfort usually subsides after you adjust to the new environment. In the meantime, don't expect to be as active as usual. Take it slow, get plenty of rest, and drink lots of fluids. If your symptoms persist for longer than five days or get much worse, return to lower ground or cooler temperatures.

WORKSHEET: EMERGENCY CONTACT SHEET FOR PREGNANT TRAVELERS

Keep this information handy in case of an emergency. Fill in the blanks, and make two copies. Keep one with you, and give the other to your mate or traveling companion.

My name:_____

MY CAREGIVER AT HOME:

Name_____

Phone_____

MY HEALTHCARE PROVIDER AWAY FROM HOME (REFERRED BY MY DOCTOR OR MIDWIFE):

Name_____

Phone_____

MY HEALTH INSURANCE:

Company name _____

Policy number_____

Phone_____

EMERGENCY CONTACTS:

Name_____

Phone_____

Relationship_____

Name_____

Phone_____

Relationship_____

PRENATAL AND MEDICAL HISTORY:

My due date _____

Most recent checkup _____

Comments _____

Allergies _____

Immunization history

_____

Medications and dosages

_____

the demands of traveling will only add to your fatigue. While you can still enjoy many of your favorite vacation activities, you'll need to slow your usual pace, keep your schedule light, and give up the idea of seeing everything. (Be sure that the person you're traveling with understands this as

BabyCenter Buzz

Comfort Strategies Away from Home

"Driving even short distances made me extremely nauseated, so I carried small kitchen-size trash bags in my car and always had one within reach. I also found it helpful to plan routes on roads with wide shoulders so I could pull over as needed." —*Anonymous*

"It helped when *I* was the driver—it forced me to keep my eyes on the road ahead of me, which is what doctors recommend to ward off motion sickness. Driving also kept me focused on the road and traffic and not on how I was feeling." —*Rachel*

"The things that helped me were Dramamine, Sea-Bands, and keeping a bottle of cold water and some snacks (peppermints, pretzels, apples) in my bag. Also, get plenty of sleep and try to stick with 'normal' food as much as possible. Finally, always find out where the closest bathroom is . . . just in case." —*Sieglinde*

"My biggest problem in the first trimester was exhaustion. I wanted to sleep 24/7. I allowed time for a nap as soon as I arrived at my destination. But what helped most was taking along my own blanket and pillow so I could get a good night's sleep in a strange bed." —*Faith*

well.) Keep your plans as simple as possible, and think *quality* rather than *quantity*. Taking an afternoon nap—or at least a rest—is an especially good way to avoid exhaustion. At your destination, set aside time each day to put your feet up and close your eyes—and be prepared to go with plan B if your original itinerary just seems too taxing.

Sleep tight. Travel can play havoc with sleep patterns. To stay rested, it's best to settle down as close to your normal bedtime as you can, unless you've crossed at least three time zones. In that case, try to adjust your sleep schedule to local time to combat jet lag. If jet lag hits anyway, spend time outside in the daylight to help reset your biological clock to the new time zone.

Ask the Experts

Does Being Pregnant Make Me More Prone to Motion Sickness?

Ann Linden, certified nurse-midwife: Motion sickness is a common travel problem. It occurs when your body's balance-sensing system—which includes your inner ear, eyes, and sensory nerves—sends conflicting messages to your brain. If your inner ear senses motion, for instance, but your eyes don't, the result is a queasy feeling that may have you reaching for an airsickness bag. There's no evidence that pregnancy *causes* motion sickness, though if you've suffered from motion sickness in the past, you're more likely to experience morning sickness—a link that researchers haven't yet fully explained. Eating frequent light, nongreasy snacks should help soothe a motion-sensitive stomach. Some women also find that sucking on ginger candy or using an acupressure wristband helps. Some mothers-to-be swear by more expensive, battery-powered wristbands, which deliver a mild electrical current to acupressure points to help curb motion sickness—as well as pregnancy-related nausea and vomiting. If you're already having nausea and vomiting or have been prone to motion sickness in the past, it's a good idea to check with your practitioner about safe antinausea medications to take with you just in case.

PART II

THE SECOND TRIMESTER: 14 TO 27 WEEKS

This trimester will mark your "coming out" as a mother-to-be. If you haven't already, now's the time to share your news with friends, family, and co-workers—but don't expect everyone in your life (particularly your boss or pals who are struggling with infertility) to be as happy about it as you are. To those outside your inner circle, your blossoming belly will soon shout your baby news for you. With your deliciously changing form may come not only relief from early pregnancy complaints like morning sickness and bone-deep fatigue, but also a spate of new symptoms—many of them welcome (the heralded "glow" of pregnancy, renewed energy, and a more serene outlook), some less so (stretch marks, back pain, and the so-called "pregnancy brain"). Take advantage of this generally carefree time to reconnect with friends and family, deepen your bond with your partner, and perhaps plan a "babymoon" trip—one last hurrah before parenthood!

Second Trimester Highlights

Welcome to the "Honeymoon Trimester"!

During this trimester, your baby will:

▶ Grow from a fragile, lemon-size thumb sucker to a foot-long, kicking dynamo capable of surviving-with medical help-outside your womb

▶ Begin thumb sucking

▶ Reveal the organs that say either "I'm a boy" or "I'm a girl"

▶ Develop hair with a distinct color

▶ Start growing bone to replace cartilage

▶ Be able to hear your voice

You will:

▶ Finally feel your baby's movements

▶ Really start to show, and your belly will announce your pregnancy for you

▶ Feel better—morning sickness and deep fatigue will probably subside

▶ Look better—many women develop a pregnancy glow in the second trimester

▶ Possibly develop new symptoms, such as back pain, heartburn, and dizziness

▶ Be offered prenatal tests, such as amniocentesis, multiple marker, and ultrasound

▶ Gain about a pound per week

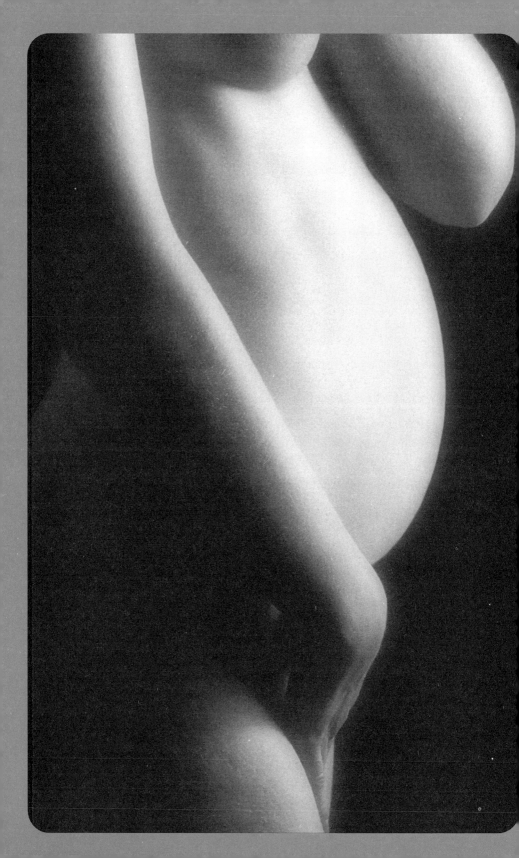

YOUR PREGNANCY WEEK BY WEEK

Your Pregnancy: 14 Weeks

Your Changing Body

Welcome to your second trimester! Your energy is likely returning, your breasts are feeling less tender, and your queasiness should be settling down now. If not, hang on—chances are good the queasies will soon be behind you (although an unlucky few will still feel nauseated months from now). While the top of your uterus is barely emerging from be-

> **HOT TOPICS**
>
> - Clothes for these "in-between" weeks (page 95)
> - What to do about excessive vaginal discharge (page 140)
> - Warning signs you should never ignore (page 147)
> - Why morning sickness may not be behind you (page 174)
> - Sex in your second trimester (page 225)

hind your pubic bone, it may be enough to cause a little tummy "pop." Starting to show can be quite a thrill, giving you and your partner visible evidence of the baby you've been waiting for. Take some time to plan, daydream, and enjoy this amazing time. It's normal to worry now and then, but try to focus on taking care of yourself and your baby—and have faith that you're well-equipped for what's ahead.

Your Growing Baby

This week's big developments: Your baby can now squint, frown, grimace, pee, and possibly suck his thumb! Thanks to brain impulses, his facial muscles are getting a workout as his tiny features form one expression after another. His kidneys are producing urine, which he releases into the amniotic fluid around him—a process he'll keep up until birth. He can grasp, too, and if you're having an ultrasound now, you may even catch him sucking his thumb.

In other news: Your baby's stretching out. From head to bottom, he measures 3½ inches—about the size of a lemon—and he weighs 1½ ounces. His body's growing faster than his head, which now sits atop a more distinct neck. By the end of this week, his arms will have grown to a length that's in proportion with the rest of his body. (His legs still have some lengthening to

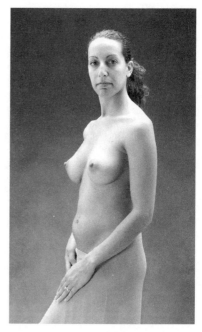

At 14 weeks, you may be feeling better physically and starting to show.

BabyCenter Buzz

What Other Women Say at 14 Weeks

"I'm starting to give in to comfort foods: chocolate, chips, and cereal." —*Jamie*

"Every morning I wake up at 4 A.M., pee, climb back in bed, and wait . . . and wait. I'm absolutely exhausted, but I can't get back to sleep." —*Rachel*

"I *hate* tight clothes, but maternity clothes seem to be made for women who are *really* pregnant. I found that stretchy drawstring pants are great now." —*Angela*

"My husband and I have stopped discussing names with others because of the comments they make. Now we just tell people who ask that we'll name the baby Gaylord if it's a boy and Phellula if it's a girl—you should see their faces!" —*Angie*

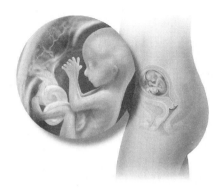

Your lemon-size baby is stretching out and becoming more flexible and active.

do, though.) He's also starting to develop an ultrafine, downy covering of hair, called lanugo, all over his body. Your baby's liver starts making bile this week—a sign that it's doing its job right—and his spleen starts helping in the production of red blood cells. Though you can't feel his tiny punches and kicks yet, your little pugilist's hands and feet (which now measure about ½ inch long) are more flexible and active.

Your Pregnancy: 15 Weeks

Your Changing Body

You've probably gained about 5 pounds by now (a little more or less is fine, too) and are well into the swing of your pregnancy, but you may still be surprised by an unexpected symptom now and then. If your nose is stuffed up, for instance, you can probably chalk it up to the combined effect of pregnancy hormones and increased bloodflow to your mucous membranes, as well as the immune system changes that pregnancy brings about.

> ### HOT TOPICS
>
> • How pregnancy may affect your hair (page 142)
>
> • All about amniocentesis (page 154)
>
> • Coping with nasal congestion (page 175)
>
> • Second-trimester dream themes (page 187)
>
> • Announcing at work (page 230)

If you're having amniocentesis, it'll most likely happen between now and week 18. This test, which can identify hundreds of genetic and chromosomal disorders, carries a very small risk of miscarriage, so it's usually offered only if you're at higher risk for these disorders. If you're stressing about the results, rest assured that more than 95 percent of women who have amniocentesis get good news about their babies—bringing welcome relief from their worries.

BabyCenter Buzz

What Other Women Say at 15 Weeks

"I'm definitely experiencing the second-trimester honeymoon phase. I have occasional sore feet and a sore back, but it's really nothing compared to the nausea, fatigue, and general blah-ness of the first trimester." —*Gypsy*

"I still have *no* relief from nausea and am throwing up every day. I need some hope that this will get better soon!" —*Erin*

"Most of my prepregnancy pants are tight (thanks to the weight I've gained in my rear, oddly enough!), but my stomach is still flat. It may be kind of silly, but I can't wait to *look* pregnant." —*Linda*

"My boss took the news really well, but other men in my group have been complaining behind my back about how 'lazy' and what a 'slacker' I've been (read: exhausted and throwing up a lot). It's better now, and my boss and I talked about it, but I'm still working hard to pull my job status back up. *Grrr!*" —*Linnea*

And don't be surprised if you and your partner are feeling a little stressed-out these days. Many expectant couples worry about their baby's health and about how they'll handle the changes ahead. But with physical discomforts on the wane and energy on the rise, this is also a wonderful trimester for most women, so do your best to enjoy it!

Your Growing Baby

Your baby now measures around 4 inches long, crown to rump, and weighs in at about 2½ ounces. She's busy moving amniotic fluid through her nose and upper respiratory tract, which helps the primitive air sacs in her lungs begin to develop. Her legs are growing longer than her arms now, and she can move all of her joints and limbs. Although her eyelids are still fused shut, she can sense light. If you shine a flashlight at your tummy, for instance, she's likely to move away from the beam. There's not much for your baby to taste at this point, but she is forming taste buds. Finally, if you have an ultrasound this week, you may be able to find out whether your baby's a boy or a girl! (Don't be too disappointed if it remains a mystery, though. Nailing down your baby's sex depends on the clarity of the picture and on your baby's position; he or she may be modestly curled up or turned in such a way so as to "hide the goods.")

Your Pregnancy: 16 Weeks

Your Changing Body

You've reached a more expansive stage of your pregnancy—both physically and emotionally. The top of your uterus is about halfway between your pubic bone and your navel, and the round ligaments that support it are thickening and stretching as it grows. You're probably looking and feeling a whole lot better as you settle into pregnancy, too. Less nausea, fewer mood swings, and "glowing" skin contribute to an overall sense of well-being. Chances are, you're probably less anxious about something happening to your baby, too, because the risk of miscarriage has dropped dramatically now.

> ### HOT TOPICS
>
> • Multiple marker screening (page 152)
>
> • Feeling your baby move (page 170)
>
> • How to handle heartburn (page 172)
>
> • Why you may need to start sleeping on your side (page 182)
>
> • Your emotional highs and lows (page 205)

Your caregiver will likely recommend that you take the multiple marker test (sometimes called the "triple screen" or the "quad screen") to find out whether your baby is at an increased risk of having certain birth defects. This blood test, which measures a protein produced by your growing baby called alpha-fetoprotein (AFP) plus the levels of two or three different pregnancy hormones, is usually done between 15 and 20 weeks, with 16 to 18 weeks being the norm.

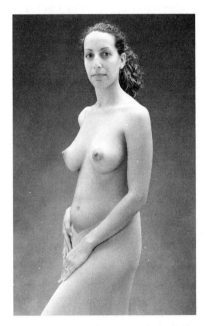

As your uterus pushes up toward your belly button, you're finally starting to show-and glow, thanks to waning nausea and the blush of increased circulation to your skin.

Soon you'll experience one of the most wonderful moments of pregnancy—feeling your baby move. While some women notice "quickening" as early as 16 weeks, most don't until 18 weeks or more. (And if this is your first baby, don't be too impatient—you may not be aware of your baby's movements until 20 weeks or so.) The earliest movements may feel like little flutters, gas bubbles, or even like popcorn popping. In the weeks that follow, they'll grow stronger and more insistent.

Your Growing Baby

Get ready for a growth spurt. In the next few weeks, your baby will double his weight and add inches to his length. Right now, he's about the size of an avocado: 4½ inches long (head to bottom) and 3½ ounces. His legs are much more developed, his head is more erect than it has been, and his eyes are closer to the front of his head (where

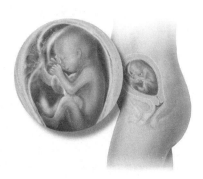

Now big enough to fill your slightly cupped hand, your baby is looking more like a tiny person, with hair, toenails, and a human-looking face. If you rest quietly in a reclining position, you may feel those first, magical movements!

they're moving—slowly—under closed lids). His ears are close to their final position, too. And some of his more advanced inner machinery, including his circulatory system and urinary tract, are now hard at work: His heart is pumping about 25 quarts of blood a day. The patterning of his scalp hair has begun, though his locks aren't recognizable yet—and he's even started growing toenails.

BabyCenter Buzz

What Other Women Say at 16 Weeks

"I wasn't sure if I could feel my baby moving, so a friend suggested that I lie down for a while. After a few minutes, I started feeling a butterfly-like sensation in my lower abdomen. It was amazing!" —Linda

"I've been having heartburn. Nothing a couple of Tums can't handle, but it's still annoying." —Kay

"I already look like I'm five or six months along! I've had two ultrasounds—and yes, there's only one baby in there—and my doctor says that the baby is growing normally and that everything looks just fine." —Heidi

Your Pregnancy: 17 Weeks

Your Changing Body

Starting to feel a bit off balance? Your center of gravity shifts upward and forward as your belly grows, so you may occasionally feel a little unsteady on your feet. Wear low-heeled shoes to reduce your risk of taking a tumble because trauma to your abdomen could be dangerous for you and your baby. You'll also want to be sure to buckle up when you're driving—keep the lap portion of your seat belt under your belly, drawn snugly across your hips for maximum protection without endangering your baby.

> ### HOT TOPICS
>
> - How your feet are changing (page 171)
> - Dealing with dry eyes (page 180)
> - Telling "good" fats from "bad" ones (page 189)
> - Handling unwelcome comments (page 229)
> - The safest way to wear your seat belt (page 247)

You may also notice your eyes becoming drier—not at all fun if you wear contact lenses. To end the pregnancy-induced drought, use an over-the-counter artificial-tears solution. (The shape of your eyeballs may temporarily change a bit, too, so if you wear hard contact lenses

BabyCenter Buzz

What Other Women Say at 17 Weeks

"I'm trying not to stress too much about my weight gain (20 pounds already!), but I feel like I have half a basketball in there!" —*Michelle*

"I've gained about 7 pounds, but I don't really look pregnant. My weight's gone to my waist and my boobs. I have great hand-me-down maternity clothes that I can't wait to wear, but they're still huge!" —*Amanda*

"Whenever I run into an acquaintance, they'll ask me, meaningfully, 'How are you feeling?' I look them in the eye and say, 'Fine.' I used to be truthful and say, 'My round ligaments are killing me, my feet are swollen, and I have to pee every 15 minutes.' That was a mistake because they'd launch into a litany of complaints about their previous pregnancy. Even men weren't safe. 'When my wife was pregnant . . . ,' they'd begin. At which point I'd have to excuse myself to go to the bathroom—or drop something heavy on my foot." —*April*

and the fit seems off, you may have to put them away until after you deliver.)

Your Growing Baby

Your baby's skeleton is changing from soft cartilage to bone, and the umbilical cord—her lifeline to the placenta—is growing stronger and thicker. Your baby weighs about 5 ounces now, and she's around 5 inches long from head to bottom—about the size of a large onion. She can move her joints, and her sweat glands are starting to develop.

Your Pregnancy: 18 Weeks
Your Changing Body

Hungry? An increase in appetite is pretty common about now. Make it count by choosing meals and snacks that are rich in nutrients (fresh fruit, veggies, yogurt, nuts), instead of empty calories (chips, French fries, pastries). You may soon begin to feel achiness around your lower abdomen; this is from your ligaments stretching as your uterus grows. Your baby's active these days—kicking, reaching, and flexing his arms and legs. You may begin to feel his movements—if not this week, then soon. Bigger, more comfortable clothes are a must now as your appetite and waistline increase. Now's the time to start shopping for (or borrowing) maternity clothes that can accommodate your expanding belly.

> **HOT TOPICS**
>
> - Finding clothes that fit your body—and budget (page 95)
> - What to expect at your ultrasound (page 157)
> - Deciding whether to learn your baby's sex (page 158)
> - Why you may be feeling dizzy (page 168)
> - Having twins or more (page 538)

Your cardiovascular system is undergoing dramatic changes, and during this trimester your blood pressure will probably be lower than usual. Don't spring up too fast from a lying or sitting position, or you might feel a little dizzy. And from now on when you do lie down, it's best to lie on your side—or at least partly tilted to one side. (When you lie flat on your back, your uterus can compress a major vein, leading to decreased blood return to your heart.) A few pillows strategically placed behind your

BabyCenter Buzz

What Other Women Say at 18 Weeks

"I wish I'd known how bad the forgetfulness and mental dullness would be. So far, my worst symptom has been stupidity!" —*Cary*

"I've been feeling consistent movement for the last two weeks. I can't wait for the kicks to be strong enough to feel from the outside so my husband can feel how amazing this is!" —*Amy*

"I have a stinging pain in my hips and my right buttock, so I've been having trouble getting to sleep while lying on my side. Moving to a firm couch has helped a lot, though." —*Kelli*

back and under your hip or upper leg will help you get comfortable in this position.

If you haven't already had one, you'll probably get an ultrasound soon. The painless procedure helps measure your baby's growth, screen for certain birth defects, check the placenta and umbilical cord, estimate your due date, and rule out twins or higher-order multiples. During the exam, you might see your baby moving around or sucking his thumb. Bring your partner along, and be sure to ask for printouts for your baby's first photo album!

Your Growing Baby

Head to rump, your baby is about 5½ inches long (the length of a large sweet potato) and weighs almost 7 ounces. He's busy flexing his arms and legs—movements that you'll start noticing more and more in the weeks ahead. His blood vessels are visible through his thin skin, and his ears are now in their final position, though they're still standing out from his head a bit. A protective covering of myelin is beginning to form around his nerves, a process that will continue for a year after he's born. If you're having a girl, her uterus and fallopian tubes are formed and in place. If you're having a boy, his genitals are noticeable now—*if* he cooperates during your ultrasound!

Your Pregnancy: 19 Weeks

Your Changing Body

Think you're big now? You'll start growing even more rapidly in the weeks to
come. As a result, you may notice some
achiness in your lower abdomen or even
brief, stabbing pains on one or both
sides—especially when you shift position
or at the end of an active day. Most likely,
this is round ligament pain. The two liga-
ments that support your uterus (one on either side) are stretching to accommodate its increasing weight. This is nothing to be alarmed about, but call
your practitioner if the pain continues even when you're resting or if it becomes persistent and severe.

> **HOT TOPICS**
> - Red palms (this page)
> - How to deal with splotchy skin (page 217)
> - Easing back pain (page 164)
> - Round ligament pain (page 176)
> - Snoring (page 319)

You may be noticing some skin changes, too: Are the palms of your
hands red? Nothing to worry about—it's from increased estrogen. You may
also have patches of darkened skin due to a temporary increase in pigment.
When these darker patches show up on your upper lip, cheeks, and forehead,
they're called chloasma, or the "mask of pregnancy." You're also likely to
notice some darkening of your nipples, freckles, scars, underarms, inner
thighs, and vulva—not to mention the line running from your belly button
to the top of your pubic bone (the "linea nigra"). These darkened areas will
most likely fade shortly after delivery. In the meantime, protect yourself from
the pigment-intensifying sun—cover up, wear a brimmed hat, and use sunscreen when you're outdoors. If you're self-conscious about your "mask," a
little concealing makeup can work wonders.

Your Growing Baby

Your baby's sensory development is exploding! Her brain is carving out spe-
cialized areas for smell, taste, hearing, vision, and touch. Some research suggests that she may be able to hear your voice now, so don't be shy about
reading aloud, talking to her, or singing a happy tune if the mood strikes
you. (Then again, don't feel compelled to talk to your growing baby if the
idea strikes you as a bit silly.) If you do hum a little tune, though, maybe
she'll wave her arms and legs (now nicely proportioned in respect to the rest
of her body) in time to the music.

Your little dancer weighs about 8½ ounces now, and she measures 6

BabyCenter Buzz

What Other Women Say at 19 Weeks

"I had terrible back pain, so my doctor suggested a maternity belt. I love how it lifts the pressure off my lower back!"   —*Anonymous*

"Last night I had my first really strong craving—for a banana split. I've hated bananas since I was 8 years old!"   —*Jessa*

"It feels like I have Mexican jumping beans in my belly. It's so weird—and wonderful!"   —*Kimberley*

"I'm pregnant with twins and haven't felt them move yet. I had an ultrasound two weeks ago and saw them moving, but I still haven't felt them. Is this normal?"   —*Stace*

"I never used to snore before, but now I sound like a Mack truck! It's gotten so loud that I even wake myself up!"   —*Nadine*

inches from her head to her bottom—about the length of a small zucchini. Her kidneys are churning out urine, which mixes with the amniotic fluid around her, and the hair on her scalp is sprouting. A waxy protective coating called vernix caseosa is forming on her skin, shielding your baby from irritating elements in the amniotic fluid and lubing her up for her eventual journey down the birth canal.

Your Pregnancy: 20 Weeks

Your Changing Body

Congratulations! You've hit the halfway mark in your pregnancy. The top of your uterus is about level with your belly button, and you've likely gained around ten pounds. Expect to gain another pound or so each week from now on. (If you started your pregnancy underweight, you

HOT TOPICS

- Choosing a childbirth education class (page 148)
- Increasing your iron intake (page 162)
- Recognizing Braxton Hicks contractions (page 166)
- Second-trimester weight gain (page 198)
- Travel tips (page 242)

may need to gain a bit more; if you were overweight, a bit less.) Make sure you're getting enough iron, a mineral you need more of now to help keep up with your expanding blood volume and to meet the needs of your developing baby and placenta. Iron-rich foods include lean red meat, poultry, fish, lentils and other legumes, prunes, dried apricots, spinach, and iron-fortified cereals.

If you haven't already signed up for one, you may want to look into a childbirth education class. Whether you're a first-timer or a pro, a structured class will help prepare you for the rigors of labor and birth and will boost your partner's comfort level and coaching ability when the big day arrives. Most hospitals and birth centers offer classes, either as weekly meetings or as one all-day session. Ask your doctor or midwife for a recommendation.

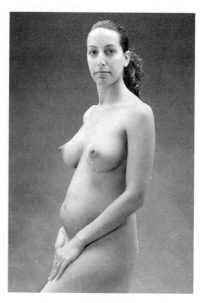

You're halfway to the finish line, and your body seems to be ripening by the minute: Not only is your belly in full bloom, but—thanks to increased pigment levels—your nipples are a deeper hue, and the normally invisible line that runs from your belly button to your pubic bone is darkening.

Your Growing Baby

By now, your baby weighs about 10½ ounces and is as long as a banana: about 6½ inches from head to bottom and about 10 inches from head to heel. (For the first 20 weeks, when a baby's legs are curled up against his torso and hard to measure, measurements are taken from the top of his head to his bottom—the "crown to rump" measurement. After that, he's measured from head to toe.) He's swallowing more these days, which is good practice for his digestive system. He's also

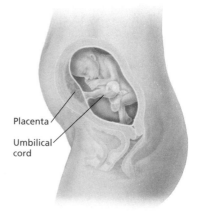

Placenta

Umbilical
cord

Starting to feel your baby kick? That's because his legs are stretching out more, instead of staying curled against his torso. As he moves and stretches, he's swallowing amniotic fluid, urinating, and processing waste in his developing digestive system—already storing it up for that first diaper delivery!

BabyCenter Buzz

What Other Women Say at 20 Weeks

"I'm already having what I think are sporadic Braxton Hicks contractions. They don't hurt, but I can feel my belly hardening and then softening. They're not frequent enough to freak out about, but it's weird that they're already here!"
—*Alicia*

"I'm a born worrier. My new fear is that my husband won't get to the hospital in time. I also worry that he'll be working in some area with bad cell phone reception and I won't get through when I call him. When it gets closer to my due date, I'm going to make a list of all the plumbers, drywallers, floor guys, and landscapers that work with him so I can call them if I can't get hold of him!"   —*Debbie*

producing meconium, a black, sticky by-product of digestion. This gooey substance will accumulate in his bowels, and you'll see it in his first soiled diaper (although a few babies pass meconium in the womb or during delivery).

Your Pregnancy: 21 Weeks

Your Changing Body

You're probably feeling pretty comfortable these days. You're not too big yet, and the usual aches and pains associated with early pregnancy are, for the most part, gone (though new ones may have taken their place!). Relax and enjoy it while you can—the third trimester may bring with it a new crop of complaints.

HOT TOPICS

- Dealing with varicose veins (page 178)
- Getting comfortable at night (page 183)
- Coping with acne outbreaks (page 215)
- Makeup tricks for moms-to-be (page 218)
- Spider veins (page 220)

That's not to say you don't have some minor malfunctions to deal with now. You may find, for instance, that your oil glands are revving up like they haven't done since junior high—resulting in regular bouts of acne. In that case, be diligent about washing with a gentle cleanser twice a day. But don't take any oral acne medications, since they're hazardous in pregnancy—

BabyCenter Buzz

What Other Women Say at 21 Weeks

"I'm feeling that out-of-my-mind kind of happiness. I can't find a single reason to complain. I'm experiencing many symptoms, but I'm just so thankful to be carrying a healthy little girl that none of it seems to matter."   —*Lisa*

"My husband felt the baby kick. His eyes got so big. He said in this amazed voice, 'I felt him!' Now he puts his hand on my belly whenever we're watching TV, hoping to feel the baby again."   —*Anonymous*

"I feel my baby's kicks, but my husband still can't feel anything. I'm hoping it happens soon because he's so looking forward to it."   —*Summer*

and be sure to check with your practitioner before using any topical acne treatments.

You're also prone to varicose veins now—especially if your mom has them. That's because pregnancy puts added pressure on the veins in your legs, and hormonal changes relax the vein walls and valves. If you start to get varicose veins, slip on maternity support hose first thing in the morning—even before you get out of bed. The hose will keep you more comfortable and may help prevent varicosities from getting worse. Getting your heart pumping with a brisk walk each day will also discourage blood from pooling in your legs, as will sleeping on your side and propping up your feet when you're sitting.

Spider veins, distant cousins to varicose veins, are areas of tiny blood vessels close to the surface of your skin that may show up on your ankles, legs, or face (and occasionally on your neck, chest, or arms). They may have little branches radiating out from the center—hence the name spider veins—or they may look like the branches of a tree. They're probably caused by the higher levels of estrogen in your system. Unsightly though they may be, spider veins don't cause discomfort, and they usually disappear after delivery.

Your Growing Baby

Your baby now measures 10½ inches long, head to heel, and weighs in at about ¾ pound—and she's starting to throw that weight around. You may soon feel like she's practicing martial arts as her initial fluttering movements turn into full-fledged kicks and nudges. You may also discover a pattern to her activity as you get to know her better. Some babies are restless in the evening, just as moms-to-be are trying to fall asleep; others get busy during the daytime. In other developments: Her eyebrows and eyelids are present now, and if she's a girl, her vagina has begun to form as well.

Your Pregnancy: 22 Weeks

Your Changing Body

At this point, you may find your belly becoming a hand magnet. It's perfectly okay to tell folks who touch your tummy that you'd rather they didn't. And if people are telling *you* that you look smaller or bigger than you should at this point, remember that each woman grows—and shows—at her own rate. What's important is that you see your practitioner for regular visits so she can make sure your baby's development is on track.

> ### HOT TOPICS
> - Sleep-well strategies (page 184)
> - All about cravings (page 196)
> - Stretch marks (page 220)
> - Comebacks to comments about your size (page 229)
> - Investigating your maternity-leave options (page 232)

With your belly in major expansion mode and your hormone levels high, you may notice that your skin is showing a little wear and tear. Some women never get stretch marks, but at least half of expectant mothers do. (And you may be in the clear now but still get them later in pregnancy.) These angry streaks range in color from pink to dark brown, depending on your skin tone, and can appear not only on your abdomen but also on your butt, thighs, hips, and breasts. Lotions won't prevent or eliminate stretch marks, but they will help your tautly stretched belly feel less itchy. Other changes in your mid-zone: Your stretched-out belly button (no longer an "innie," alas!) is flattening and may even be popping out. (It'll revert to its usual shape after your baby is born.)

Your Growing Baby

At 11 inches and almost a pound, your baby is starting to look like a miniature newborn. His lips, eyelids, and eyebrows are becoming more distinct, and he's even developing tiny tooth buds beneath his gums. His eyes have formed, though his irises (the blue or brown orbs you'll be getting lost in a

BabyCenter Buzz

What Other Women Say at 22 Weeks

"I've become the biggest klutz! I can't go a day without spilling something." —*Julie*

"I'm having trouble sleeping at night. I don't fall asleep until 6 A.M., so my days are shot. I have 18 weeks to go, but I'm so anxious to get to my due date!" —*Anonymous*

"I'm starting to get a big ol' belly. I hate how stretched out I'm getting, but it's for a good cause." —*Anonymous*

"It's 9:30 in the morning. Why am I craving spaghetti?" —*Anonymous*

"My baby likes to toy with me: Once every 20 minutes, it jumps up—and then comes crashing down on my bladder!" —*Susie*

few months from now) still lack pigment. If you could see inside your womb, you'd be able to spot the fine hair (lanugo) covering his body and the deep wrinkles on his skin, which he'll sport until he adds a padding of fat to fill them in. Inside his belly, his pancreas—essential for helping his body produce needed hormones—is developing steadily.

Your Pregnancy: 23 Weeks
Your Changing Body

You may notice that your ankles and feet are starting to swell a bit, especially at the end of the day or during the heat of summer. Sluggish circulation in your legs, coupled with pregnancy-induced water retention, is to blame for this condition, known as edema. Your body will get rid of the extra fluid after you have your baby (which is why you'll probably pee frequently and sweat a lot for a few days after delivery). In the meantime, put your

HOT TOPICS

- Staying hydrated (opposite page)
- Easing edema (page 176)
- Healthy snack ideas (page 193)
- Staying focused when you have "pregnancy brain" (page 326)
- Helping your mate bond with the baby (page 470)

feet up when you can, stretch out your legs when you sit, and avoid sitting—or standing—in one place for long periods. Also, try to exercise regularly to increase circulation, and wear support stockings and roomy, comfortable shoes. You may be tempted to skimp on liquids to combat fluid retention, but you need to drink plenty of water because staying hydrated actually helps *prevent* swelling. (If you notice severe or sudden swelling in your hands and face, be sure to call your midwife or doctor; it may be a sign of a serious condition called preeclampsia, page 531.)

Your Growing Baby

Feeling pretty good? Turn on the radio and sway to the music. With her sense of movement well-developed now, your baby can feel you dance. And now that she's over 11 inches long and tips the scales at more than a pound, you may even be able to *see* her squirm underneath your clothes. Blood vessels in her lungs are developing to prepare for breathing, and the sounds that your baby's increasingly keen ears pick up are preparing her for entry into the outside world. Loud noises that become familiar now—such as your dog barking or the roar of the vacuum cleaner—probably won't faze her when she hears them outside the womb.

BabyCenter Buzz

What Other Women Say at 23 Weeks

"I almost fall over putting on my pants each morning, and my husband thinks it's the funniest thing he's ever seen." —*Jen*

"My ligaments are stretching like crazy-every time I move, I feel like I'm tearing my abdomen! Luckily, it's just a quick, sharp pain and it doesn't last long." —*Michelle*

"I've gone from never being hungry to feeling starved all the time. I went to the grocery store yesterday to stock up on healthy snacks because if I keep eating chocolate cookies and ice cream all day, I'm going to get huge!" —*Anonymous*

"I'm already having concentration problems at work. I've started taking my vitamins more regularly, and I'm trying to get more sleep, but this is becoming a minute-by-minute battle! Luckily, I have a great boss." —*Carole*

Your Pregnancy: 24 Weeks

Your Changing Body

In the past few weeks, the top of your uterus has risen above your belly button and is now about the size of a soccer ball.

Most women have a glucose screening test sometime between now and week 28. This test checks for gestational diabetes, a pregnancy-related high-blood-sugar condition. Untreated diabetes boosts your chances of having a difficult vaginal delivery or needing a cesarean section (because it causes your baby to grow too large) and raises your baby's odds for other complications, like having low blood sugar right after birth. A positive result on your glucose screening doesn't necessarily mean you have gestational diabetes—but it does mean you'll need to take a different test, called the glucose tolerance test, to find out for sure.

Finally, if you don't already know how to spot the signs of preterm labor, now's the time to learn. Get in touch with your caregiver immediately if you notice any of the following symptoms: a change in your vaginal discharge (if it's watery, mucousy, pink, blood-tinged, or much more copious than normal); vaginal bleeding or spotting; abdominal pain or menstrual-like cramping; more than four contractions in an hour; an increase in pelvic pres-

HOT TOPICS

- Gestational diabetes screening (page 159)
- Simple ways to power up on protein (page 191)
- Warning signs of preterm labor (page 297)
- Taking time to pamper yourself (page 328)

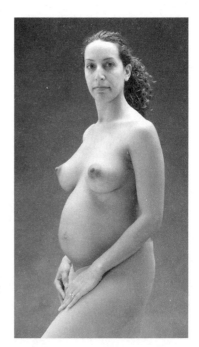

Your skin has a lot of stretching to do now to accommodate your ever-expanding uterus. To prevent itchiness, use mild soap and moisturizers. A warm oatmeal bath and wearing loose cottom clothing can help, too.

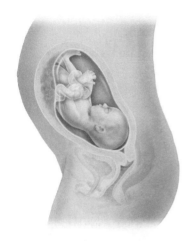

As you may have suspected from your own expanding middle, your baby's in major growth-spurt mode. At just over a pound, he's still relatively lean for his less-than-12-inch frame, but he'll soon add more body fat to balance out his rapidly growing brain, limbs, and lungs.

sure; or lower-back pain that you haven't had before.

Your Growing Baby

Your baby is growing steadily, having gained about 4 ounces since last week. That puts him at just over a pound. Since he's almost a foot long, he cuts a pretty lean figure at this point, but his body is filling out proportionally and he'll soon start to plump up. His brain is also growing quickly now, and his taste buds are continuing to develop. His lungs are developing "branches" of the respiratory "tree" as well as cells that will produce surfactant, a substance that will help his air sacs inflate once he hits the outside world. His skin is still thin and translucent, but that will start to change soon.

BabyCenter Buzz

What Other Women Say at 24 Weeks

"I've never felt so energized. Maybe I'll start slowing down in a couple of weeks?" —*Shannon*

"I feel good, but I don't think I look good anymore. My husband seems to be more in the mood, though, so maybe he's finding the big belly sexy." —*Amber*

"My maternity pants all seem to slide down my belly. I walk around all day, too, so I'm constantly pulling my pants up." —*Bonnie*

"I'm making friends with every bathroom I see—only to realize I don't really have to go after all! I hope this is just a passing phase." —*Anonymous*

Your Pregnancy: 25 Weeks
Your Changing Body

You may find you're having lots of "good hair days" now, thanks to pregnancy hormones. Those fuller, more lustrous locks (and possibly thicker body hair as well) aren't due to extra hair *growth* but to a lack of shedding. Because of hormonal changes, the hair that would normally come out in your brush each day is sticking around longer than usual. Enjoy the fullness while you can; the extra hair will fall out after you give birth.

HOT TOPICS

• Choosing a baby name (opposite page)

• How to modify your exercise regimen (page 81)

• Anemia (page 162)

• Why you need more iron now (page 190)

You may also notice that you can't move around as gracefully as before. Unless your caregiver has advised you otherwise, it's fine to continue to exercise, but use common sense: Don't work out when you're feeling overly tired, and stop if you feel pain, dizziness, or shortness of breath. Don't lie flat on your back or do any exercise where you're apt to lose your balance. Be sure to drink plenty of water, and make time for both warm-up and cooldown periods.

When you have your glucose screening test, your practitioner may also take a second tube of blood to check for anemia. Although your blood

BabyCenter Buzz

What Other Women Say at 25 Weeks

"Strangers are starting to notice that I'm pregnant now, and asking me if it's a boy or a girl and when I'm due. It's new now, so it's still exciting—but I imagine all this public questioning will get pretty tiresome before long!" —*Maria*

"I'm feeling good, overall: large in front, enjoying lots of kicks and flutters. But I'm sick of insensitive people telling me I'm huge." —*Anonymous*

"I saw my first 'belly roll' last night! It was right before I went to sleep, and I happened to look down from my book and saw the baby moving from one side to the other. It was awesome!" —*Kristin*

volume is increasing dramatically, the number of red blood cells doesn't increase as rapidly as the amount of plasma does—possibly leading to anemia. If your blood tests signal iron deficiency anemia, your caregiver will likely recommend an iron supplement in addition to your prenatal vitamins.

Have you started thinking about baby names yet? Choosing a name is an important decision, but it should be a fun one, too. Look to family history (Great-Grandpa Harry), favorite locations (Venice, where you honeymooned), or cherished book or film characters (Meg or Atticus, for example). Check out a couple of baby-name books to help you brainstorm, too.

Your Growing Baby

Head to heels, your baby now measures about 13½ inches. Her weight—1½ pounds—doesn't sound like much, but she's beginning to exchange her long, lean look for some baby fat. As she does, her wrinkled skin is starting to smooth out, and she's looking more and more like a newborn. She's also growing more hair—and if you could see it, you'd now be able to discern its color and texture.

Your Pregnancy: 26 Weeks
Your Changing Body

Are you rushing around, trying to get to childbirth classes and prepare your baby's room while still taking care of all your other daily tasks? Make sure that you also continue to eat well and get plenty of rest. Around this time, your blood pressure may be increasing slightly as it returns to its normal, prepregnancy range. (It was at a low from 22 to 24 weeks.) And though the condition most often occurs in the third trimester, this is a good time to be aware of the warning signs of preeclampsia, a complication that strikes 3 to 7 percent of pregnancies. Call your caregiver right away if you notice swelling in your face, puffiness around your eyes, or excessive swelling in your feet or ankles. Be alert for these symp-

HOT TOPICS

- Protein pointers for vegetarians (page 68)
- The benefits of prenatal massage (page 167)
- Spotting the warning signs of preeclampsia (page 177)
- Relaxation tips (page 185)
- Shopping for baby gear (page 343)

BabyCenter Buzz

What Other Women Say at 26 Weeks

"I've been feeling slower than usual lately—probably because of how much bigger I'm getting." —*Milena*

"We tried having sex last night-for the first time in weeks—and it made my sciatic nerve act up big-time! I told my poor hubby that we probably won't be doing it again until after the baby's born because I was very uncomfortable." —*Shelley*

"Has anyone else turned into a snot-manufacturing plant? I'm going to buy stock in Puffs! I think I'm single-handedly keeping them in business." —*Lisa*

"Ugh. I have acne all around my chin—even though I never had it as a teenager." —*Faith*

toms as well: rapid weight gain, severe or persistent headaches, vision changes—like seeing double, blurriness, seeing spots, or vision loss—intense abdominal pain or tenderness, or vomiting.

If your back seems a little achy, you can thank both your shifting center of gravity and the pregnancy hormones that are loosening up your joints and ligaments. Standing or sitting for long periods can put a strain on your back, as can bending or lifting. A warm bath or cool compress might bring relief.

Your Growing Baby

The network of nerves in your baby's ears is better developed and more sensitive than before; he may now be able to hear both your voice and your partner's as you chat with each other. His lungs are developing now, too, as he continues to take small breaths of amniotic fluid—good practice for when he's born and takes that first gulp of air. And, of course, he's continuing to put on baby fat, approaching the 2-pound mark as his length nudges up to about 14 inches from head to heel. If you're having a boy, his testicles are beginning to descend into his scrotum—a trip that will take two or three days.

Your Pregnancy: 27 Weeks

Your Changing Body

The second trimester is drawing to a close, but as your body gears up for the final lap, you may notice some new symptoms. Along with an aching back, your leg muscles might cramp up now and then. They're carrying extra weight, after all, and your expanding uterus is

HOT TOPICS

- Birth control after baby (page 146)
- Easing leg cramps (page 173)
- Dealing with sleep problems (page 182)
- Checking out the hospital or birth center (page 369)

putting pressure on the veins that return blood from your legs to your heart, as well as on the nerves leading from your trunk to your legs. Unfortunately, the cramps may get worse as your pregnancy progresses. Leg cramps are most likely to occur at night, but you can also get them during the day. Flexing your foot (by pointing your toes forward and then flexing them back toward your shin) stretches your calf muscles and should give you some relief. Walking for a few minutes or massaging your calf may help, too.

BabyCenter Buzz

What Other Women Say at 27 Weeks

"I dream about water. I think it's because my bladder is full and I need to wake up and use the bathroom." —*Joan*

"I had horrible insomnia in the first trimester—and now it's coming back. What can I do to get to sleep? I've been up since 2 A.M.!" —*Anonymous*

"I get off the sofa as if I'm 102 years old. My husband literally has to push my butt just to help me up. I told him to get used to it, 'cause this is what things will be like for us in another 60 or so years." —*Karen*

"I'm feeling great, actually! I feel energized and have been walking daily, which has boosted my self-esteem. I hope I won't get so uncomfortable in the last trimester that I can't enjoy all the things I'm enjoying now." —*Carissa*

And while it may be the furthest thing from your mind right now, it's not too soon to think about family planning. You'll want to have made some decisions about postpartum birth control before your baby arrives. In some states, if you're considering a tubal ligation during your hospital stay, laws require that you sign a consent form at least a month before delivery day. (Even if you sign one now, you can still change your mind later.)

Your Growing Baby

Your baby is bulking up as she prepares for her grand entrance. This week, she weighs in at almost two pounds and measures 14½ inches long with her legs extended. She's *acting* more like a newborn, too: sleeping and waking at regular intervals, opening and closing her eyes, and perhaps even sucking her fingers. With more brain tissue developing, your baby's brain is very active now. Also, while her lungs are still immature, they're capable of functioning—with a lot of medical help—if she were to be born now. Chalk up any tiny rhythmic movements you may feel to a case of hiccups (your baby's), which may be common from now on. Each episode usually lasts only a few moments, and it doesn't bother her, so just relax and try to tolerate the tickle.

Symptoms You Should Never Ignore in the Second Trimester

If you have any of these complaints, call your caregiver immediately:

- Decrease in fetal movement from your baby's usual level of activity (once he begins moving regularly)
- Vaginal bleeding or spotting
- An increase in vaginal discharge or a change in the type of discharge—if it becomes watery, mucous-like, or bloody (even if it's only pink or blood-tinged)
- Menstrual-like cramping, abdominal pain, or more than four contractions in one hour (even if painless)
- Increase in pelvic pressure (a feeling that your baby's pushing down)
- Lower back pain, especially if it's a new problem for you
- Persistent or severe headache
- Severe or persistent abdominal pain or tenderness
- Blurred or double vision, or seeing spots or "floaters"
- Swelling in your face or around your eyes, more than slight swelling in your hands, or severe and sudden swelling of your feet or ankles
- Rapid weight gain (more than 4 pounds in a week)
- Persistent or severe leg or calf pain that doesn't ease up when you flex your ankle and point your toes toward your shin, or one leg is significantly more swollen than the other
- Pain or burning when you urinate, or little or no urination
- Severe or persistent vomiting, or any vomiting accompanied by pain or fever
- Chills or fever over 100 degrees F
- Fainting, frequent dizziness, rapid heartbeat or palpitations
- Difficulty breathing or coughing up blood
- Persistent itching all over
- Trauma to your abdomen
- Any worsening health problem that you'd ordinarily call your practitioner about even if it's not pregnancy related—like a cold

If you're not sure whether a symptom is serious, or you're uneasy—trust your instincts and call your healthcare provider.

YOUR HEALTH

Baby, you're on your way! Some of the thrilling firsts you can expect over the next few months: Hearing your baby's heartbeat, seeing him (or her!) during your ultrasound, and feeling those first fluttering movements. You're likely to have lots of questions about your baby's development and concerns about new symptoms you may be feeling—including a few that (literally) may be keeping you awake at night.

Prenatal Checkups

Typically, you'll visit your practitioner once every four weeks during this trimester. But the exact number of appointments you'll have depends on your medical history and whether you have any illnesses, complications, or previous obstetric problems that call for more frequent checkups. At each visit, your practitioner will:

Gather information. She'll probably start by reviewing your chart and following up on issues that were raised at your last prenatal visit. She should let you know about any test results that have come back unless she called you about them. Ask if she doesn't bring them up. She'll also ask specific questions (Are you still nauseated? Are you feeling the baby move yet? And, later on, Is your baby moving as often as before? Have you been leaking fluid or had any vaginal spotting or bleeding? Have you felt any contractions?) and want to know how you're feeling in general. Whether she asks you or not, these visits are your opportunity to bring up any questions, concerns, or symptoms you have. Don't suffer in silence. Your healthcare provider can help you, and your symptoms may signal a problem you're not aware of.

Provide education and counseling. Sometime during this trimester, your practitioner should talk to you about childbirth education classes. Ask her opinion about the classes offered in your community or at the hospital where you plan to deliver. Also get the scoop on breastfeeding classes and infant CPR so you can cross them off your list in time for your baby's arrival.

And if it hasn't been addressed already, your midwife or doctor should discuss your options for prenatal genetic screening. Toward the end of this trimester, she'll advise you about the warning signs of preterm labor. (She may also discuss the signs of preeclampsia then.)

At the end of each appointment, your practitioner may briefly review her findings to let you know if everything's looking fine or if she has any special concerns. She should also let you know what changes you might expect in the interval until your next visit, and what lab tests may be coming up.

Check your weight. Though your baby's growth is partly affected by your weight-gain pattern, there's a fairly wide range of "normal." Some mothers-to-be find getting weighed at every checkup nerve-racking-especially as the numbers on the scale creep up into digits you've never seen before. If hopping on the scale bothers you, try not to look during weigh-ins. Just tell your provider you'd prefer to know your weight only if it's problematic. And take off your shoes and bulky clothing so your clothes won't be a factor and you'll get a more accurate picture of your actual weight gain.

Check your urine and blood pressure. Protein in your urine can be a sign of a urinary tract infection or, if it's accompanied by high blood pressure, a sign of preeclampsia. An occasional, small amount of sugar can be normal, but a high or persistent amount may signal gestational diabetes and blood testing will be needed. If your blood pressure alone increases, you could have gestational hypertension (page 140).

Listen to your baby's heartbeat. Checking your baby's heartbeat will become a routine part of every prenatal visit from here on out. Bring your partner along so he can share in the thrill of hearing this dramatic sign of the life you've created together.

Examine your belly. Your practitioner will feel your abdomen to get a sense of your growing uterus's size. From midpregnancy on, she'll use a tape measure to determine your fundal height—the distance between your pubic bone and the top of your uterus—to estimate your baby's size and growth rate. From 20 weeks until late in your third trimester, the measurement (in centimeters) should roughly correspond to how many weeks pregnant you are; so if you're 24 weeks pregnant, your fundal height should measure about 24 centimeters. Your practitioner will also check your hands and feet for swelling.

Just the Facts

Does Heart Rate Hint at Your Baby's Sex?

A fetus's normal heart rate ranges from 120 to 160 beats per minute. Although folk wisdom says that female fetuses' hearts beat at the higher end of this range, while males' tend to beat at the lower end, scientific research doesn't support the claim. So you'll have to wait until your ultrasound appointment to get clues about which color to paint the nursery.

How to Get the Most out of Prenatal Visits

Many women look forward to their monthly prenatal appointments but are dismayed to discover that they're in and out of the office in 10 minutes. Take heart: A quick visit is actually a sign that everything is progressing normally. If you leave feeling frustrated, though, try these tips:

Write down your concerns. Between visits, note your questions and your partner's. Bring the list to each appointment so you can run through it with your practitioner. And if anything else is bothering you, speak up. Your caregiver isn't a mind reader.

Get the go-ahead. Before you use any herbal teas, nutritional supplements, or over-the-counter medications, bring them with you (or a list of their ingredients) so your doctor or midwife can read their labels and let you know if they're safe.

Be flexible. If your practitioner really doesn't have time to talk as long as you'd like, ask to see a nurse or someone else in the practice who can address your concerns. Whatever you do, don't tolerate a provider who brushes you off without giving you complete answers, doesn't show compassion, or barely looks up from your chart. You and your baby deserve more than that.

MEASURING LARGE

There are a variety of reasons your fundal height might measure larger than expected. Among the possible explanations are your particular physical attributes: your height and shape or having looser abdominal muscles as a result of an earlier pregnancy. You may also be measuring large because your due date was figured incorrectly or you have uterine fibroids, or because you're carrying twins or more. Later in pregnancy, you might measure large for dates if you have too much amniotic fluid. You may also measure larger if your baby is positioned high above your pelvis as might be the case with a breech baby or if you have a placenta previa. Or you may simply be carrying a big, perfectly healthy baby. Occasionally, though, having a bigger-than-normal baby can signal a problem such as gestational diabetes, and you'll be tested to rule that out. If you measure large for dates, your provider will most likely schedule an ultrasound to find out why.

MEASURING SMALL

If your fundal height is more than two centimeters less than what's normal for your stage of pregnancy, your provider will most likely do an ultrasound to confirm your due date and rule out problems such as intrauterine growth restriction or too little amniotic fluid. Many times, a baby who seemingly measures "small for dates" is just fine. Your size, shape, and the condition of your abdominal muscles can throw off the initial measurement. And some babies are simply small because their parents are small, not because of any problems.But if it turns out that your baby isn't growing like he should be (page 526), you'll have another ultrasound in a few weeks to check on his growth and frequent monitoring to assess his well-being.

Prenatal Tests

Several tests may be offered to you this trimester: You'll likely have a mid-pregnancy ultrasound to check your baby's development. Unless you al-

Ask the Experts

I'm Measuring Large for My Stage—Is Something Wrong?

Doctors Joyce and Marshall Gottesfeld, obstetricians: Most likely everything is fine. Although your fundal height is usually within 2 centimeters of the week of pregnancy you're in, this measurement can vary depending on your size and shape. If you measure larger than expected early in pregnancy, it could be due to twins, an incorrect due date, or uterine fibroids. Later in pregnancy, it could indicate excessive amniotic fluid, a large baby (especially if you're diabetic), or just an error in measuring. If you're large to begin with, your provider will likely watch for a trend—growth of about a centimeter a week after 20 weeks—rather than focus on an absolute number. But generally, practitioners are more concerned when the fundal height is too *small*, which could signal that your baby isn't growing properly.

ready had prenatal genetic testing in your first trimester, you'll also be offered the multiple marker screening, a blood test that gives an estimate of your *risk* of having a baby with a neural tube defect or certain chromosomal abnormalities. (If you had a first-timester screening, you'll likely get only the AFP test now.)

If you're 35 or older (or otherwise at higher risk of having a baby with a chromosomal or other genetic abnormality), you will also be given the option of having amniocentesis, an invasive test that can definitively tell if your baby has certain chromosomal abnormalities or a number of other genetic problems.

Toward the end of this trimester (between 24 and 28 weeks), you'll likely have a glucose screening test. And if you're Rh negative, a blood test called an antibody screen will be done prior to your receiving an injection of Rh immunoglobulin at 28 weeks.

Multiple Marker Screening

WHAT: This screening test measures blood levels of a substance called alpha-fetoprotein (AFP), plus two or three hormones-human chorionic gonadotropin (hCG), and unconjugated estriol (uE3), and sometimes inhibin-A. It won't tell you if your baby has a problem, but it will give you an estimate of your *risk* of having a baby with a neural tube defect and a few other malformations, Down syndrome (the most common chromosomal abnormality), and trisomy 18 (a relatively rare chromosomal abnormality). Multiple marker screening is also sometimes known as the "triple screen" or—if the test measures inhibin-A—the "quadruple screen." (Adding inhibin-A increases the detection rate of babies at risk for Down syndrome and trisomy 18.)

WHO: All pregnant women without known risk factors for having a baby with a genetic abnormality. If you'll be 35 or older on your due date or have other risk factors for having a baby with a genetic problem, you'll be given the option of having amniocentesis, though you may still opt to start with the multiple marker to learn more about your risk profile before making a final decision. (No matter how old you are, the multiple marker screening won't be offered if you're carrying twins or more because it's difficult to interpret the results for more than one baby.)

WHEN: Between 15 and 20 weeks (16 to 18 weeks is the norm).

WHY: The main advantage of the multiple marker is that it's a simple

BabyCenter Buzz

My Multiple Marker Results Were Positive

"When my multiple marker test came back positive, we were shocked and terrified—and had to have some heart-wrenching discussions about what we'd do if our baby had major problems. We were on pins and needles the entire time we waited for the results of our follow-up amnio, and it turned what had been a joyous time into a terrible one. Luckily, the amnio showed that our baby was just fine." —*Caroline*

"My quad screen showed an increased risk for a neural tube defect. I was very scared, and it turned out that our daughter did have severe problems. Even if you'd never think of ending your pregnancy, early diagnosis will help you and your doctors modify your care or line up specialists to treat the baby. The more information available to you, the better prepared you'll be." —*Diana*

blood test that gives you information about the likelihood of certain birth defects without the risk of miscarriage associated with amniocentesis or chorionic villus sampling. But keep in mind that it's just a screening test-it can provide only an *estimate of risk*, and only for certain abnormalities. So the multiple marker can identify you as "high-risk" even if your baby is fine (so-called false-positive results), or it can miss a problem altogether (false-negative results). (Unlike amniocentesis or CVS, it can't tell you if your baby actually has—or doesn't have—these problems). Another factor to consider: Certain results may also mean that you're at increased risk for problems such as preeclampsia, premature birth, or placental abruption. Knowing this will put your practitioner on high alert for future signs of trouble.

Before having the multiple marker test, consider whether you'd opt for the next step—amniocentesis—if your results signal an increased risk for problems. Some women who are opposed to abortion skip the multiple marker altogether because they're sure that even if it indicated a possible problem, they still wouldn't have an amnio. Since they wouldn't act on the results, they simply don't want to know. Most women, though, do opt for a screening test—though their feelings about how they'd proceed in the face of a positive result vary considerably. Some are sure that they'd have an amnio and end the pregnancy if their baby had a major problem, while others would follow up a positive screen with an amnio to find out more so they could prepare—if necessary—for a child with special needs. And a number of women really aren't sure *what* they'd do next; they just want to take it one step at a time. No matter what the particulars of your situation, discuss the risks and benefits of the screening with your doctor or midwife or ask for a referral to a genetic counselor if you still have unanswered questions.

HOW: A technician will draw blood from your arm to send to a lab for analysis. The lab analyzes the various components of the sample to determine whether they fall within a "normal" range for this stage of your pregnancy, based on your age, weight, race, and health conditions such as diabetes. Having too much or too little of these substances is considered a "positive," or abnormal, result. Even so, this doesn't necessarily mean there's a problem; in fact, in the majority of cases with positive results, the baby is just fine. That's why positive readings—which are quite common—are followed up with further tests.

If you have an abnormal multiple marker result, the first thing that will happen is that you'll have a detailed ultrasound to confirm your baby's age or to look for twins. And if it turns out that your due date is off, your risk estimate will be recalculated according to this new information. The ultrasound will also include a careful look at your baby's spine and the rest of his body.

Some of the problems your multiple marker may have hinted at—like neural tube defects—can usually be diagnosed with a detailed ultrasound. But the chromosomal abnormalities that the multiple marker screens for Down syndrome and trisomy 18 can only be definitively diagnosed, at this point, with amniocentesis. Still, babies with chromosomal abnormalities often have abnormal ultrasound findings, so it's one more piece of useful information that you can factor in.

Understanding the meaning of a "positive" result can be difficult, even if you're adept at math and statistics. It's also emotionally trying. If your test reveals that you're at high risk of having a problem and you need help deciding whether you want to pursue further testing, or if a problem is actually diagnosed on ultrasound and you don't know what to do next, meet with a genetic counselor. She can't make decisions *for* you, but she can help you get a better handle on the situation and explain the pros and cons of your options.

Amniocentesis

WHAT: Amniocentesis can identify chromosomal abnormalities (like Down syndrome and many others), several hundred types of genetic disorders (including cystic fibrosis, sickle-cell disease, Tay-Sachs disease, and Huntington's disease), and neural tube defects (such as spina bifida and anencephaly). The report will also reveal your baby's sex—so if you don't want to know, tell your provider.

WHO: Amniocentesis is usually offered to women who are at increased risk of having a baby with a chromosomal or genetic defect. You may be in this category if:

- You'll be 35 or older on your due date. The risk of having a child with a chromosomal defect increases as you age. At age 35, the chance that you're carrying a baby with Down syndrome, for instance, is about 1 in 270—compared to 1 in 1,250 at age 25.

- You've had a screening test—such as a multiple marker, an ultrasound, a nuchal fold scan, or a "combined screening"—that signaled an increased likelihood of a problem.

- You've previously been pregnant with a child with a birth defect.

- You or your partner has a chromosomal abnormality, has a genetic disorder, is a carrier for an inherited disorder like cystic fibrosis or sickle-cell disease, or has a family health history that puts your child at increased risk for genetic problems.

WHEN: Between 15 and 20 weeks, but most often at around 16 weeks.

WHY: If you've been offered an amnio, you'll need to weigh your desire to know more about your baby's health against the slight risk that the test could lead to miscarriage. Even if you're sure that you'd never terminate a pregnancy for *any* reason, knowing in advance that your

---

BY THE NUMBERS

Amnio Safety

Risk of miscarriage from amniocentesis: **1 in 200**

Source: *Centers for Disease Control and Prevention*

QUICK TIP

Minimizing the Risks of Amniocentesis

The more experienced the physician performing your amniocentesis, the lower your risk of complications. Find someone who does at least 50 amnios a year. Ask your practitioner or genetic counselor for a referral. Make sure that an experienced, registered diagnostic medical sonographer provides continuous ultrasound guidance during the procedure. This greatly increases the odds that the doctor can collect enough fluid on the first try. Also, when continuous ultrasound guidance is used, injuries to the baby from the amnio needle are very rare.

baby may have special needs will give you time to prepare for the challenges ahead. You might want to switch to a better-equipped hospital with pediatric specialists, for instance. Your medical team could monitor your pregnancy and bring a neonatologist or pediatric surgeon on board to help your baby after delivery. And a few problems can even be treated in utero.

HOW: Before you have your amnio, you'll have an ultrasound to measure your baby and to check his basic anatomy. This may happen on the same day as the amnio or a few days or weeks beforehand. Also, most centers require that you meet with a genetic counselor so you clearly understand the risks and benefits of amnio before you consent to the procedure.

For the amnio itself, you'll lie on an exam table and have your belly cleaned with alcohol or an iodine solution. A doctor or technician will use ultrasound to pinpoint a pocket of amniotic fluid a safe distance from both your baby and your placenta. Then the doctor will insert a long, thin hollow needle through your abdominal wall and into the sac of fluid around your baby. She'll withdraw a little more than a tablespoon of amniotic fluid and then remove the needle. (Don't worry; your baby will quickly make more fluid to replace what's taken out.)

You may feel some cramping, pinching, or pressure during the procedure. The amount of discomfort varies among women and even from one pregnancy to the next. Afterward, your doctor will listen to the baby's heartbeat for reassurance. You'll want to take it easy for the rest of the day and avoid any heavy lifting or strenuous activity for the next two days. You may have some minor cramping for a day or so. A very small number of women (about 1 to 2 percent) have heavy cramping, temporary vaginal spotting, or leaking amniotic fluid. Call your practitioner right away if you have any of these symptoms—or a fever—because they could be signs of impending miscarriage.

After the procedure is done, the fluid sample will be sent to a lab, where a technician will collect some of your baby's sloughed-off cells and allow them to multiply for a week or two. Then she'll test the cells for chromosomal abnormalities or evidence of certain genetic birth defects. You should have the full results

> ## QUICK TIP
>
> ### Rh Precautions
>
> If you're Rh negative, you'll need a shot of Rh immunoglobulin after amniocentesis to prevent Rh sensitization because it's possible that your baby's blood may have mixed with yours during the procedure.

within two weeks, though some labs can provide preliminary results in as little as eight days.

Ultrasound

WHAT: An ultrasound (sometimes called a sonogram) is a noninvasive diagnostic test that uses sound waves to create a visual image of your uterus, baby, and placenta that helps your practitioner gather information about the progress of your pregnancy and about your baby's health.

WHO: Most women are offered a routine ultrasound during the first half of their second trimester.

WHEN: Between 16 and 20 weeks.

WHY: Your practitioner may recommend a second-trimester ultrasound to check on:

The number of babies. If you or your caregiver suspects that you're carrying more than one baby, an ultrasound will help confirm it.

Your baby's heartbeat. Your practitioner or the ultrasound technician will measure the number of beats per minute.

Your baby's size and age. The sonographer will measure your baby's length, across and around his skull, along his thighbone, and around his abdomen to make sure he's about the size he should be. If this is your first ultrasound and there's a discrepancy of more than two weeks between your due date and your baby's size, you'll be given a new due date. And if your practitioner has any concerns about how your baby is growing, she may order a series of follow-up ultrasounds to check his progress (though after the first trimester, ultrasound isn't as accurate in this regard).

Location of the placenta. If the placenta is covering the internal opening of your cervix (a condition known as placenta previa) and it stays there, it can cause painless but severe bleeding later in pregnancy. If you have placenta previa, your practitioner will order a follow-up scan toward

QUICK TIP

Experience Counts

Sonograms done at state-of-the-art academic hospitals can detect abnormalities up to 80 percent of the time, while at sites such as doctors' offices—which tend to have lower-tech equipment and less experienced personnel—the detection rate can dip to as low as 13 percent. Consider requesting that a "registered diagnostic medical sonographer" or a doctor who's highly skilled at interpreting the results administer your ultrasound, especially if other tests have raised suspicions about possible problems.

Just the Facts

Ultrasound Safety

Numerous large studies done over the last 35 years have concluded there's no evidence to date that ultrasounds harm a developing baby or that there's a cumulative effect from having multiple scans. And reports from some small studies suggesting that the procedure increases the risk of low birthweight, speech and hearing problems, and left-handedness haven't been borne out by other, more rigorous research.

the end of this trimester to see if the placenta has moved as your uterus has grown. In the meantime, don't panic! Only a small percentage of placenta previas detected on ultrasound before 20 weeks persist until delivery.

Amniotic fluid volume. Too much or too little amniotic fluid can signal a problem. If the amount looks abnormal, you'll have a complete workup to see if the cause can be identified, as well as repeat scans to monitor what's going on.

Physical abnormalities. Your sonographer will look closely at your baby's anatomy, including his head, neck, chest, heart, spine, stomach, kidneys, bladder, extremities, and umbilical cord to see if they're developing the way they should. In many cases, the technician will do an even more thorough ultrasound, called a level II scan, to check for signs of specific birth defects. And because a fair number of babies with chromosomal abnormalities also have physical abnormalities that can be spotted on ultrasound, some practitioners routinely offer detailed scans in conjunction with the multiple marker. (Amniocentesis is still needed for a definitive diagnosis, though.)

HOW: You'll lie on an exam table with your belly exposed. The sonographer will squeeze some gel on your abdomen to improve sound conduction, and then she'll slide a sound wave-emitting transducer

BY THE NUMBERS

Boy, Girl—or Big Surprise?

75% of mothers-to-be want to find out if they're having a boy or a girl ahead of time

18% want to save the surprise for delivery day

7% haven't made up their minds

Source: A BabyCenter.com poll of more than 267,000 women

Just the Facts

3-D Ultrasounds

You may have heard about the new 3-D ultra-sounds, which use special equipment to show a view of your baby that's almost as detailed as a photo-graph. The technique allows more detailed evalua-tion of problems such as spina bifida and cleft palate. Some parents-to-be also find that the highly realistic image heightens their bond with their baby. But the new technology does require a more skilled sonographer and isn't yet available in many places. Expect it to become an increasingly common addi-tion to 2-D ultrasound technology—but not to re-place it anytime soon. A word of warning: Be wary of centers that advertise 3-D ultrasounds done solely to create keepsake photos or videos. The personnel at such centers may not be qualified to counsel you if your ultrasound reveals a problem—and since the scan is for "entertainment only," the results may be falsely reassuring.

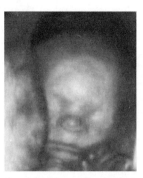

New 3-D ultrasound technology gives parents a much more life-like peek at their growing baby than the grainy images of a tra-ditional reading.

(which looks a bit like a handheld microphone) back and forth over your belly. As a computer translates the resulting echoes into pictures on a nearby monitor, your baby will appear on the screen before your eyes. During the scan, the sonographer will record your baby's measurements and take still pictures or video for your caregiver to interpret. (At some centers, a physician who's a specialist in obstetric sonography will come in and watch—or do—part of the exam.) If you'd prefer not to know your baby's sex, tell the sono-grapher that up-front. While you'll be eager to know what the technician is seeing, don't be surprised if she refuses to answer your questions. Your doctor or midwife will need to review the results before discussing them with you.

Glucose Screening

WHAT: Like any screening test, the glucose challenge test (GCT) isn't used to actually *diagnose* gestational diabetes, a condition that affects between 2 to 5 percent of expectant mothers. Rather, it's a way to spot women who need to undergo the more cumbersome three-hour diagnostic test for diabetes.

WHO: All pregnant women.

WHEN: Between 24 and 28 weeks.

BabyCenter Buzz 🐻

Why We Did—or Didn't—Want to Know Our Baby's Sex

"We found out that our baby was a boy and had his name picked out at five months. We spoke to him by name, and by the time he was born, he was an established family member." —*Rima*

"Not knowing the sex of my babies was the only thing that got me through labor. It gave me extra incentive to push. I can't wait for that shocked, excited feeling to wash over me again." —*Trixie*

"Waiting gives your husband a glorious moment to shine. He gets to be in the spotlight and announce the sex to the grandparents and everyone in the waiting room." —*Stefanie*

"I'm too busy *not* to know! I'd like to be able to shop ahead of time, decide on names, and fix up the baby's room. We can always keep the gender a secret from our friends or family if we choose." —*Mary*

"Once you get past Santa Claus and the Easter Bunny, there are so few real surprises in life. This is one that can be cherished. Why open your present before it gets here?" —*Anonymous*

WHY: Because gestational diabetes rarely causes any obvious symptoms, the GCT is the best way to figure out if you need the diagnostic test.

HOW: You'll be given a sugar solution that contains 50 grams of glucose. The stuff tastes like a very sweet soda pop, and you have to down it all in five minutes. (Some centers keep it chilled or let you pour it over ice and drink it cold.) An hour later (bring a book or magazine because you can't leave the office), your practitioner or a technician will take a blood sample from your arm to check your blood sugar level. Some women feel a little nauseated after drinking the glucose solution, and a few even throw up. You may find that it helps to eat something a few hours before the test.

Expect the results in a few days. If your blood sugar level is too high, you'll have to come back for the glucose tolerance test.

Glucose Tolerance Test

WHAT: The glucose tolerance test (GTT) is a follow-up to the glucose challenge test. It's used to definitively diagnose gestational diabetes after a positive glucose screening.

WHO: Any pregnant woman whose GCT signaled an elevated blood sugar level.

WHEN: Soon after the GCT results are noted.

WHY: If your GCT signaled a possible blood sugar problem, this test can tell for sure if you've developed gestational diabetes. The sooner the problem is identified and treated, the fewer problems you and your baby will have.

HOW: For three days before the test, you'll need to eat at least 150 grams of carbohydrates a day (adding an extra piece of bread to each meal should do the trick). And for eight to 14 hours before the test, you can't eat or drink anything but sips of water, so you'll want to schedule it for first thing in the morning.

When you arrive, a technician will take a blood sample to measure your "fasting blood glucose level" and then have you drink either a more concentrated dose or a larger volume of the glucose solution that you drank for the screening. Not surprisingly, more women feel nauseated during the GTT than during the GCT. Brace yourself for three more arm pricks as the technician draws blood every hour for the next three hours. (You'll definitely need some light reading or another source of distraction, since you'll have to stay in the waiting room between drawings. And bring something to eat right after your final blood sample is drawn because you'll likely be famished.)

Just the Facts

Blood Sugar: How High Is Too High?

Practitioners standards vary when determining whether your blood sugar level in the glucose challenge test is high enough to merit further testing. Some say that if your one-hour level is 140 milligrams of glucose per deciliter of blood plasma (mg/dL) or more, you need to take the glucose tolerance test. Others set the cutoff at 130 mg/dL to catch more women who may have gestational diabetes, even though there are likely to be more false positives this way. If your glucose level is higher than 200 mg/dL, most practitioners will diagnose gestational diabetes without proceeding to the three-hour test.

Just the Facts

Abnormal Readings

This chart shows the levels that the American Diabetes Association considers abnormal at each interval of the glucose tolerance test.

Interval	Abnormal reading
Fasting	95 mg/dl or higher
1-hour	180 mg/dl or higher
2-hour	155 mg/dl or higher
3-hour	140 mg/dl or higher

If one of the readings is abnormal, you may have to take another test later in your pregnancy or make some changes in your diet and exercise routine. If two or more of your readings are abnormal, you'll be diagnosed with gestational diabetes and need to work out a treatment plan with your practitioner.

Why You'll Feel Better and Worse

They call this the honeymoon stage of pregnancy for a reason. Most women get a boost of energy and an emotional lift in their second trimester as bothersome symptoms such as nausea and fatigue recede. Still, it may not be *all* smooth sailing from now on. Some early-pregnancy symptoms may continue to plague you, and new ones may crop up. From the top of your head to the tips of your toes, you're starting to see and feel just how completely pregnancy has taken over your body. Your growing belly is only the most obvious sign that you're expecting; everything from your bra size to your shoe size is likely to change, too.

Most midpregnancy aches and pains are related to the extra work your body is doing to accommodate your growing baby. While some symptoms are barely noticeable, others can be downright painful. And one change, feeling your baby move for the first time, is wondrous and exhilerating. Here, a rundown of what's happening and why—plus what you can do to stay comfortable.

Anemia

Although the total amount of blood in your body (your blood volume) is rising rapidly, the increase in your red blood cells usually doesn't keep pace

BabyCenter Buzz

What's Happening to My Body?!

"It feels like my hips and bones are stretching apart." —*Diane*

"Nosebleeds—ugh. I sat up at 4 this morning, and blood came gushing out. I've had some bleeding in the past due to dry sinuses, but this is ridiculous." —*Anonymous*

"My breasts have started to leak. I didn't know that could happen so soon!" —*Anonymous*

"I'm extremely congested. As a result, I can't sleep, and my husband says I've been snoring a lot. So now *both* of us can't sleep." —*Antonella*

"I have a terrible taste in my mouth most of the time—and there doesn't seem to be anything I can do about it." —*Anonymous*

"With all the constipation and flatulence I've been having, my husband's convinced that someone kidnapped his 'real' wife!" —*Anonymous*

with the increase in plasma, sometimes resulting in anemia. Your practitioner probably screened you for the condition at your first prenatal visit, but because anemia is most common later in pregnancy, you can expect another blood test between 24 and 28 weeks.

Iron deficiency is the most common cause of anemia, though it's also possible to develop anemia from not getting enough vitamin B_{12} or folic acid. Anemia can also be triggered by blood loss or by inherited blood disorders, such as sickle-cell anemia or thalassemia.

Without a blood test, you might not even know you're anemic because you might not have any symptoms. Plus, one of the early symptoms is fatigue, which is common in pregnancy. Other symptoms include looking pale or having decreased color in your fingernail bed or the lining of your eyelids. If you're very anemic, you may be short of breath, have heart palpitations, or feel weak or faint. (Some severely anemic women have an unusual desire to eat ice or even nonfood substances, like clay, a condition known as pica. Don't give in to those cravings, and let your caregiver know.)

To combat anemia, your doctor or midwife may recommend iron supplements or iron-rich foods. Though high-dose supplements can cause some unpleasant side effects—such as constipation and an upset stomach—it's important to take them, since untreated anemia may not only make you feel weak but also increase your odds of needing a transfusion if you lose a lot of blood during delivery.

Backache

As pregnancy hormones loosen your joints and the ligaments that attach your pelvic bones to your spine, it's not unusual to feel some back pain when you're walking, standing, sitting for long periods, bending, twisting, or lifting. Your expanding uterus is also starting to stretch out and weaken your abdominal muscles, altering your posture and putting additional strain on your back. Another cause of lower-back pain may be your baby and growing uterus pressing on a nerve. You're more likely to notice back pain if you've had back problems in the past, are overweight, have poor abdominal muscle tone, are carrying twins or more, or have been pregnant before.

During your pregnancy, you may get one or both of the following types of back pain: lumbar pain (so-called because it occurs in the area of the lumbar vertebrae in your lower back) and posterior pelvic pain (pain in the back of your pelvis).

Lumbar pain is like the lower-back pain that you may have had before you were pregnant. You'll feel it over and around your spine around the level of, or a little above, your waist. You might also have pain that radiates to your legs. It's usually aggravated by sitting for long periods, standing, or lifting, and tends to be worse at the end of the day.

Even more pregnant women get posterior pelvic pain, which is lower on your body than lumbar pain. You may feel it deep inside your buttocks, on one side or both. You may also have pain in the backs of your thighs. You'll likely find that it's triggered by activities such as walking, climbing stairs, getting in and out of the tub or a low chair, rolling over in bed, or twisting and lifting. Positions in which your hips are bent—such as sitting in a chair and leaning forward while working at your desk—may make posterior pelvic pain worse.

While this type of pain is often confused with a condition called sciatica, true sciatica affects only about one in 100 pregnant women and causes severe symptoms in a much smaller number. (Sciatica can be caused by a herniated, or bulging, disk in the lower part of your spine.) Generally, if you have sciatica, your leg pain will be worse than your back pain, it will radiate

BabyCenter Buzz

My Back Is Killing Me!

"Swimming is the only thing that eases my back pain. The pain is especially bad when I sit at my desk at work." —*Bonnie*

"I've had horrible lower-back pain for a few weeks now . . . and I'm barely even showing! By the time I get home from work and lie on the couch, I'm almost in tears. I wore heels to work one day and felt it in the worst way for the next few days." —*Karla*

"I use heat and ice to reduce the pain to where it's tolerable and have found that walking seems to help if I do at least a little bit every day or every other day." —*Anonymous*

below your knee, and you'll feel numbness or a tingling, "pins and needles" sensation in your legs. With severe symptoms, you may even have trouble urinating. (If you think you have sciatica, see your healthcare provider; if it's combined with loss of bladder sensation, see her *immediately*.)

There are many things you can do to squelch back pain before it starts.

Try sleeping on your side with a pillow between your legs, or use an adjustable pregnancy wedge to support your back and belly. Take care when getting out of bed: Bend your legs at your knees and hips when you roll to the side, and use your arms to push yourself up as you dangle your lower legs over the side of the bed.

Start an exercise program that includes stretches to strengthen muscles that support your back and legs, including your abdominals. Swimming is ideal because it strengthens your abdominal and lower-back muscles without putting stress on your joints and ligaments. Water aerobics is also a good way to exercise during pregnancy. Don't do anything that hurts, and avoid all high-impact exercise.

Stand up straight. This gets harder to do as your belly expands, but try to keep your pelvis tucked in and your shoulders back. Pregnant women tend to slump their shoulders and arch their backs as their bellies grow, which puts more strain on the spine.

If you sit all day, make sure to sit up straight and raise your feet with a footstool or other low object. Don't sit for long periods; every hour or so, get up and walk around or step outside for a break.

Wear comfortable shoes, and skip the high heels for now. As your belly grows and your balance shifts, heels will throw your posture even more out of whack than it already is (and boost your odds of stumbling and falling).

Always bend from your knees and lift from a crouching (rather than stooped) position, to minimize back stress. Let someone else haul heavy objects; this is *not* the time to risk throwing your back out completely. Don't reach for high objects, either, and try not to twist your back.

But if pain already has you in its grasp, relief may be found in some simple ways.

Soak in a warm bath. A hot pack can work wonders, too. (Try a cold pack if heat doesn't work for you.)

Relaxation techniques may help you cope with the discomfort and may be especially handy at bedtime if back pain is just one more thing that makes it hard to get to sleep.

Avoid activities, like vacuuming and mopping, that require you to bend and twist at the same time. If there's no one else to do these chores, move your whole body with the mop rather than twist or overreach to get to out-of-the-way spots.

If you have posterior pelvic pain, try to limit activities like stairclimbing that may make the pain worse, and avoid exercise that requires extreme movements of your hips or spine. If you sit for long periods, try to use an adjustable chair and slightly tip the front downward. And talk to your caregiver about using a "sacral belt"—for some women it seems to help lessen the pain when walking (though for others it doesn't help at all, and for a few it may even increase pain).

For lumbar pain, try doing pelvic tilts, which can ease back pain by stretching your muscles and, over time, by strengthening them as well.

Braxton Hicks Contractions

Toward the middle of your pregnancy, you may start to notice the muscles of your uterus randomly and painlessly tightening for 30 to 60 seconds at a time. These are called Braxton Hicks contractions. You may find that they tend to come a little more often when you do physical activity like lugging groceries from the car or step up your pace to catch a bus.

If you feel them at all at this point in your pregnancy, they should be painless and very sporadic. Within a few weeks of your due date, Braxton

Just the Facts

The Benefits of Prenatal Massage

A rubdown by a trained prenatal massage therapist can relieve tense shoulders, an aching neck, and lower-back pain; increase mobility; and help you feel more relaxed. Prenatal massage therapists are specially trained to understand the changes a pregnant woman's body goes through. They often use a special table or pad with hollowed-out areas to accommodate the pregnant belly and perhaps the breasts as well, so you can comfortably lie facedown while you're getting your aches and pains massaged away.

Hicks contractions can become more frequent, intense, and longer lasting. At that time, they can become so uncomfortable that you think you're in labor, even though you're not. If you start having frequent contractions (even painless ones) now, it may signal preterm labor—so don't *assume* they're Braxton Hicks. Lie down, drink some water, and pay close attention. If they continue, call your midwife or doctor right away.

Carpal Tunnel Syndrome

Pain and numbness in your hands and fingers is most likely caused by carpal tunnel syndrome (CTS). Although you probably associate CTS with jobs requiring repetitive hand movements (such as data processing, computer programming, and assembly-line work), certain physical changes that happen during pregnancy make it a relatively common problem for expectant mothers in just about any line of work.

The general swelling and fluid retention of pregnancy can increase the pressure in the carpal tunnel, a relatively narrow bony canal formed by your wrist bones on three sides and a ligament that runs across your wrist on the other. This in turn compresses the median nerve, which runs through the tunnel, and may cause numbness, tingling, burning, pain, or a dull ache in your fingers, hand, wrist, and, rarely, up your arm to your shoulder. If you're like many pregnant women, your

BY THE NUMBERS

Wrist Watch

Pregnant women who develop symptoms of carpal tunnel syndrome: **1 in 4**

symptoms will usually show up at night or when you first wake up in the morning. Strategies for minimizing the pain:

• Whenever you feel a twinge, shift your sleep position and try to prop your arm up with a pillow or two.

• Don't sleep on your hands. If you wake up with pain or numbness, try gently shaking your hands until it goes away.

• When you're working at a computer, adjust your chair height so your arms are straight from elbow to fingertips as you type, consider trying a special ergonomic keyboard, and remember to take breaks to stretch your hands.

• If you can, avoid tasks that require forceful, repetitive hand movements. Though they may not have *caused* your carpal tunnel problems, they can certainly aggravate your symptoms.

• If you have a lot of discomfort, consider wearing wrist or hand braces (available at medical supply stores and some larger drugstores). These hold your wrist in a way that slightly opens the carpal tunnel.

• Consider doing yoga, which can help relieve the pain and increase hand strength.

• Let your practitioner know if the pain and numbness interfere with your sleep or daily routine.

The symptoms usually go away gradually after delivery as pregnancy swelling subsides. (If the pain persists after your baby is born, mention it to your practitioner so she can refer you to an orthopedist.)

Dizziness and Light-Headedness

Most of the time, your cardiovascular and nervous systems are able to adjust to the many changes taking place in your body. But occasionally they can't, and it can make your head spin. Here are some of the most common causes of dizziness or light-headedness during pregnancy—and advice for avoiding them.

Standing up too fast. When you stand up suddenly or stand or sit for long periods, blood pools in your feet and lower legs. As a result, you may not get enough blood returning to your heart from your legs, and you'll have a rapid decrease in blood pressure, which can leave you feeling light-headed and faint.

Lying on your back. Your growing uterus can slow bloodflow by compressing the inferior vena cava (the large vein that returns blood from the lower half of your body to your heart) and your pelvic veins. Lying flat on your back can exacerbate this problem.

Not getting enough to eat or drink. When you don't eat enough, you can end up with low blood sugar, which can make you feel dizzy or faint. Some dehydration can have a similar effect.

Anemia. Because women with anemia have fewer red blood cells carrying oxygen to their brain and other organs, this condition can lead to light-headedness.

Getting overheated. Spending time in a very hot room or taking a hot bath or shower causes your blood vessels to dilate, lowering your blood pressure and making you woozy.

Hyperventilation. Because they cause you to breathe quickly and shallowly, anxiety and rigorous exercise can sometimes make you feel faint.

Vasovagal response. Some pregnant women get dizzy when they strain to cough, urinate, or have a bowel movement. These actions can prompt a "vasovagal" response (the effect of the vagus—a major nerve that runs from your head to your abdomen—on your circulatory system): a decrease in your blood pressure and heart rate, which leads to dizziness and fainting. Dehydration, anxiety, or pain can also trigger this type of fainting. It's often preceded by light-headedness and other warning signs, such as a feeling of warmth, paleness, sweating, nausea, yawning, and hyperventilation.

Avoid the "spins." No matter what the cause of your light-headedness, stop what you're doing and lie down as soon as you feel it, to keep from falling and hurting yourself. Lying on your left side will maximize bloodflow to your heart and thus to your brain and will likely relieve the sensation of light-headedness altogether. (If you're in a place where it's impossible to lie down, sit down and put your head between your knees.) When you're ready to get up, sit up slowly and stay sitting for a few minutes with your legs dangling over the side of the bed. Then slowly rise from sitting to standing.

If you're standing in one place for a long time, move your legs to promote circulation, and wear support stockings to aid circulation in the lower half of your body.

Avoid hot, crowded places and wear clothing in layers so you can shed some as needed. Remember to stay well-hydrated by drinking at least eight glasses of water a day—more if you're exercising or if it's hot.

Take warm—not hot—showers or baths, and try to keep the bathroom cool by turning on the fan or cracking a window.

BabyCenter Buzz

How I Deal with "the Spins"

"I was cooking dinner and started to feel hot and weak. I splashed cool water on my face and slowly fanned myself, which helped a lot."   —*Aggie*

"When I fainted, my doctor told me to eat frequent, small meals with extra protein. It turns out that I had severe low blood sugar."   —*Nickole*

"A change in temperature, the motion of the subway, being in a car too long, leaning back, and stress can all trigger dizzy spells and passing out for me. My doctor told me to drink a *lot* of water. I also keep a box of raisins in my purse and pop a few when I feel a spell coming."   —*Mary*

Some exercise is good, but be careful not to overdo it if you're feeling fatigued. Start out slowly. If you begin to feel light-headed or dizzy, stop and take a breather.

Try to keep your blood sugar from dipping by eating small, frequent meals during the day, instead of three large ones. Carry healthy snacks with you so you can eat when you get hungry, and take an iron supplement or a prenatal vitamin with iron if your caregiver prescribes it.

Fetal Movements

Feeling your baby's first, fluttering movements, also known as "quickening," is a thrilling milestone. While an ultrasound can identify fetal movement as early as 7 or 8 weeks, you probably won't *feel* your baby move until sometime between 16 and 20 weeks (some women don't feel movement until 22 weeks). Though thin women and women who've already had a baby are likely to have quickening a littler earlier than others, there's really no predicting when you'll first feel the sign of life inside you.

Remember, the initial sensations you'll notice won't feel like real kicks—instead, some women describe the sensation as being like "popcorn popping" or "butterflies in the stomach." You're more likely to feel these early, barely perceptible movements when you're sitting or lying quietly.

At this point, you may notice your baby moving only now and then,

BabyCenter Buzz

The First Time I Felt My Baby Move

"I've spent most of the day at my desk in awe of the movement I'm finally feeling! The best way I can describe it is like tiny vibrations."   —*Tarns*

"I was lying in bed and noticed something that felt like popcorn popping in my stomach. It wasn't gas, so I know it was my baby. It was so exciting!"   —*Melissa*

"The first movement I felt was like a wing fluttering across the inside of my belly. It was very faint, but unlike anything I'd ever felt before."   —*Holly*

"I'm almost at week 19 and just felt the first kicks. I've been worried about it and focusing on my belly every night to try to feel something—to no avail. But today while I was at work, I felt two gentle taps right below my belly button and knew instantly that it was my little boy. I'm so excited!"   —*Chandra*

but toward the end of this trimester, these reassuring movements will be stronger and you'll feel them throughout the day (and night!).

Foot Growth

Shoes getting a little tight? Swelling is partly responsible for this anti-Cinderella syndrome, but pregnancy hormones are also loosening the ligaments in your feet, causing your foot bones to spread apart. While foot *swelling* generally subsides within a month after delivery, foot *spreading* is permanent.

Avoiding Big-Foot Frustrations

• If your shoes are too tight, buy a few pairs of comfortable, versatile shoes. You may need them a half or whole size larger than the ones you wear now. There should be room for future spreading or swelling—but they shouldn't be so loose that you might trip.

• Some moms-to-be find that if they take their shoes off—especially late in the day—they can't get them back *on*. Keep a pair of roomy backup shoes in your trunk or in your desk drawer or locker at work for just such emergencies.

BabyCenter Buzz

My Shoes Don't Fit!

"I don't know where I'd be without my clogs. It doesn't matter how wide my feet get; I can slip them on without worry—plus, I don't have to bend over to fool with laces or a zipper!" —*Jocelyne*

"I've gone ahead and invested in a pair of expensive but super-comfortable walking shoes. I tried them on with extra-thick socks so if my feet get wider, they should still fit." —*CeCe*

"Fortunately, I've been able to walk around in flip-flops all summer and haven't had to worry about squeezing into my fall shoes—yet." —*Anonymous*

Heartburn

For some women, the second trimester marks the onset of heartburn, also known as acid indigestion or acid reflux. You'll feel a burning sensation that extends from the bottom of your breastbone to the back of your throat and that may be accompanied by an acid taste in your mouth. Hormonal and physical changes are to blame: Progesterone relaxes smooth muscles and impedes digestion by slowing the wavelike contractions of your stomach and intestines. It also relaxes the valve that separates your esophagus from your stomach, allowing gastric acid to seep back up and cause the uncomfortable sensation of heartburn. This problem is compounded as your growing uterus begins to push upward on your stomach.

To avoid heartburn or help ease it when it strikes:

• Pass up carbonated beverages; alcohol (off-limits during pregnancy anyway); caffeine; chocolate; acidic foods, like citrus fruits and juices, tomatoes, mustard, and vinegar; mint products; processed meats; and spicy, highly seasoned, fried, and fatty foods—all of which can make the problem worse.

• Eat small, frequent meals, and chew your food slowly and thoroughly.

• Chew gum after eating, to stimulate your salivary glands. Saliva can help neutralize acid that's seeped up into your esophagus.

• If you haven't already, quit smoking.

• Give yourself two or three hours to digest before lying down. Sleep with extra pillows, to keep your head and upper body propped up about 6

inches from the mattress. You can try sleeping semi-upright in a comfy recliner, too.

- Wear clothes and sleepwear that fit loosely around your abdomen
and waist.

- Bend at the knees instead of at the waist.

- If the problem persists, try an over-the-counter antacid with
calcium—ask your caregiver for a recommendation.

Leg Cramps

Leg pains may start to plague you now and get worse as your pregnancy progresses and your girth increases. While these sudden, sharp, painful cramps
may strike during the day, they usually happen at night-jolting you out of
bed, and often out of a sound slumber. They can be aggravated by circulation problems in your legs that may develop as your uterus expands and puts
pressure on the blood vessels. Compression of the nerves that extend from
your trunk to your legs may be a factor, too.

You may have heard that getting too little calcium or potassium can
bring on leg cramps, or that getting too much phosphorus (found in
processed meats, snack foods, and soda) can have the same effect because it
keeps you from absorbing enough calcium. While these theories have yet to
be borne out by research, it's a good idea to increase your intake of calcium
now anyway.

To keep leg cramps at bay:

- Avoid standing or sitting with your legs crossed for long periods of time.
- Stretch your calf muscles (by straightening your legs, flexing your
toes back toward your shins, and rotating your ankles) regularly during the
day and several times before you go to bed.
- Rotate your ankles and wiggle your toes when you sit, eat dinner,
or watch TV.
- Try to take a walk every day (unless your midwife or doctor has ad-
vised you not to exercise).
- Avoid getting too fatigued. Rest by reclining on your left side, to im-
prove circulation in your legs.
- Stay hydrated by drinking at least eight glasses of water a day.
- Try a warm bath before bed, to relax your muscles.

- If you get a cramp, immediately stretch your calf muscles: Straighten your leg, heel first, and gently flex your toes back toward your shins. It might hurt at first, but the pain will gradually go away. You can relax the cramp by massaging the muscle or warming it with a hot-water bottle. Walking around for a few minutes may help, too.

- Ask your caregiver about taking a magnesium supplement in addition to your prenatal vitamin—there's some evidence it might help. (Always check with your practitioner before taking *any* kind of supplement.)

Morning Sickness: What to Do If It Persists

No one knows exactly why, but nausea can sometimes last well into the second and even third trimesters. Though you may just have to tough out an extended bout of morning sickness, let your doctor or midwife know if you continue to feel nauseated so she can rule out any complications—and perhaps consider prescribing medicine to treat the problem. Also let her know if you have nausea and vomiting that *starts* in the second trimester so she can search for a cause other than garden-variety morning sickness.

Nasal Congestion

Believe it or not, it's common to develop a chronically runny or stuffy nose during pregnancy. This condition, called rhinitis of pregnancy, often starts in the third month and can last until delivery or even a few weeks afterward.

What's to blame? Increased levels of pregnancy hormones like estrogen cause swelling in the mucous membranes lining your nose, and may even spur the production of more mucus. What's more, the increase in your blood volume and the expansion of your blood vessels to accommodate all that extra fluid can lead to swollen nasal membranes as well.

That said, a stuffy nose may just mean what it usually means—that you have a cold or allergies. If your stuffy nose is accompanied by sneezing, coughing, a sore throat, or mild aches and pains, you probably have a virus. Check with your practitioner before taking any cold or allergy remedies to see which ones are safe during pregnancy.

Pregnancy can also aggravate your allergies or increase your sensitivity to allergens and other irritants. Whether you think your congestion is allergy-related or not, it helps to avoid any potential irritants, such as cigarette smoke, aerosols, and sudden temperature changes.

BabyCenter Buzz

I Thought Morning Sickness Would Be Over by Now

"Everyone kept telling me that I'd feel better after week 13—but I don't! I can at least function somewhat now, but the nausea still lingers." —*Michelle*

"I'm at week 17, and still vomiting in the morning and feeling sick at night. It isn't typical, but from all that I've heard and read, it does happen." —*Jen*

"I'm at the end of my second trimester—and I still throw up every morning like clockwork. It's awful. My doctor prescribed Phenergan so I can function for the remainder of the day, though I'm trying to wean myself off it now." —*Anonymous*

Here are some strategies for relieving a stuffy nose:

• Steam can be very effective at relieving congestion. So take a warm shower before bed. Use a humidifier or vaporizer to put more moisture into the air, and keep it near your head at night. For serious stuffiness, cover your head with a towel and lean over the humidifier for ten to 15 minutes a few times a day. (Keep the humidifier very clean so it doesn't become a breeding ground for bacteria. For a low-tech alternative, use a bowl of steaming-hot water instead, or simply turn on the hot-water tap and lean over the sink.)

• Drink plenty of fluids, and keep your head elevated at night.

• Try saline drops or a buffered saline nasal spray, available over the counter at the drugstore. Spritz or drip a bit into each nostril, and within five or ten minutes, you should be able to blow your nose more easily.

• If congestion still makes you miserable and keeps you from getting a good night's rest, ask your practitioner which decongestants are safe. Avoid overusing decongestant nasal sprays, though, since they can cause rebound congestion and make the problem worse.

Nosebleeds

Inconvenient and embarrassing as they can be, nosebleeds are perfectly normal now. Pregnancy causes the blood vessels in your nose to expand, and your increased blood supply puts even more pressure on those delicate veins. The membranes inside your

BY THE NUMBERS

The Nose Blows

Mothers-to-be who have congestion without any other cold symptoms: **30%**

nose may also dry out, especially in cold weather, air-conditioned or heated rooms, airline cabins, and other dry environments. These changes can cause your nasal veins to rupture easily, leading to minor nosebleeds. A nasal or sinus infection can also bring on nosebleeds.

Here are some tips on preventing nosebleeds:

- Drink extra fluids to help keep your mucous membranes moist.
- Blow your nose gently. Aggressive blowing can lead to nosebleeds.
- Try to keep your mouth open when you sneeze.
- Avoid dry air, especially in wintertime or in dry climates, by running a humidifier inside your house and by not overheating your bedroom.
- Use a lubricant to prevent nasal dryness. Some experts recommend petroleum jelly, while others suggest a special water-based nasal lubricant made for this purpose (available over the counter). Saline nasal sprays or drops can help, too.

Round Ligament Pain

Been alarmed by a brief sharp, stabbing pain or a longer-lasting dull ache in your lower abdomen or groin? Most likely, that's round ligament pain. The round ligaments support your uterus in your pelvis, and as your womb grows, these ligaments stretch and thicken to accommodate your new girth.

You may feel round ligament pain as a quick jabbing sensation if you suddenly change position—when you're getting up from a bed or chair, say, or when you cough, roll over in bed, or get out of the bathtub. Or you may feel it as a dull ache after a particularly active day, such as when you've been walking a lot or doing some other physical activity. The pain may extend from the side of your abdomen to deep inside your groin, and you may feel it on one or both sides. The area where you're likely to feel round ligament pain follows the bikini line on a high-cut bathing suit.

When round ligament pain strikes, sit down and relax. Flexing your knees toward your abdomen may make you feel better. Or lie down on your side with one pillow under your belly and another between your legs. A warm bath may help, too. If you're more prone to round ligament pain when you're active, cut back a little to see if that helps.

Swelling

Swelling (or "edema" in medical parlance) happens when fluid collects in your tissues. Due to your new tendency to retain excess water, it's normal to have a certain amount of swelling during the second half of pregnancy—especially

Call Your Caregiver If You Have . . .

- Swelling in your face or puffiness around your eyes, more than slight swelling of your hands, excessive or sudden swelling of your feet or ankles, or rapid weight gain (more than 4 pounds in a week)
- Severe or persistent headache
- Vision changes, including double vision, blurriness, seeing spots or flashing lights, light sensitivity, or temporary loss of vision
- Intense pain or tenderness in your upper abdomen
- Nausea or vomiting

These are possible signs of preeclampsia, a potentially serious condition (see page 531 for more information).

in your feet and ankles. Your growing uterus also puts pressure on your pelvic veins and your inferior vena cava, a large vein that returns blood from your lower limbs to your heart. This pressure slows your circulation and causes blood to pool in your legs, forcing fluid from your veins into the tissue there. Plus, rising levels of progesterone cause the walls of your blood vessels to relax, compounding the problem. This swelling tends to be worse in the summer, at the end of the day, and as your pregnancy progress. Later in pregnancy, you may also notice a small amount of swelling in your fingers. (*Hint:* If you wear a wedding band, you might want to pry it off your ring finger soon and put it away for safekeeping or showcase it on a delicate chain around your neck.) But more than a little swelling of your hands or any facial puffiness (including swelling about your eyes) should prompt a call to your caregiver.

To prevent puffiness:

- Drink plenty of water (at least eight glasses a day). This actually helps flush excess fluid from your body.
- Eat a diet rich in fruits and vegetables and avoid junk food, especially super-salty snacks. Processed and fast foods often contain tons of sodium, which can lead to fluid retention.
- Wear waist-high maternity support hose to compress the tissues in your legs and help force the water back into your circulatory system; put the hose on before you get out of bed in the morning, so blood and fluid don't have a chance to pool around your ankles.

- Don't wear socks or stockings with tight bands around your ankles or calves; this will further inhibit circulation.
- Don't cross your legs when you sit (this, too, cuts off your circulation), and elevate your feet on a stool or a pile of books stacked under your desk.
- Stretch your legs regularly while you're sitting: Extend your leg, heel first, and gently flex your foot to stretch your calf muscles. Then rotate your ankles and wiggle your toes.
- Take breaks; get up and go for a short walk every so often (even if it's only to the bathroom or the water cooler) to keep your blood pumping.
- Kick back and prop your feet above the level of your heart, or lie on your side to relieve pressure on your vena cava.
- Use cold-water compresses on swollen areas.

Varicose Veins

Varicose veins often show up for the first time or get worse in pregnancy because rising progesterone levels cause your vein walls and valves to relax. This is compounded by your growing uterus, which puts pressure on your pelvic veins and inferior vena cava, inhibiting circulation in your lower body. Depending on the severity of your varicose veins, you may feel intense discomfort or only occasional itching or mild achiness at the end of a long day.

BabyCenter Buzz

My Legs Are Killing Me

"My doctor didn't take my varicose veins seriously until I repeatedly complained about the pain. He finally sent me to a vascular surgeon, but all he could do was tell me that they'd go away after I gave birth." —*Anonymous*

"I'm pregnant with my fourth child. My legs were bad with my third, but now they're awful! I live in my support hose—they help, but at the end of the day, it hurts just taking the support hose *off*." —*Dana*

"I have a major varicose vein running down my left leg, and more in my vulva. The one in my leg runs all the way from the top of my bikini line down to my calf. I'm wearing support stockings and trying to stay off my feet, which seems to be helping. The ones that are causing the most discomfort, though, are the ones in my vulva—they constantly throb and ache. My doctor says they won't prevent a vaginal delivery, which is some comfort, at least." —*Anonymous*

You're most likely to notice varicose veins on your legs, though you can get them other places, such as your vulva. Hemorrhoids, in fact, are simply varicose veins of the rectal area.

Whether you'll get varicose veins depends on several factors, though genetics is usually the most important one. Women who stand all day, are carrying multiples, are older, or are overweight are also more prone to varicose veins. Sometimes varicose veins will subside on their own within three or four months after delivery. But if they stick around after that and become too uncomfortable to live with or you're unhappy about how they look, you can have them surgically removed or chemically treated. If your main concern is cosmetic, though, you should probably wait until you've had all the children you want before consulting a dermatologist or plastic surgeon because unfortunately varicose veins tend to worsen and multiply with each pregnancy.

To keep the pressure off:

• Talk to your caregiver about buying prescription-only "graduated-compression" support hose, which keep blood from pooling in your calves and lend support to surface veins. For best results, put them on first thing in the morning.

• Exercise daily—even a brisk walk around the block will keep your blood moving (and not pooling in your veins).

• Rest and elevate your feet and legs whenever you can: Keep a stool or a box under your desk, and prop up your feet on a pillow when you're kicking back at home.

• Don't cross your legs when you're sitting down, and don't stay on your feet for long periods of time—both of which can impede circulation in your legs.

• Sleep on your left side, with your feet on a pillow, to improve bloodflow.

Call your caregiver if you experience either of the following:

• Your legs are significantly swollen, the skin near varicose veins has changed color, or there are sores on these veins that won't heal. These symptoms signal a more serious circulation problem.

• Your vein feels hard and ropelike or the area around it is reddened, hot, tender, or painful, which can be a sign of a blood clot. Unlike clots deep in your leg (which you can't see), these superficial clots are usually not serious but still need to be checked out.

Vision Changes

Pregnancy hormones and fluid retention can also affect your eyes. Your corneas thicken, just like the rest of your body, which means that you might not see as well as you did prepregnancy. These vision changes are probably slight, and you likely won't need your optometrist to tweak your prescription, because your vision should return to normal after you have your baby If you have a big problem, though, have your eyes checked.

Even if your eyesight isn't affected, you may find that your eyes are drier and more irritable than usual, possibly making contact lenses feel torturous.

To relieve dry eyes:

- Try using lubricating drops (available over the counter at the drugstore).
- If you have contact lenses, wear them for shorter stretches of time.
- If all else fails, switch to glasses until you have the baby.

Yeast Infections

If you've been getting more yeast infections than normal, you're not alone. Increased estrogen levels during pregnancy cause your vagina to become richer in a substance called glycogen, creating an environment in which yeast thrives. Some researchers think estrogen also has a direct effect on yeast, causing it both to grow faster and to adhere more easily to vaginal walls.

Although it's uncomfortable for you, a yeast infection won't affect your developing baby. (If you have an infection when you go into labor, there's a small chance that your newborn will contract it as he passes through your

Ask the Experts

What About LASIK Eye Surgery?

Dr. Marguerite McDonald, ophthalmologist tells us: It's not likely to be unsafe for your baby, but there are other good reasons not to do it now. First, pregnancy can throw off your vision. Pregnant women tend to get more nearsighted than normal, though some get more farsighted. Plus, you need drops to dilate your eyes before and during surgery, and though they're probably safe for the baby, we don't know for sure (a little of every drop gets into your bloodstream). After surgery, you need steroids and antibiotic drops, and again, we're just not sure if they're safe. Finally, pregnancy hormones dry out your eyes, which is why most pregnant women can't wear contacts. If you start surgery with dry eyes, you won't heal as well.

Just the Facts

Red Flags for Yeast

The symptoms of a yeast infection include:

- Itchiness, irritation, burning, redness, soreness, or sometimes even swelling in your vaginal area
- An odorless white, creamy, or cottage-cheesy vaginal discharge
- Pain during sex

birth canal, resulting in a condition called thrush, which is easily treated.)

If you have a yeast infection, your practitioner will recommend a prescription or over-the-counter antifungal cream or suppository that's safe during pregnancy. The medication should bring relief within a few days (though you'll need to continue the full seven-day course of treatment to make sure the infection is truly gone; the one- or three-day treatments you may have used in the past don't work as well in pregnancy). In the meantime, soothe your itching with an ice pack or a ten-minute soak in a cool bath.

You can't prevent all yeast infections, but you can make it harder for one to develop.

- Wear breathable cotton underwear, and avoid panty hose, leggings, and tight pants, particularly those made from synthetic materials.
- Sleep without underwear, to "air out" your genital area at night. (A nightgown without underwear allows more air circulation than pajama bottoms.)
- Skip the perfumed soaps, bubble baths, overlong soaks in the tub, scented laundry detergent, and feminine hygiene sprays. Clean your genital area gently with warm water (not soap) and *never* douche during pregnancy.
- Eat yogurt that contains live *Lactobacillus acidophilus* bacteria, which may help restore the balance of "good" bacteria in your vagina.

Second Trimester Sleep: Enjoy It While You Can

Chances are, you feel much more rested now than you did during your first few months of pregnancy, and you likely won't need to spend as many hours in the sack as you did in your first trimester. No one knows for sure what causes early pregnancy fatigue to lift, but it's a welcome—if not entirely understood—relief.

More good news: Morning sickness has probably passed, too—or at least started to fade. (Hey—this isn't called "the honeymoon trimester" for nothing!) Take advantage of your newfound sense of well-being to start an exercise program—a strategy that will give your mental and physical health a boost and help you sleep well at night. And spend plenty of time resting now, before your bulging belly and other physical discomforts again make sleep a challenge.

Second-Trimester Sleep Problems— and Solutions

Despite the improvement in your slumber, things aren't all rosy. After all, you *are* still pregnant. Though the total amount of time you actually snooze this trimester will be close to that of your prepregnancy days, you're spending less time in the restorative stages of *deep* sleep. Some common second trimester sleep-snatchers, and how best to handle them:

Heartburn and Indigestion

As important as progesterone is to maintaining a healthy pregnancy, it does have a few less-welcome side effects. For one, it relaxes the valve that separates your esophagus from your stomach, allowing gastric acids to seep back up and produce that uncomfortable sensation of heartburn. The hormone also slows the wavelike contractions of your stomach, making digestion sluggish.

There's no sure-fire way to avoid gastric discomforts at night, but you can take steps to minimize them. First of all, avoid foods and drinks that trigger your heartburn. Eat small, frequent meals and chew your food slowly and thoroughly. Then give yourself two or three hours to digest before going to bed. When you do hit the hay, prop up your head and chest with extra pillows or even try sleeping semi-upright in a comfy recliner. Wear sleepwear that's loose around your abdomen and waist. If the problems persist, talk to your doctor or midwife about an over-the-counter antacid that's safe to use during pregnancy.

Leg Cramps

Some of the physical changes of pregnancy can cause your leg muscles to cramp in protest, sometimes so painfully that you're jarred from a deep sleep to clutch at your knotted calf.

Trouble Getting Comfortable

Getting—and staying—comfortable in bed may be one of your greatest challenges during pregnancy, particularly if you're used to sleeping on your stomach or your back. Your larger breasts and abdomen will probably rule out sleeping facedown, and sleeping on your back puts too much weight on a major vein and impedes circulation.

Many pregnant women feel most comfortable lying on their side with their knees bent and a pillow between their legs. Arrange additional pillows under your belly and behind your back for extra comfort and support. (If you find that lying on your side puts too much pressure on your hips, buy a soft egg-crate-style foam mattress pad to go under your sheet for added cushioning.) Though lying on your left side is best, it's fine to alternate between your left and right side during the night to stay comfortable.

Waking Up Hungry

No matter how much or how often you eat, you may still feel ravenous night and day. That's not surprising. After all, your metabolic rate is rising and the person growing inside you has caloric needs of his own.

To avoid hunger pangs during the night, never go to bed starving—but don't stuff yourself close to bedtime or eat unhealthy foods, either. Sugary snacks such as chocolate, cookies, or candy before bed may leave you feeling revved up or restless. Instead, have a glass of milk, a piece of cheese, or some crackers before you hit the hay. Likewise, if you wake up craving a middle-of-the-night snack, try to choose something that packs a nutritional punch

QUICK TIPS

Easing a Leg Cramp

- If you do get a cramp, immediately stretch your calf muscles: Straighten your leg, heel first, and gently flex your toes back toward your shins. (It might hurt at first, but it *will* ease the spasm.)

- Massage the muscle or warm it with a hot-water bottle.

- Walk around for a few minutes.

- If your muscle pain is constant or if you notice swelling or tenderness in your leg, call your practitioner right away. In rare cases (one in 2,000) a pregnant woman develops a blood clot, which requires immediate medical attention.

Ask the Experts

Why is sleeping on my side best now?

Dr. Mary O'Malley, sleep medicine specialist: Once you get to the halfway point in your pregnancy, it's wise to avoid sleeping on your back, a position that puts the full weight of your uterus on your spine, back muscles, intestines, and the inferior vena cava (the vein that transports blood from your lower body to your heart). Back-sleeping can also put you at risk for backaches, hemorrhoids, indigestion, impaired breathing and circulation, and blood-pressure changes. For some women, it causes a drop in blood pressure that makes them feel dizzy; for others, it causes an unwanted increase in blood pressure.

Instead, lie on your side, preferably your left side. Though there's no harm in sleeping on your right side, lying on your left side is actually *beneficial* for you and your baby: It improves the flow of blood and nutrients to the placenta and it helps your kidneys eliminate waste products and excess fluid. That, in turn, reduces swelling in your ankles, feet, and hands. (To make side-sleeping more comfortable, consider investing in a pregnancy wedge pillow and/or an egg-crate foam mattress pad.) If you wake up at night and find yourself on your stomach or back, don't worry—you haven't done any harm to your baby. Just roll back onto your side.

---

as well as satisfying your hunger pangs: a bowl of cereal with milk, toast with peanut butter, or a few crackers with cheese.

Sleep Aids

Sometimes it takes a little extra ammunition to get some shut-eye. A few remedies to help you get the sleep you crave:

MATERNITY PILLOWS

Using pillows to support your belly and back in bed can mean the difference between a sleepless night and a peaceful slumber. Regular pillows work fine, but you may want to splurge on one of these specialty pregnancy pillows:

• **Single or dual pregnancy wedge.** These wedge-shaped pillows support your belly when you lie on your side. You can also use them to prop yourself up to a semi-reclining position when you're on your back. The dual pregnancy wedge is two pillows attached with adjustable Velcro tabs that provide simultaneous support in front and back.

• **Full-length body pillow.** These mega pillows are at least 5 feet long and are designed to support your back and cradle your belly.

• **Bean pillow.** This sleep accessory supports your belly and your back, and makes a good nursing pillow later.

EATING SMART

What you eat—and when you eat it—can affect the quality of your sleep. Some sleep-inducing snacks:

• **Warm milk.** Drinking a glass of warm milk before bed is a time-tested way to bring on sleep. Experts believe the amino acid L-tryptophan (found in milk and foods such as turkey and eggs) makes your eyelids heavy by raising the level of a chemical in your brain called serotonin. Others suggest the somnambulant effects of warm milk may be all in your head. But if it helps you snooze, does it really matter? (*Note:* Do *not* take tryptophan supplements—they're not safe during pregnancy.)

• **Protein-packed snacks.** If bad dreams, headaches, or full-body sweats are disturbing your sleep, you could be suffering from low blood sugar. To fix the problem, try a high-protein snack before bed, such as a few cheese cubes, an egg, some peanut butter, or a slice of turkey on bread to keep your blood sugar up during the night.

RELAXATION TECHNIQUES

If you're tense, anxious, or overtired, sleep can seem as hard to grab as your own shadow. Try these simple, time-tested techniques to help calm your mind, relax your muscles, and put sleep within your grasp:

• **Yoga and stretching.** In addition to helping you relax, yoga and stretching have the added benefit of keeping you toned and flexible. Although you don't want to work up a sweat too close to bedtime, gentle stretching can make falling asleep easier.

• **Massage.** Getting a massage relaxes tense, tired muscles. If you visit a massage therapist, make sure he or she has experience working with pregnant women and uses a table and pillow designed for that purpose. Professional massage can be expensive, but getting a foot, hand, or neck massage from your mate is a perfect way to wind down before bed.

• **Deep breathing.** Breathing deeply and rhythmically eases muscle tension, lowers your heart rate, and helps you fall asleep faster. Lie down on your side on the carpet or your bed. Place a pillow between your legs for support or wedge a pillow partly under the right side of your back so you're tilted slightly to the left. With your mouth closed, breathe in slowly through your nose, feeling your stomach rise as you gradually fill your diaphragm and lungs with air. Hold for one second before exhaling through your nose to the count of four. Repeat this slow, deep breathing for several minutes.

• **Progressive muscle relaxation.** Release tight muscles by first tensing and then completely relaxing them. It may take several weeks to master the technique, but once you do, it can really help you wind down. Lying on your bed or on the floor, focus on one group of muscles at a time and alternate between your right and left side. Start by tensing and releasing your hand and forearm muscles, followed by your biceps and triceps, face and jaw, chest and shoulders, stomach, thighs, and so on until you reach your feet.

• **Guided imagery.** Picture yourself in a quiet, relaxing scene—lying on a warm, sandy beach or walking in a field of wildflowers. Now imagine every detail of the scene, including the sounds, smells, tastes, and textures around you. If you can't picture a relaxing setting, use an image from a photograph or magazine and fill in the missing details. It may take some practice, but guided imagery can calm your restless mind and help you slip into a deep sleep.

EXERCISE

Regular exercise during pregnancy makes you healthier both physically and mentally, and it can help you sleep better, too—provided you don't exercise vigorously within four hours of bedtime. Working out too close to lights-out will rev you up and even rob you of deep sleep by interfering with your natural sleep cycle. Instead, work up a sweat in the morning, afternoon, or early evening.

SLEEP MEDICATIONS

Ideally, you should avoid all medications and herbal remedies (page 566) now, since most haven't been tested on pregnant women and their affect on your developing baby may be unknown. But if you're so exhausted from insomnia that you're having a hard time functioning, your practitioner may recommend a prescription or over-the-counter drug to help you sleep. Nonprescription diphenhydramine hydrochloride and doxyalamine (Benadryl, Sominex, or Unisom) are generally considered safe during pregnancy. Never take any medication without first consulting your doctor or midwife, though, and never drive or operate machinery after taking a drug to help you sleep.

What's in a Dream? Second Trimester Dream Themes—and What They *Really* Mean

You thought your first trimester dreams were weird? Don't be surprised if the crazy night-visions continue now—though their imagery and meanings may change as your pregnancy progresses. Here, BabyCenter dream expert, clinical psychologist, and *Women's Bodies, Women's Dreams* (Ballantine) author Patricia Garfield takes a look at some common second-trimester dreams and offers possible interpretations:

BabyCenter Buzz

"What I'm dreaming about now"

"I dreamed I was in the doctor's office, and he asked if I wanted to see my baby. Without hesitation, I said, 'Yes!' So he reached into my vagina and pulled on a small thread, which was attached to a balloon with my baby inside. He put the balloon in my arms and I could see my baby's face and that it was a boy. I gave the baby back to the doctor, who told me that I still had 20 weeks to go, then stuck the balloon back through my cervix." —*Anonymous*

"I was in water, though I can't swim in real life. There were two ducklings. I wasn't allowed to touch them, but had to help them get across the pond. Next thing I knew, they changed into two babies. It was only when I guided them to the other side of the pond that I could pick them up and hold them." —*Steph*

"I've been dreaming of nursing my cat! I look down and expect a baby, and it's my kitty. I always wake up right after that." —*Melissa*

"I'm dancing with my husband on a crowded dancefloor. A mystery man standing behind me makes seductive contact. My husband encourages me and I turn around and let him grope me. He then picks me up and invites my husband to join us. We go to a room, and my husband watches the two of us together." —*Anonymous*

"I've been having dreams about trying to save my children. I end up hanging from something with one arm, with fire and lava beneath me, and grasping onto my 3-year-old daughter with the other arm. I have no idea where my unborn child is." —*Anonymous*

"Last night I dreamed that I had my baby early. I wanted to cart the baby around with me while I did errands, but didn't have a baby carrier. So I cut arm- and leg holes in a cereal box. I glued Velcro strips on the back of the box and on the front of my shirt. Away I went with a baby in a cereal box attached to the front of my shirt." —*Nikki*

Just for Dad

What *You* May Be Dreaming About

During your partner's second trimester, your own dreams will probably become less sexual and more protective and nurturing, according to dream expert Patricia Garfield. You may find yourself dreaming about your own parents or even of being pregnant and giving birth yourself. Despite your mate's unique role as child bearer, it's natural to want to share in her pregnancy experience as fully as possible. It's common for dads-to-be to feel a bit left out at this stage of pregnancy, which can lead to dreams of being excluded and alone. Confiding troublesome dreams to your partner will help you overcome feelings of loneliness, while trading happy dreams will increase your confidence and intimacy with your mate.

• **You're caring for baby animals.** During the second trimester, a pregnant woman's dreams typically contain cuddly, baby-like animals, such as puppies, chicks, and kittens. You may find that the animals in your dreams develop from sea creatures to land mammals, retracing the journey of our primitive ancestors. Friendly creatures in your dreams are generally thought to signify a good relationship between you and your instincts. Menacing animals, on the other hand, may represent ambivalence about the strange new creature coming into your life.

• **You have a sexy encounter with an old flame.** The farther along you are in your pregnancy, the more likely you are to have erotic dreams. Many mothers-to-be are concerned about their changing figure and its effect on their sex life—while many others feel more sexually charged than ever. Both feelings are often reflected in your dreams. Not only do erotic dreams offer comforting reassurance—"Don't worry—you're still hot"—but they may mirror the sexiness you feel during your waking hours, too.

• **Your mate is straying.** If you dream that your partner hooks up with an ex-girlfriend or a total stranger, it can signal insecurity about holding his love and attention through a time of great change. Right now, you're dependent on the goodwill and support of those around you, especially your partner. Fearing his loss is a common emotional reaction to being pregnant. For most women, happily, the insecurity is unfounded and soon passes.

YOUR NUTRITION AND FITNESS

Three to Grow On:
The Most Important Nutrients Now

If you had a tough time stomaching the idea of food during your first trimester, you may be pleasantly surprised to find your appetite returning in full force over the next few months. The trick now is to get the extra calories you and your baby need from the freshest, most nutritious food that you can.

A healthy, well-balanced diet is important throughout pregnancy, of course. But certain nutrients are star players at different points in your baby's gestation. For instance, while folic acid is important throughout pregnancy, it was vital in the very early days and weeks after conception, when your baby's neural tube was forming. Now that her focus is on growth, take steps to get plenty of the nutrients that will fuel that development and keep *you* healthy: protein, iron, and calcium.

Power Up on Protein

Protein is essential for healthy growth, which is why it's more important than ever now that your baby is starting to bulk up. You'll want to get enough of this important nutrient (you need about 71 grams a day now) to meet *your* increased needs, too.

The Inside Skinny on Fats

There are four types of fats in food: monounsaturated, polyunsaturated, saturated, and hydrogenated. Monounsaturated fats—found in olive, canola, and peanut oils, as well as in nuts and nut butters—are considered "good" fats because they're best at lowering cholesterol.

Dining Out—without Filling Up on Fat

Watch out for hidden fats when you're eating in a restaurant, particularly if you eat out a lot or are gaining a lot of weight. Tip-off words and phrases include "pan-fried," "crispy," "creamed," "fried," "au gratin," "hol-landaise" (which you should avoid anyway because it's made with raw eggs), "escal-loped," and "buttery." In-stead, choose grilled, baked, or steamed menu selections—or ask your waiter if the chef can either use a "good" fat like olive oil or skip the oils and other high-fat ingredients when he prepares your dish.

Polyunsaturated fats are beneficial, too. They include the omega-3 fatty acids, found in some fish, and omega-6 fatty acids, found in corn oil, among others. The omega-3 fatty acid docosahexaenoic acid (DHA), in particular, lowers your risk for depression, aids your baby's brain and vision development, and even helps regulate his sleep patterns as a newborn.

Saturated and hydrogenated fats (also known as trans fats) fall into the "bad" category. Saturated fats are found in high-fat meats (such as liver), whole milk, and tropical oils (such as palm oil). Hydrogenated and partially hydrogenated fats are found in margarine and in most packaged crackers, cookies, chips, common brands of peanut butter, microwave popcorn, and many commercially fried foods. A diet high in saturated and hydrogenated fats can raise *your* cholesterol and may eventually put you at risk for heart disease and cancer.

The key to fat consumption during pregnancy is balance. Remember that no more than 30 percent of your daily calories should come from fat. But don't beat yourself up if you indulge in a bag of chips or a plate of fried chicken on occasion—you can make up for it by trying to stick to lower-fat foods the next day. You should get about four servings of fat a day (ideally from the monounsaturated and polyunsaturated groups). A serving equals about 1 teaspoon of butter, margarine, mayonnaise, or oil; ten peanuts; or one slice of bacon.

Why Iron Is Key

The amount of iron you need each day has gone up significantly since you conceived (you now need about 27 milligrams). What's more, many mothers-to-be are diagnosed with iron deficiency anemia during the latter half of pregnancy, so it's important to pay attention to your iron intake now.

To pump up your iron intake, cut back on coffee and black or green tea because natural substances in these beverages reduce the amount of iron your

BY THE NUMBERS

Protein Powerhouses

Lean meats, eggs, and dairy products are great sources of protein, as are beans and soy products like tofu. Fish is also a good protein source, though due to concerns about contamination, you'll need to be careful about how much and what type of fish you eat. A look at how much protein you'll get from various foods:

DAIRY	SERVING SIZE	PROTEIN
Cheese, Parmesan	3 Tbsp	6 g
Cheese, Swiss or Cheddar	3 oz	22 g
Cottage cheese, low-fat	1 cup	28 g
Eggs, large	two (or three large egg whites)	12 g
Milk, fat-free	1 cup	8 g
Tofu	7 oz	16 g
Yogurt, low-fat, plain	1 cup	12 g

BEANS, NUTS, AND LEGUMES		
Almonds	1 oz (about 23)	6 g
Beans, kidney or garbanzo	1 cup	13 g
Peanut butter	2 Tbsp	8 g

MEAT AND FISH		
Chicken, turkey, beef, lamb, pork, or veal	3 oz (about the size of a deck of cards)	18 to 30 g (depending on the meat and cut)
Crabmeat	3 oz	10 g
Fish fillet	3 oz	22 g
Lobster meat	3 oz	17 g
Shrimp	3 oz (about 17 baby shrimp or 2 jumbo prawns)	18g

body absorbs. If you continue to imbibe, drink coffee and tea between—and not *with*—meals or supplements.

Cook in a cast-iron skillet to get even more of the mineral. Moist, acidic foods like tomato sauce absorb the most iron. But because some iron is lost in cooking (as is the vitamin C needed to absorb iron in vegetables), don't overcook vegetables, and use only a small amount of water.

Meat, poultry, and fish sources of iron (called heme iron) enhance the absorption of other types of iron, so putting a bit of beef in a pot of vegetable

Buying Calcium Supplements

- Look for calcium carbonate or calcium citrate. Calcium carbonate has a high concentration of elemental calcium, is well-absorbed when taken with meals, and is inexpensive. Calcium citrate is somewhat better absorbed than calcium carbonate and less likely to cause gas, but it has half as much elemental calcium (so you'll need to take more pills), and it is more expensive. (Avoid calcium phosphate because it's difficult to absorb. Pass on the calcium lactate or calcium gluconate, too, because they have very low concentrations of elemental calcium.)

- Avoid "natural" calcium supplements made from bonemeal, dolomite, or oyster shells—they're more likely to contain lead, which can be harmful to your growing baby. "Refined" calcium tablets may contain a small amount of lead, too. Look for tablets marked "lead-free" or "purified," or ask your practitioner or pharmacist to recommend a brand.

- Take calcium supplements with food to aid your body's absorption of the mineral.

chili or lentil soup can boost the amount of iron you get from vegetables and legumes. If you're cooking the meat alone, add cooked juices back into your sauce or pour them over meat (after you skim off the fat) to retain the iron lost from meat during cooking.

Calcium decreases iron absorption, so if you're also taking calcium supplements (or an antacid), don't take them at the same time you take your iron supplement. Likewise, don't take your iron supplement with a glass of milk or while you're eating dairy products and other high-calcium foods. To maximize absorption, take your supplements or eat iron-rich foods from plant sources with a glass of orange juice or other vitamin C-rich fare, such as other citrus fruits or juices, strawberries, or sweet peppers.

High-dose iron supplements can cause constipation, so eat more fiber and drink more liquids to help you stay regular—but not at the same time you take your pill. Take it at bedtime to avoid mixing it with foods that can inhibit iron absorption, and to minimize tummy troubles.

Are You Getting Enough Calcium?

Your baby needs calcium for a host of things, including the formation of his bones and teeth. He'll take what he requires from *your* body, so getting enough calcium (1,000 milligrams a day; 1,300 milligrams if you're under 19) is vital to keep your own bones healthy. If you pay attention to your diet and consume dairy products regularly, you'll be able to reach that number without too much trouble. (If you're lactose intolerant or don't eat dairy products, you'll need to carefully select other foods high in calcium and possibly take a calcium supplement.)

BabyCenter Buzz

How to Fit Healthy Eating into a Hectic Schedule

"Plan ahead. If you keep cut-up fruits and veggies in the fridge, it's easy to throw them in a bag before work. Packing healthy snacks kept me away from the candy machine at the office." —Jodie

"When you have time to prepare healthy meals, make several servings and freeze them for later. And if you must eat fast food, ask for a salad instead of fries." —Soo Jin

"Make quick, nutritious snacks. I'm hooked on peanut-butter-and-banana sandwiches on multigrain bread. Taking string cheese, carrots, and those single-serve microwave bowls of oatmeal to work is easy, too." —Anonymous

"I made a simple chart of the basic food groups and posted it on the refrigerator. At the end of the day, I checked off what I had eaten. Then, for my bedtime snack, I tried to pick something that would fulfill whatever category was lacking—yogurt (or a bowl of ice cream!) if I needed more dairy, for example, or an orange if I needed more fruit." —Anonymous

Healthy Eating on the Go

It's hard to stick to a healthy meal plan when you're trying to keep on top of a hectic schedule. Eleven snack foods to keep on hand that not only taste good, but are good *for* you:

1. Single-serve fruit bowls or fresh fruit. These handy little 4-ounce fruit cups count as one serving of fruits and vegetables. Choose varieties packed in their own juice rather than in sugary syrup. Apples, tangerines, and bananas are also easy to keep on hand and eat on the go.

2. Soy milk. Your soy milk options include 8-ounce servings of plain, chocolate, and vanilla flavor. Stash one in your purse or briefcase (they don't need to be refrigerated). One bottle supplies a third of your

BY THE NUMBERS

Calcium Champs

Bread, calcium-fortified, two slices:	**300 mg**
Cheese, Cheddar, 1 oz:	**202 mg**
Cottage cheese, 2 cups:	**300 mg**
Juice, orange, calcium-fortified, 8 oz:	**300 mg**
Milk, 8 oz:	**about 290 mg**
Sardines, 3 oz:	**300 mg**
Tofu, firm, 4 oz:	**166 mg**
Tortillas, corn, 3:	**150 mg**
Yogurt, low-fat, 1 cup:	**414 mg**

daily calcium and vitamin D requirement.

3. Raisins. A 1-ounce box provides 2 grams of fiber, 4 percent of your daily iron requirement, and 1 gram of protein.

4. Yogurt. This classic nutritious *and* convenient snack provides 25 percent of your daily calcium requirement—plus protein and several other necessary vitamins and minerals. (Be aware that some brands are loaded with sugar—check the label. Or get plain and add a bit of sugar or jam, and fruit, nuts, or seeds.)

5. Trail mix. Toss a handful of shredded-wheat-type cereal together with a handful of dried cherries and almonds. Keep a Ziploc bag in your desk or car for a handy crunchy snack.

6. Salad. Some fast-food joints and many grocery stores and cafeteria-style restaurants have salad bars where you can serve yourself practically a whole day's worth of fruits and vegetables. Load up on spinach, carrots, tomatoes, celery, cucumbers, zucchini, raisins, and nuts. Add chickpeas or kidney beans for a protein boost. Keep in mind, though, that in order to steer clear of dangerous bacteria, you'll need to avoid raw sprouts, unpasteurized or soft cheeses (including blue cheese and Roquefort dressing), and any deli meats or prepared deli salads.

7. Baby carrots. Available in single-serving bags or packs, carrots are full of beta-carotene and fiber. Dip them into fat-free yogurt mixed with a little ranch dressing for an extra dose of nutrition. Look for other prewashed and prepacked veggies like broccoli, cauliflower, and spinach.

8. String cheese. If you don't know about string cheese now, just wait until your baby is a toddler—this food will become a snack staple. Low-fat mozzarella sticks are chock-full of calcium and have some protein, too.

9. Orange juice boxes. Now available in many grocery stores, a four-ounce serving of calcium-fortified OJ provides half of your daily requirement of vitamin C and about 15 percent of your calcium quota.

10. Unsweetened cereal or instant oatmeal. Stash a few single-serve boxes of healthy breakfast cereal (not the sugar-coated kind) or oatmeal packets in your desk at work for a quick healthy snack. Almost all breakfast cereal is fortified with essential vitamins and minerals.

BabyCenter Buzz

What I Crave

"I'm craving salty and spicy foods now: dill pickles, barbecued potato chips, salsa, pizza with jalapeños on it, Thai food, etc. My husband and I went out for Mexican food the other night, and it never tasted better!"   —*Aimee*

"I want carbs all the time! Bread, bagels, pasta, rice, cereal. I also crave those mini doughnuts that come in six-packs from the grocery store in chocolate or powdered sugar, but I only give in to *that* urge about once a month."   —*Anonymous*

"All I crave is mashed potatoes with gravy. I think I could go through the rest of my pregnancy eating just that!"   —*Valerie*

"Peanut butter and jelly. Last time, it was shrimp."   —*Anonymous*

"This is my third pregnancy, and I can't get enough tomatoes. With my first pregnancy, it was Granny Smith apples by the bag, and during my second pregnancy, it was more about what I *didn't* want to eat than what I did."   —*Deb*

11. Cottage cheese cups. Stock up on single-serve low-fat cottage cheese containers, available in the dairy section of your grocery store, and get almost a quarter of the way toward your daily protein goal with each 4-ounce serving.

Whether you're tipping the scales a bit too much, or staying within your healthcare provider's recommendations, here are five foods to cross off your shopping list:

1. Ramen noodles. They may taste good, but they're packed with salt, fat, and . . . little else.

2. Soda. Fill up on empty calories and sugar, and you won't have room for more nutritious drinks. Low-fat milk, carbonated water, or juices (in moderation) are a good substitute.

3. Prepackaged lunches. They may be a quick fix for hunger pangs, but preservatives, salt, and fat make them a bad choice. Even more important, you should avoid deli meats (unless you reheat them so they're steaming hot) because they can be a source of listeria.

4. Almost all prepared frozen meals. They tend to have astronomical amounts of salt and fat. Instead, pop a potato in the microwave, then top it with cheese and steamed broccoli for a fast, healthy meal. If you can't avoid the occasional frozen meal, look for organic brands or those low in salt and fat.

5. Iceberg lettuce. If you're going to eat a salad, choose a green, such as romaine, that has twice the fiber and also provides A, B, and C vitamins, folate, calcium, and potassium (iceberg lettuce has only trace amounts of these nutrients). And add other veggies, such as spinach, bell peppers, and broccoli, to give your salad a nutritive boost.

Food Cravings

Yearning for a particular type of food is an undeniable part of carrying a baby. In fact, about 85 percent of expectant mothers report at least one major food craving. These cravings often seem to come out of nowhere and have an overpowering ferocity. Experts are still mystified about exactly what causes the phenomenon—no one knows for sure whether cravings are related to hormonal changes, cultural norms and lore, emotional issues, some combination of these, or something else altogether.

How to Indulge Your Cravings Healthfully

While a few pregnant women have been known to pine for broccoli, spinach, bananas, or oatmeal, most reach for ice cream and chocolate. If your urge for sugar and fat is just too powerful to resist, go ahead and indulge occasionally. But think, too, of your growing baby and the nutrients he needs—and try to work them into your sugar or salt fix. Five tips for keeping your cravings under control:

Eat breakfast every day. If you do, you'll be less susceptible to midmorning junk-food snack attacks. A winning combination: a glass of calcium-fortified orange juice, yogurt and fresh fruit, and an egg on whole wheat toast.

Exercise regularly. Working out is an excellent way to curb cravings for unhealthy foods (and the boredom or anxiety that can lead to excessive snacking).

Get the emotional support you need. The hormonal roller coaster of

BabyCenter Buzz

How I Satisfy My Sweet Tooth (without Going Overboard)

"I love ice cream, and if I buy a pint, I can't resist it and eat the whole thing! So instead of keeping it in the house, I go out and get a cone with one scoop." —*Ann*

"Root beer for dessert!" —*Kelli*

"I try to eat fruit when I crave something sweet: strawberries, blueberries, pineapple, apples, oranges. If I'm *really* craving sugar, I put whipped cream on top." —*Kenna*

"Sometimes just sucking on a piece of hard candy is all I need to get over a sweet craving. I keep a bag stashed in my desk at work." —*Laura*

pregnancy can make you more vulnerable to mood swings. You may turn to food when what you *really* need is someone to talk to.

Train yourself to think small. Try a few spoonfuls of ice cream rather than a whole bowl, or one square of chocolate instead of the entire bar. Or if you find those mini portions are just too much of a tease, have a real portion, but do so less often.

Substitute healthy stand-ins for your less virtuous cravings. Here are a few suggestions:

Instead of:	Try:
Ice cream	Fat-free frozen yogurt, sorbet, or sherbet
Soda	Mineral water with fruit juice or a squeeze of lime
Doughnut or pastry	Whole grain bagel with jam
Cake	Low-fat banana-nut or zucchini bread (If you must have cake, try angel food topped with fresh strawberries.)
Sugary cereals	Whole grain cereal or oatmeal topped with brown sugar
Potato chips	Low-fat chips, microwave popcorn, pretzels
Sour cream	Fat-free sour cream, fat-free plain yogurt
Sundae toppings	Fresh berries or sliced bananas (If you crave crunch, throw on some crispy rice cereal or granola.)
Canned fruits in sugary syrup	Fresh fruit, unsweetened frozen fruit
Chocolate	Fat-free hot cocoa made with fat-free milk, or trail mix made with raisins, dried fruits, nuts, and a small handful of chocolate chips
Cookies	Graham crackers with a little peanut butter for added pizzazz
Cheesecake or another creamy dessert	Cheese on whole wheat crackers, or low-fat rice or vanilla pudding

Healthy Weight Gain

How Your Weight Will Change in the Second Trimester

On average, women can expect to gain between 12 and 14 pounds this trimester. But how much you'll actually gain depends on a number of factors, including your prepregnancy weight, whether you're carrying twins or more, and your diet.

Worried about Your Weight? How to Stay on Track

Too many pregnant women deal with weight gain in one of two ways: Either they use impending motherhood as an excuse to throw caution to the wind and eat as much as they want, or they go in the opposite direction and fret over every morsel because they're worried about gaining too *much*. Neither approach is healthy. Unless you're very underweight, you and your baby don't need the extra fat all those late-night pints of Ben & Jerry's will pack on, and gaining too *little* may rob your baby of the nutrients that he needs to grow.

The range of pregnancy weight gain that's considered normal is fairly wide, so you shouldn't feel terrorized by the scale. Still, you'll want to avoid extremes of weight gain because it can have an influence on your baby's birth weight and your health. For instance, if you don't gain enough weight, particularly if you started out underweight or at average weight, you'll increase your risk for preterm birth and for having a too-small baby.

BabyCenter Buzz

I Can't Seem to Gain Enough Weight

"I had horrible morning sickness early in my pregnancy and lost 16 pounds. Now I eat like crazy, but I haven't gained much." —*Court*

"At 20 weeks, I've gained only 5 pounds. I'm not *trying* to eat less; in fact, I've upped my calcium and protein intake and have been eating more than normal. I guess every person is different." —*Sunny*

"As soon as I got pregnant, I started losing weight in my arms and legs. Now, at 27 weeks, I've gained about 7 pounds. I eat whole-milk products and have a snack every two hours or so, but I just can't seem to gain much weight. I was a little overweight to begin with, and my midwife says she's not concerned. This is just what my body is doing." —*Jessica*

BabyCenter Buzz

I'm Gaining More than I'm Supposed To

"I've already shed tears over the weight I've gained, even though I've been watching what I eat and trying to exercise. But perhaps some of us are *meant* to gain more weight during pregnancy than others . . ."   —*Anonymous*

"The extra weight is hard to deal with. I gain an average of 50 pounds per pregnancy (this is my fourth). My doctor doesn't seem too concerned because this high weight gain seems 'normal' for me and I lose it all afterward. (Fingers crossed it will be the same this time!)"   —*Anonymous*

"I thought I'd gain only 25 pounds because I exercise six days a week and eat fairly well. I was wrong. I'm trying very hard to surrender to this reality and trust that my body will allow me to lose the weight after I have the baby. (P.S. I feel much better since throwing out my scale!)"   —*Deanna*

"I'm a little alarmed at how big and bumbling I already feel. I've never gained so much weight so quickly, and I hate how big my butt and thighs are getting. Two things keep me from getting too depressed, though: Knowing that this weight gain is normal and good for my baby, and that my husband loves my extra padding!"   —*Georgie*

And if you gain too much, you'll increase your risk for having a larger-than-normal infant and a difficult delivery, or of having a c-section—especially if you were heavy at the start of your pregnancy. Also, if you put on excess pounds, it can be difficult to lose them after you give birth, increasing your risk for long-term obesity (and related health problems like heart disease and diabetes).

Your caloric needs now depend on a variety of factors, including your metabolism, activity level, prepregnancy weight, and how many babies you're carrying. Unless your doctor or midwife advises otherwise, all you need to support your growing baby are an extra 300 calories a day (that's just one glass of low-fat milk and one piece of buttered whole wheat toast). And those extra calories shouldn't come from junky snacks like chips, soda, candy, cookies, or French fries. Instead, pack in a dose of nutrition along with your bonus calories by eating more servings of vegetables, whole grains, and low-fat dairy products. Of course, every mother-to-be needs at least some indulgences, so enjoy them in moderation.

How Weight Gain Will Affect Your Body

Some of the aches and pains you'll feel during your pregnancy are at least partially related to your changing body shape and the increased weight of your womb, which causes a shift in your center of gravity. As your belly grows and you begin to carry extra weight up front, you may begin to have occasional backaches. Your rapidly changing body may make you feel clumsy and more prone to falls—which is why you'll want to be extra careful when walking on wet or icy surfaces and why you may need to modify your fitness routine. And your increasingly lax joints, combined with the added load they're carrying, are another thing you'll want to take into account when you do physical activity so you don't injure yourself. Finally, sometimes your growing belly and breasts—and the added weight you may be putting on elsewhere—can be too much for your skin to handle, resulting in stretch marks. But the only harm *this* change can do is to your vanity.

Staying Fit

Now that your old get-up-and-go is back, it's a good time to recommit to a regular fitness routine. If you're not there yet, aim to work up to a half-hour or more of moderate exercise a day—it'll keep your heart and lungs in top condition, tone your muscles, help relieve some common pregnancy discomforts, aid sleep, and improve your mood and body image.

Sport-Specific Safety Strategies

Bicycling

Cycling provides a good cardiovascular workout with minimal strain on your joints, but as your balance begins to change, your risk of falling increases. So try stationary cycling instead, and use a bike with upright handlebars so you don't strain your back.

Low-Impact Aerobics

Remember that it may be harder to keep your balance as your belly expands, so use caution as you move across the floor. You may want to switch to a prenatal water aerobics class now if one is offered in your community. You'll get a great workout—without the stress on your joints.

Just for Dad

The Couple That Works Out Together...

Your support can make all the difference when it comes to your partner's starting—and sticking with—a fitness routine. Increase your share of housework so she can carve out a little extra time for herself to go for a swim or attend an exercise class. Also, plan to work out together on occasion and kill two birds with one stone: Enjoy exercise *and* relaxed couple time. You might take a walk after dinner every night, for instance, or go for a long hike on weekends. You can also find ways for each of you to do your own thing while still being together. Head over to the track at the neighborhood high school where she can walk laps and you can run. Or visit the Y together and play a game of racquetball while she swims or takes a prenatal yoga class. By the time the baby arrives, you'll *both* be fitter.

Swimming

You probably won't need to do much to modify your swimming routine because it's impact-free and relatively easy on expectant moms. One caution you should take now, though, is to climb or walk rather than dive into the pool, since the impact of the water on your growing belly isn't safe. You'll find a maternity swimsuit more comfortable as your belly expands, too. It can be tough to find one at the mall, especially off-season, so start your search at a specialty maternity shop or online.

Walking

A bigger belly may cause you to arch your back, so pay attention to your posture when you walk to avoid straining your back. Keep your head straight, your chin level, and your hips tucked under your shoulders, to avoid a swayback pose. Keep your eyes on what lies ahead, too, and swing your arms for balance and to intensify your workout.

Weight Training

Starting this trimester, lift weights while you're sitting down rather than standing—thanks to changes in your circulatory system, blood can pool in your legs when you stand still, leaving you lightheaded. But *don't* lift weights above your head or while you're lying on a bench—or in any position that leaves your belly vulnerable to a falling weight. And take care not to strain your lower back muscles; your stretched-out abdominal muscles can't protect your lower back as well as they did before. Finally, use good technique (ask a friend or your partner to spot you) and lighter weights.

Yoga

Be more cautious now because of your loosening joints—and because your slowly expanding waistline can throw off your balance. Don't try to hold poses for a long time, and remember to sink into yoga positions slowly and carefully, to avoid injury. Take your time if you have to, and don't overdo it. Choose a side-lying relaxation pose instead of lying flat on your back in Savasana, too, to keep blood flowing properly through your body. Look for a yoga class specifically designed for pregnant women.

Five Great Stretches

These simple moves will help keep you limber. Use them to cool down after a workout—or when you just need to relax. Breathe deeply and regularly as you stretch, and for stretches done in a standing position, remember to move your legs around between sets.

Shoulder Circles

- While you're standing or seated, rotate your shoulders forward, up, back, and down in the largest circle you can make.
- Repeat four times.
- Reverse the direction, and repeat four more times.

Arm Stretch

- Stand and lace your fingers together behind your lower back.
- Pull your arms up toward the ceiling as far as they can go; then lower them toward your buttocks.
- Release and repeat eight to ten times.

Wall Pushup and Calf Stretch

- Stand about 2 feet from a wall with your arms extended forward from your shoulders.
- Reach your hands to the wall and lean forward, bending your elbows as your body tilts.

- Keep your heels on the floor to stretch your calf muscles. (Don't do this exercise in socks or slippery shoes; you want your feet to stay put.)
- Push slowly away from the wall to straighten up.
- Repeat eight to ten times.

Thigh Stretch

- Sit on the floor with your legs extended straight out in front of you.
- Bending your right leg, cross your right ankle over your *left* knee.
- Use your left hand to pull your *right* thigh to the left, stretching the outside of your right leg.
- Increase the twist by looking over your right shoulder. Hold for one minute. (As your belly grows, make adjustments accordingly. Do what feels comfortable.) Repeat eight to ten times.
- Switch sides, and repeat eight to ten times.

Leg Stretch

- Lie on your left side with your head on a pillow or a folded towel.
- Bend your left leg at the knee while keeping your right leg straight. Use your right hand on the floor as a brace.
- Stretch your right leg as you lift it toward the ceiling. Then lower it to the floor.
- Repeat four times; then switch sides.

Kegel Exercises

Kegels are pelvic floor exercises that strengthen the muscles supporting your urethra, bladder, uterus, and rectum. Get in the habit of doing them now. Not only will they prime your pelvic floor muscles for child-birth—possibly making for a shorter, easier labor—but doing regular Kegels now will also help prevent urine leaks during (and after) pregnancy and increase circulation to your rectal and vaginal areas, keeping hemorrhoids at bay and speeding healing after an episiotomy or a tear during labor. (*Bonus:* Keeping Kegels up after giving birth will help you maintain bladder control and encourage a stretched-to-its-limit vagina to regain its tone, making postpartum sex more enjoyable.) Unlike with certain other exercises, *everyone* can do Kegels. What's more, you can do Kegels anytime and anyplace—at work, while you're watching TV, or even in line at the grocery store. In fact, you can do them right now.

Imagine that you're trying to stop yourself from passing gas and trying to stop the flow of urine in midstream at the same time (don't actually do this while you're urinating, though—it's just a check of your technique). The feeling is one of "squeeze and lift"—a closing and drawing up of the front and back passages. (*Hint:* Insert a clean finger into your vagina before doing a Kegel. If you feel pressure around your finger, you're on the right track. Or try a Kegel during lovemaking and ask your partner if he can feel it—if you're doing it correctly, he'll be able to.)

Make sure that you squeeze and lift without pulling in your tummy, squeezing your legs together, tightening your buttocks, or holding your breath. (In other words, only your pelvic floor muscles should be working.) Though you may have trouble using these muscles in isolation at first, it gets easier with practice. It might help to place a hand on your belly while you're doing your Kegels to make sure that it stays relaxed.

Hold for eight to ten seconds before releasing and relaxing for a few seconds before doing the next one.

Start with a few Kegels at a time throughout the day, and gradually increase the number you do and the length of time you hold each one, eventually working up to three sets of ten, done three times a day.

Chapter 9

YOUR EMOTIONS

There's no doubt that pregnancy is a thrilling experience for most women. But that doesn't mean it isn't fraught with emotional lows as well as highs. Knowing what lies ahead will help you weather the storms. And if you find that you need outside help maintaining your equilibrium, by all means seek it out. Still, as the troublesome physical symptoms of the first trimester—not to mention the shock and worry you may have felt when you discovered your pregnancy—fade, most women find that their second trimester is filled with excitement and enthusiasm about expanding their family.

Ups and Downs: The Wild Ride Continues

Many women find that their emotions are less fragile in the second trimester than they were earlier in pregnancy. Still, you may sometimes find yourself feeling moody, vulnerable, and super sensitive. Besides raging hormones, the dawning realization that your life is about to change in a big way may be responsible for your weepy—or short-tempered—state of mind. Try to remind yourself that emotional upheaval is normal right now. Clueing your partner in about how you're feeling and reassuring him that you still love him will help him avoid taking your outbursts personally.

What You May Be Worrying About Now

Pregnant women are champion worriers. Even when all is well, it's common to latch on to *something* to fret about: Am I eating right? Gaining too much weight? Too little? Is my baby okay? Chalk it up to your developing protec-

BabyCenter Buzz

How I Handle Mood Swings

"I've found that yoga works really well for me. And if all else fails, it always makes me feel better to get my hair done or to get a manicure or pedicure." —*Amanda*

"It helps if you laugh about it, especially if you laugh with the person who was dealing with your emotional outburst at the time. As long as you and everyone else around you remember that this is normal for expectant mothers, it's easier to deal with." —*Anonymous*

"To calm myself down, I usually take a warm bath or shower or just lie down, close my eyes, and think about why I'm upset. Sometimes a good pep talk with my husband cheers me up. A little affection—not to mention sex—helps, too!" —*Anonymous*

"It's so important to sit down, cool off, and take a deep breath before getting yourself worked up, because you have to think of what all that chaos and adrenaline does to the baby." —*Leigh*

"I've learned that what helps sometimes is to let it out. Go to a private place and just cry it out. Don't be so hard on yourself because it's not you—it's pregnancy." —*Cheryl*

"I started a diary. When I have a bad day, I write down all the positive things that are happening in my pregnancy and how excited we are about our little one's arrival. It gives me a sense of hope and excitement." —*Anonymous*

tive instinct. Even though you might not feel like a mother yet, your body knows otherwise. You're responsible for the safety and well-being of your baby, and as a result, you're more attuned to potential dangers.

To help calm these fears, don't be shy about talking openly with your pregnancy provider and getting all your health questions answered. And there's nothing like a good heart-to-heart with a friend—especially one who's been through pregnancy herself—to get you over the rough spots, which can include:

Test results. This trimester, you'll likely have an ultrasound, a multiple marker screening, and perhaps amniocentesis to check on your baby's well-being. Anticipating the procedures themselves, then awaiting the results, is anxiety provoking. Chances are that everything will be fine, so don't jump immediately to worst-case scenarios. Take it one step at a time. If something does come up, review your options with your practitioner, and take time to weigh these options with your partner. Remind yourself that a positive result for a screening such as the multiple marker doesn't necessarily mean there's a problem—it merely signals a need for more testing. So do your best to stay positive until the final results are in.

Body image. With our culture's emphasis on slimness, it can be tough to accept your growing body as beautiful. You may find yourself resisting your partner's amorous advances because you feel self-conscious. Or you may be marveling at the wonders of your pregnant body and feel more confident than ever before, making *you* the one who's in the mood—and him the one who's reluctant. If that's the case, don't automatically assume that he's put off by your new curves. The fact is that most men find their partner's growing body to be the essence of femininity, and therefore quite attractive. If your mate is shying away from sex, he may be worried about harming you or the baby—something he needn't worry about. Talk to each other frankly about your feelings. Even if sex isn't high on your agenda right now,

BabyCenter Buzz

I'm Disappointed about My Baby's Sex

"When the technician said that we were having a girl, my mind went numb. I thought, 'What am I going to do with a girl? Play Barbies? I think not. Have tea? Not likely.' I had visions of taking my boy to games, playing sports in the yard, going to see dumb boy movies, and taking him to Cub Scouts. I felt horribly guilty for thinking that. It took me a few hours to really wrap my mind around 'girl.' Now I'm gung-ho about it." —*Dave*

"I wanted a little girl. I cried the whole way home when I learned I was having a boy. But now I'm happy—the baby's healthy, and I realize that's what's important." —*Adrianne*

"I wanted a boy and was so disappointed when the tech said, 'It's a girl.' Then I started thinking about how daughters usually end up being 'Daddy's girl,' and how much I wanted to teach everything I've learned about the world to my daughter." —*Anonymous*

"I was secretly hoping for a little girl, but when we saw that telltale penis, we were just as happy. It's okay to *hope* for a particular sex, but recognize that what matters in the end is having that precious little bundle—no matter what kind." —*Andrea*

BabyCenter Buzz

My Worries about My Older Child

"I look at my daughter, who'll soon be 2, and think about how much I adore her. It scares me to death to have feelings of guilt over baby number two." —Anonymous

"I'm afraid that I'm going to lose a part of my daughter when the new baby comes. I love her so much, and it's hard for me to think that I could love anyone else that much. I just don't want her to think that she doesn't have all of my heart." —Carol

"I was afraid I couldn't love another child the way I loved my first. When everyone told me it would happen, I just nodded my head and smiled. Well, they were right. He's now 2½ and I adore him, as does his 6-year-old brother." —Anonymous

cuddling, back rubs, and other forms of physical affection will help both of you feel loved and appreciated.

Looming life changes. As your belly grows and the reality of your pregnancy finally settles in, you're likely to be struck by what a milestone this represents in your life. Many moms wonder how they'll handle the loss of freedom, the sleepless nights, and the responsibility of caring for another person. And well-meaning friends who point out that your life will never again be the same aren't exactly helping matters. It's true; having a child will change your existence dramatically. But maintaining a network of friends, especially other new moms, will keep you from feeling isolated. Also, keeping up—within reason—with activities you enjoyed before you got pregnant, whether it's going to the gym or checking out new music, will help you stay connected with your own needs. There's no reason your old life needs to disappear. It just needs to adapt.

Your relationship with your firstborn—and your new baby. If you're already a mom, you'll probably find that pregnancy brings up bittersweet feelings about your older child, who soon won't be your "baby" any longer. Many moms struggle with sadness and even guilt at the thought of another child's coming into the family. Reassure yourself that these feelings are normal. And though the new baby *will* take a big chunk of your time and attention, you'll find ways to maintain—and even deepen—your bond with your firstborn. And even if this baby will be number

Just for Dad

What *You* May Be Worried about Now

As a father-to-be, you're going through a major attitude adjustment of your own. Don't be afraid to let your partner know that sometimes you yourself need a shoulder to lean on. (It's probably best not to bring this up while she's in the middle of a crying jag, though.)
Some issues you may be contending with:

- **Your mate or child's health.** It's easy to let your imagination conjure up scary scenarios, such as losing the baby or even losing your partner and having to raise your child alone. Going to prenatal visits with her can help keep your worries at bay and reassure you that everything is under control.

- **The foreignness of "women's medicine."** Men aren't used to the ob-gyn establishment. It's foreign, it's sometimes cold, and it's something you don't understand well. As observers, many men feel embarrassed and inhibited around stirrups and gynecological exams. Exam rooms aren't always made comfortable for dads-to-be. Men may also feel in the dark about some aspects of pregnancy or become shy about participating and asking questions. When you encounter all this, it's normal to feel clobbered by it. Being prepared—reading up on pregnancy issues and talking with your partner about her care—will help you feel more at ease.

- **Being squeezed out by the baby.** Men often fear that their significant other will love the new arrival more than anyone on earth—and they'll be the odd man out in that relationship. And it's true: Some mothers *do* become so wrapped up in their newborn that Dad winds up feeling like an outsider. To prevent this, take an active role in your baby's life right from the start—and even before. Join in your partner's pregnancy and baby preparations as much as possible. Fantasize together about what life will be like as new parents. "Talk" to your baby in her womb. Help peruse baby names and decorate the nursery. And while you can't breastfeed once the baby arrives, you *can* change diapers and soothe him during fussy spells. The more you interact with your newborn, the more adept you'll become at reading his signals and knowing how to keep him happy (and the more energy your partner will have left over for *you*). Not only will you reap the benefits of this special bond with your child, but your mate will continue to see you as an equal partner—in parenting and in life.

three (or more), you'll still feel torn about how your relationships with your other children will be affected. Although you know from experience that things will work out eventually, you may worry more than you did before because your time and attention will be spread even thinner. Rest assured, though, there's no limit to your love. You will adore the new baby every bit as much as you do your other children. As the saying goes, your heart will simply grow to accommodate the love you feel for *all* your children.

Depression During Pregnancy

Though pregnancy is portrayed as a time of great joy, that's not the reality for all women. In fact, depression is surprisingly common among mothers-to-be. Learn more about how to tell if you're at risk for the blues, how to recognize them when they strike, and how to get help.

Risk Factors for Depression

For years, experts mistakenly believed that pregnancy hormones protected against depression. The thinking was that only after the baby was born and hormone levels plunged did depression become a threat. But in fact the hormonal changes of pregnancy themselves may play a role in sparking depression. At least one in ten pregnant women suffer from bouts of depression. Some experts think that it might be the rapid increase in hormone levels at the start of pregnancy that disrupts brain chemistry, sometimes leading to a bout of depression. What's more, past and current circumstances in your life can make you especially susceptible to becoming depressed during pregnancy. Some common risk factors:

Personal or family history of depression or anxiety. If you've struggled in the past with depression or extreme anxiety (or, to a lesser extent, if depression runs in your family), you're more likely to become depressed now that you're expecting. Even if you've never experienced a full-blown bout of depression or anxiety but have a tendency to get down or anxious during stressful or uncertain times, you may be more susceptible to depression now.

Relationship difficulties. If you're in a troubled relationship, and talking things out as a couple isn't working, get counseling. (And if you're in an abusive relationship, get help immediately—page 98) Don't make the mistake of assuming that your baby's arrival will make everything rosy. A newborn will only add to the strain on your relationship—so don't put off seeking professional advice on repairing your relationship now. If you're young or single or have an unplanned pregnancy, your risk of depression is also higher.

Fertility treatments. If you had trouble getting pregnant, chances are you've been under a lot of stress. And if you've gone through multiple fertility procedures, you may still be dealing with the emotional side effects of months or even years of treatments and anxiety-laden waiting. On top of that, now that you're pregnant, you may be terrified of losing the baby you worked so hard to conceive. All of these make you more prone to depression.

Just the Facts

Signs of Depression

Talk to your doctor or midwife if you have any of the following symptoms for more than two weeks:

- A sense that nothing feels enjoyable or fun anymore
- Feeling blue, sad, or "empty" for most of the day, every day
- Decreased ability to concentrate
- Extreme irritability or agitation or excessive crying
- Trouble sleeping, or sleeping all the time
- Extreme or unending fatigue
- A desire to eat all the time, or not wanting to eat at all
- Inappropriate guilt or feelings of worthlessness or hopelessness
- Suicidal thoughts or recurrent thoughts of death
- Mood swings with cycles of depression alternating with periods of an abnormally high spirits—including increased activity, little need to sleep or eat, racing thoughts, inappropriate social behavior, or poor judgment. These are signs of a serious condition called bipolar disorder. Bipolar disorder requires immediate attention, so call your caregiver right away if you have these symptoms for more than a few days.

Granted, some of these hallmarks of depression mimic normal pregnancy symptoms, but when they're combined with a sense of sadness or hopelessness or interfere with your ability to function, depression is probably at least partly to blame. Don't be shy about letting your caregiver know if you feel low; your emotional health is every bit as important as your physical health. (And in fact, it can *affect* your physical health. Research has shown, for instance, that depression and anxiety can increase your risk for preterm labor.) Just like diabetes or high blood pressure, depression is an illness, which can—and should—be treated for you and your baby's well-being.

Guard Against Postpartum Depression *Now*

The single most important thing you can do for yourself and your baby is to treat any depression that develops during your pregnancy.

- Build a support network (made up of friends, family members, your partner, your healthcare practitioner, and your therapist) so that your helpers will already be in place when the baby arrives.
- Talk with your partner about how you're going to divide the household responsibilities and care for each other as well as for your baby.

Previous pregnancy loss. If you've miscarried or lost a baby in the past, it's no wonder you're worrying about the safety of this pregnancy. And if the loss was recent or if you've miscarried several times in the past year, you may not have had time to fully recover emotionally or physically. And as with fertility treatments, if you're dealing with health restrictions, you're more vulnerable to depression and anxiety.

Problems with your pregnancy. A complicated or high-risk pregnancy—one that requires weeks of bed rest or numerous genetic tests, for instance—can take an emotional and physical toll. (Women who are pregnant with twins or more often fall into this category, as well.) The strain of having to endure difficult procedures, combined with fear about your baby's well-being, is often difficult to shoulder. Likewise, not being able to work or do other things you're used to doing makes it tougher to maintain your emotional balance. Because you're at increased risk for prenatal depression and anxiety, talk to

Just the Facts

Signs of Anxiety

Tell your caregiver right away if you're experiencing:

- Panic attacks. These can come on with no warning and include a racing heart, light-headedness or faintness, sweaty palms, breathlessness, and feeling like you are having a heart attack or are about to pass out.
- Frequent, recurrent concerns about your or you baby's health or a frequent feeling that something terrible is about to happen.

Therapy, medication, or a combination of the two can be very effective at putting extreme anxiety to rest.

Ask the Experts

Will My Depression Harm My Baby?

Dr. Diana Dell, obstetrical psychiatry specialist: Research suggests that when you're depressed, your body generates chemicals like the stress hormone cortisol, which can have an adverse effect on your baby. What's more, extreme stress is linked to a higher rate of miscarriage and preterm birth. It may also make your baby less able to cope with stress later in life. Finally, being depressed may get in the way of taking proper care of yourself while you're pregnant, in terms of eating right, getting plenty of rest, avoiding drugs and alcohol, and getting proper prenatal care.

But genetics plays a role, too, as does environment. Since babies' brains continue to develop after they're born, they can compensate for those prenatal influences. Growing up in a supportive, loving family has a major impact on a child's development. Still, because depression might affect your baby in the womb, early recognition and treatment will help minimize that risk.

your caregiver about your emotional as well as physical well-being. Taking steps now will also reduce your risk for problems after giving birth—and help you to better enjoy the baby you've worked so hard to bring into the world.

Stressful life events. Financial worries? Relocating? Contemplating switching jobs? Any major concerns or life changes such as these—or a breakup, the death of a close friend or family member, or a job loss-can send you into a serious funk.

Past history of abuse. Women who've survived emotional, sexual, physical, or verbal abuse may have low self-esteem, a sense of helplessness, or feelings of isolation—all of which contribute to a higher risk for depression. Pregnancy can trigger painful memories of your past abuse, and the loss of control over your changing body may mirror the helplessness you experienced when you were abused.

Getting Help

Healthcare professionals often misdiagnose or disregard depression in expectant mothers, chalking it up to the usual emotional upsets and physical symptoms that come with pregnancy. But clinical depression goes beyond moodiness, and if left untreated, it can impair your ability to take care of your-

Call Your Caregiver If . . .

You're finding that you're unable to handle your daily responsibilities, you're having panic attacks, or if thoughts of harming yourself cross your mind. Seeing a therapist or psychiatrist isn't an indication of weakness. On the contrary, it shows that you're willing to take the steps necessary to keep your baby and yourself safe and healthy.

....

self and your developing baby. If you're depressed, it's vital to get the treatment you need, whether it's psychotherapy or antidepressant medication or both.

If you've been feeling low for two weeks and nothing you've tried seems to lift your spirits, seek professional help. Ask your doctor or midwife for a referral to a psychologist or psychiatrist, or check with your insurance company for a list of mental health providers. About half of women suffering from depression during pregnancy go on to develop postpartum depression, but treatment during pregnancy can reduce that number dramatically. Whatever you do, don't try to treat yourself by taking Saint-John's-wort or other remedies. The safety of these remedies during pregnancy is unknown, and they're not an effective substitute for professional help.

Keep in mind that hormonal and coming life changes can make you feel more anxious than usual, too, and that excessive anxiety during pregnancy is a condition that can and should be treated.

THE REST OF YOUR LIFE

How Pregnancy Affects Your Looks

The "bloom" or "glow" of pregnancy isn't just a saying. Your skin is retaining more moisture now, which plumps it up, smoothing out fine lines and wrinkles. The glow that makes you look so radiant comes from the increased amount of blood pumping through your body and the increased blood flow to your skin. All that extra blood can make you look—and feel—flushed at times. But not all skin changes are welcome ones. Here is a look at some common skin conditions during pregnancy, and advice on what to do about them.

Acne

Pregnancy sometimes brings on the kind of breakouts you haven't seen since junior high. Higher levels of hormones called androgens can boost production of a substance called sebum—the oil that keeps your skin supple. This extra sebum, combined with the shed skin cells that line your hair follicles, blocks your pores and creates fertile ground for bacteria—resulting in acne, greasy skin, and pimples. Your skin will likely clear up after delivery, but if your acne is severe, you may need treatment now. Because some acne medications are dangerous during pregnancy, let any practitioner you see know that you're pregnant.

CLEAR-SKIN STRATEGIES

To banish pregnancy pimples:

• Wash gently with a mild cleanser a few times a day, and use an oil-free moisturizer. Don't scrub your face with a washcloth because it can make the problem worse; instead, use your hands to gently wash your face.

215

Call Your Caregiver If . . .

• Changes in skin pigmentation are accompanied by pain, tenderness, redness, or bleeding or if you notice changes in the color, shape, or size of a mole.

• if you develop itchy eruptions on your belly or blistering lesions (page 302).

• If you have intense itching all over your body; this can be a sign of a liver condition called intrahepatic cholestasis.

• Pat your skin dry; rubbing it can irritate acne.

• Don't squeeze or pop your pimples—both will make the problem worse and could lead to scarring.

• If you wear makeup, opt for products that are water- (not oil-) based as well as those labeled "noncomedogenic" or "nonacnegenic"— meaning they won't clog your pores and cause breakouts. Always wash off your makeup before going to bed, too.

• Ask your doctor or midwife about using medicated gels or lotions. (If your acne is severe, you may need to see a dermatologist.) There are a number of over-the-counter and prescription products that help clear up acne, but some of the ingredients haven't been well-studied in pregnancy—so don't use *any* acne preparation without your caregiver's okay. It's particularly important to avoid the oral prescription drug isotretinoin (Accutane), which can cause serious birth defects. (Avoid using topical tretinoin—like Retin-A—as well.) Prescription antibiotic creams containing erythromycin or clindamycin are safe, but stay away from those with tetracycline, which can discolor your baby's teeth (page 552) and affect your baby's bones.

Chloasma: The "Mask of Pregnancy"

It's normal to develop areas of darker skin (known as chloasma or melasma) on your face and body during pregnancy, especially if you have a darker complexion. These hyperpigmented splotches can show up on your upper lip, nose, cheeks, and forehead, sometimes in the shape of a mask (think: the

Lone Ranger), as well as on your forearms and other parts of your body that are regularly exposed to the sun.

You may also find that your nipples, areolas, freckles, scars, underarms, and even inner thighs and vulva have darkened since you became pregnant. All of these changes are due to the temporary (and harmless) increase in your body's production of melanin, the natural substance that colors your hair, skin, and eyes.

Dry, Itchy Skin

Do your growing breasts and belly feel itchy? Join the club. Not only is your skin stretching to accommodate your increasing girth, but pregnancy hormones may also be making you itch. (In fact, some pregnant women also find themselves with red, itchy palms—and sometimes soles—a condition likely caused by an increase in estrogen.) If you have naturally dry skin or eczema, you may also find that it worsens now. As with most pregnancy complaints, this itchiness usually disappears after delivery.

HOW TO TAKE THE EDGE OFF YOUR ITCH

• Skip steaming showers and baths, which dry your skin. Instead, bathe in warm—not hot—water. If you can't bear to turn the water temperature down, limit your showers to just a few minutes.

• Use a mild, moisturizing soap, and be sure to rinse your skin well and towel off gently.

• Slather on moisturizer—preferably a fragrance-free variety, since some perfumed additives can cause irritation. Moisturize your skin while it's still damp after a bath or shower.

- Try an occasional warm oatmeal bath; premixed preparations are available in most drugstores.

Fast-Growing Fingernails

If your nails are growing faster than usual, credit pregnancy hormones. While some women's fingernails become harder, other women develop softer or brittler nails. You may even notice tiny grooves forming along the base of the nail. These changes are temporary, and your nails should return to normal within a few months after giving birth.

Hair Changes

One of the perks of all those pregnancy hormones is thicker, more lustrous locks. (You're not actually growing more hair; you're just *losing* less than normal due, of course, to those ubiquitous pregnancy hormones.) Some women also notice that the texture of their hair changes or that their mane becomes shinier. If you normally have a thick head of hair and worry that any more will be unmanageable, you may find a shorter cut easier to deal with now (or ask your stylist to thin it out at your next cut). But don't do anything dramatic that you may regret; you're going through enough transformation as it is. Work with your stylist to find a cut that suits you, or play around with clips, barrettes, and combs to enhance your existing style.

Hairiness

You may have been expecting thicker hair on your head during pregnancy, but is the new growth on your chin, upper lip, jaw, and cheeks throwing you for a loop? It may be unsightly, but the extra hair is harmless, and it will likely go away after your baby's born. Pregnancy-induced hair growth is

---

QUICK TIP

The Power of Makeup

Makeup is a fun, relatively inexpensive pick-me-up. Beauty basics to keep on hand during your pregnancy include:

- Concealer for blotches, blemishes, spider veins, and dark under-eye circles (*Hint:* Let the concealer sit on your skin for a minute or two before blending for a smoother, more natural look.)

- A lightweight foundation that matches your skin tone, to even out blotchy areas

- Blush (Go easy on it, though, because your cheeks may already be flushed.)

- Your favorite lip color

BabyCenter Buzz

Why I Like My Pregnant Body

"The combination of my expanding belly and breasts feels feminine and sexy to me. My hair and nails are growing faster as well. My husband loves the changes, which really helps me feel good about my new body." —*Shelly*

"It's an announcement to the whole world that I'm carrying our bundle of joy. It's like I get to tell everyone about the most important thing that's happened to my husband and me, without saying a word." —*Allison*

"I usually work so hard to suck my belly in. For the first time in my life, I can just let it hang out, and I feel great about it." —*Anonymous*

"I've always been too skinny, and I like how my chicken legs have filled out and my arms aren't so tiny now." —*Kim*

"I love the fact that I've gone from an A cup to a C! I also love how sexy I feel— maybe it's because my husband is always telling me how sexy I *am*." —*Karen*

caused by an increase in sex hormones known as androgens. In addition to new facial hair, you may notice stray hairs on your breasts, belly, arms, legs, and back.

To get rid of the hair, you can safely tweeze, wax, or shave. (No one knows for sure if topical creams or lotions to remove hair or slow hair growth, or bleach to lighten its appearance are totally safe during pregnancy; see page 576). And the new moisturizers that claim to reduce hair growth are soy-based, which means they may contain plant-based hormones; until more is known about them, it's wise to err on side of caution and avoid them.)

As for permanent hair-removal techniques—laser and electrolysis— these procedures can be painful, and you may decide that you already have enough discomfort to deal with during pregnancy. So the final option is to be patient: Most of this unwanted hair should be gone by three to six months after you deliver.

Linea Nigra

The dark line that you may have noticed running from your belly button to the top of your pubic bone is called the linea nigra (literally "black line"). Before your pregnancy, you had an unnoticeable, lighter line (called the linea alba) in the same place. The increased production of melanin that causes chloasma's dark facial splotches is responsible for this, too—and as with chloasma, the line usually fades a few months after your baby arrives.

Skin Tags

As your pregnancy progresses, you may start to notice tiny pieces of loose skin showing up where two areas of skin rub against each other, such as under your breasts, in your armpits, or in your groin. These little tags (called acrochordon) are common during pregnancy and completely harmless. Although they won't go away after your baby is born, you can ask a dermatologist to remove them if they bother you.

Spider Veins

Spider veins—so-called because they look like spider webs, though they can also have a sunburst pattern—are common in pregnancy, particularly if you're already prone to them. They are tiny, dilated blood vessels that lie close to the surface of your skin. Though they're most likely to show up on your legs and face, they can appear anywhere and are caused by your increased blood volume and hormone levels. In most cases, the veins will fade once your hormone levels settle down after delivery. If they don't, you can have them removed by a dermatologist.

Stretch Marks

Caused by tiny tears in the supportive tissue that lies just beneath your skin, stretch marks are small, depressed streaks of differently textured skin and can be pink, reddish, or dark brown, depending on your skin tone. These

Just the Facts

The Truth about Stretch Mark "Miracle" Creams

Unfortunately, there's little proof that any of the costly creams, salves, and oils that claim to prevent stretch marks actually *work* (though keeping your belly well-moisturized will at least make it less itchy). In fact, there's no guaranteed way to prevent stretch marks at all—you're either genetically predisposed to them or you're not (ask your mom for clues). Still, gaining no more than the recommended amount of weight, and gaining it slowly, may help reduce the number and severity of stretch marks.

striations usually appear in the second half of pregnancy as your belly expands to accommodate your growing baby—though they can also show up on your butt, thighs, hips, or breasts.

Whether you get stretch marks depends on how naturally elastic your skin is. But women who quickly gain a lot of weight, who carry multiples or especially big babies, or who have excess amniotic fluid are more likely to get stretch marks than others, and at least half of all expectant mothers get them. Stretch marks appear less frequently in women with darker skin.

The sight of fresh stretch marks can be depressing, but the good news is they usually fade considerably by six months to a year after birth. Chances are they'll become lighter than your surrounding skin so you won't notice them as much (though the texture remains the same). If you're wondering what they'll look like, ask a friend who has a child over age 1 to show you hers. While these light streaks will always be there, try not to feel bad about them-instead, view them as badges of honor for bringing your child into the world. (If, a year or so down the line, you truly can't bear the sight of your pregnancy battle scars, a dermatologist may be able to diminish their appearance with laser or microdermabrasion. Treatment with isotretinoin gel (Retin-A) can help, too, but it's not safe to use while you're pregnant. Afterward, it's most effective if used soon after delivery, while the marks still have their darker pigmentation—but this treatment also isn't an option if you're breastfeeding.

> ## BY THE NUMBERS
>
> **How Expectant Moms Feel about Their Form**
>
> **49%**   revel in most of the physical changes that came with pregnancy.
>
> **22%**   have mixed feelings— they loved some things and couldn't stand others.
>
> **19%**   love every inch of their voluptuous new form.
>
> **10%**   really dislike their pregnant body.
>
> Source: *A BabyCenter.com poll of more than 10,700 women*

You and Your Partner

For months now, you and your growing baby have been joined at the hip, so to speak. But to your partner, the reality of your pregnancy may not have completely sunk in. Now—with your new shape as visible proof—expect it to finally hit home. Treat your mate's new awareness as an opportunity to plan together for the big event. Have fun fantasizing together about the baby, sharing the big news with friends and family (if you haven't spilled the beans already), readying the nursery, choosing a name, and working on a birth plan (page 378). Make time to share interests *other* than the baby, too. You're still a couple, after all, not just parents-to-be—and it's this connection that will keep your relationship—and your family—healthy in the years ahead.

Make the Most of Couple Time Now

Becoming parents needn't and *shouldn't* spell the end of time together for just the two of you—but there's no denying that it will pose logistical challenges. So enjoy the chance for alone time now, while the getting is good. Shed your roles of parents-to-be for a few hours, and just enjoy being a couple. Some ideas for keeping the spark in your relationship:

Make dates. It's easy to get so caught up in work, baby preparations, and other responsibilities that intimacy starts to slide. Set aside a regular time each week for each other. See a movie, go out for dinner, or simply take a

BabyCenter Buzz

How Pregnancy Has Changed Our Relationship

"At 20 weeks, I was at my wit's end. My husband had no idea how to relate to me. But now he's made an about-face. I think it just took him a little while to get over being freaked-out once the pregnancy suddenly became 'real' to him." —*Anonymous*

"My husband was great before we got pregnant, but now he's just unbelievable. He's forever cleaning the house, cooking dinner, running errands—and has never once complained. I don't know what I'd do without him."   —*Anonymous*

"My husband is normally great, but since I've been pregnant, things have been off in our relationship. He's been drinking quite a bit, smoking (which he never did before), and buying lots of toys—even a sports car. It's like a midlife crisis." —*Anonymous*

"Pregnancy can make some hard decisions clearer. When I was pregnant and in a terrible marriage, my father said something that stuck with me: 'The only thing that baby needs for the first 5 years of her life is *you*.' We've been on our own—and happy—ever since."   —*Anonymous*

Just the Facts

When Arguments Cross the Line

If fights with your partner ever include physical aggression or intimidation, or verbal threats, your relationship is abusive. (See page 98 for info and advice on getting help.) And while people sometimes say cruel things to each other during arguments, it crosses the line to abuse if your partner often calls you names or constantly criticizes and humiliates you.

stroll. If you'd rather stay in, rent a video, pop some popcorn, and snuggle on the couch.

Take a vacation. If you can, enjoy a prebaby getaway (some people call it a "babymoon"). Now's the perfect time: You're feeling better, your due date is still several months away, and you don't yet have weekly prenatal checkups keeping you close to home.

Be spontaneous. Surprise him at his office for lunch, show up at bedtime in sexy lingerie that highlights your juicy new figure (or skip the maternity merry widow and adopt a sexy *attitude*), call him just to say "I love you," or write him a note reminding him why you love him. In other words, treat him like you would if you just fell in love—it'll come back to you in spades.

Fighting Fair: What to Do When You Disagree with Your Mate

There's no such thing as a conflict-free relationship. You *will* disagree—sometimes loudly. In fact, if you don't have an occasional quarrel, one of you is probably holding in something that would be better off expressed. But there are constructive and destructive ways to fight. The next time you're itching to take your gloves off with your mate, try these fair-fighting tactics.

Agree on *how* you'll disagree. Most couples who fight effectively have recognized the inevitability of conflict and established guidelines for dealing with it. When you're not in the heat of the moment, talk about how you want to handle arguments. You might vow never to go to bed angry, for instance, or agree that when a disagreement arises, you'll take a time-out to cool down if emotions become too heated.

Just for Dad

How to "Be There" for Your Pregnant Partner

Truth be told, women often feel that their mates just don't "get it" when it comes to pregnancy. And let's face it; your perspective is understandably different from hers. Nobody who's not pregnant can fully comprehend the minute-by-minute, close-to-the-heart, kick-in-the-gut reality of carrying a baby inside your body. But that doesn't mean you need to be a mere bystander in the process. There are plenty of things you can do to participate in the pregnancy experience right alongside your partner.

Be enthusiastic. Show your interest in the momentous changes going on. Caress her belly, feel those little legs kicking, read up on fetal development, and talk to your baby—he or she really *can* hear you from inside the womb.

Accompany her to appointments. Try to make it to at least some of your partner's many prenatal checkups, especially for the important tests, and don't be shy about asking questions. Whatever you do, don't miss the chance to get a glimpse of your growing baby during the ultrasound. And, of course, attend childbirth classes so you can play an active role on the big day. *Bonus:* Besides making your mate happy, learning more about what's going on will help alleviate any anxiety *you* might be feeling.

Get healthier, too. As your mate tries to modify her diet and kick bad habits, support her by sharing these lifestyle changes. Swear off junk food. Eat nutritious meals along with her. Cut down on or eliminate alcohol. Don't smoke—not just to help *her* abstain but because secondhand smoke can harm your developing baby. Spend time walking or exercising together.

Love her changing body. Ask your mate if she wants you to take a photo of her in profile each month to document her progress. Be sensitive to the fact that as her pregnancy progresses, she may feel unattractive at times. Keep reassuring her that she's beautiful. If your sex life gets a PG rating for a while, be patient. What with hormone changes, back pain, fatigue, and an understandable preoccupation with the stirrings of life, sex can take a hit. But don't hold back on your affection. She needs hugs and kisses now more than ever.

Go the extra mile. Your partner may have become intensely demanding since she got pregnant. Go with it. She's doing all the heavy lifting, so to speak, so a little pampering is in order. Shop for groceries, mop the floor, send her flowers, and do your best to indulge her 11 P.M. demands for cottage cheese and strawberry jam—with a smile.

Fight nice. It's essential to avoid belittling your partner during an argument. Don't call names, lay blame, or drag others (especially kids) into the argument—there are no winners in these situations.

Don't digress. Avoid bringing up past grievances when you argue. Instead, focus on the immediate issue at hand ("After I cooked that big meal, I wish you'd offered to help with the dishes") rather than a general situation ("You never notice how tired I am"). And next time around, if your partner doesn't volunteer, *ask* for help instead of quietly going it alone and ending up furious.

BabyCenter Buzz

How I Get the Support I Need

"At first my husband didn't seem to want anything to do with my pregnancy, so I made sure he came along to all my prenatal appointments and ultrasounds. It made a big difference once he saw our son's image on the monitor." —Amber

"My husband's on the road Sunday through Thursday every week. He got a cell phone with a nationwide plan and a *lot* of minutes, and he makes a point to call me every night." —Julie

"My boyfriend is overseas in the army. Since I've been pregnant, his family has become an unexpected life raft for me. At first it bugged me that they checked up on me so much, but now I'm so grateful that they're involved." —Trina

"My husband's on call for work 24 hours a day. It's hard, but having a network of friends really helps. They're a support group I can call on when I need them." —Anonymous

"Instead of helping with the housework (which is what I *really* need), my husband is working overtime. I finally told him that I miss him and that I'd rather have him around than have the extra money!" —Anonymous

Take time out. When things heat up, take a break. This will help you avoid moving into the realm of the irrational. Later, when you've both cooled down, talk it over and ask, "How do we resolve this?"

Make up. Be sure to reach an understanding that you both can live with, whether it's a meeting of the minds, a compromise, or simply agreeing to disagree. Unresolved hurt feelings and frustrations will only fester.

Sex in the Second Trimester

After the exhaustion and nausea of the first trimester finally fade, it's not uncommon to feel your sexual desire skyrocket after months of being grounded. You can thank the increased bloodflow to your pelvic area and the heightened sensitivity to stimulation this brings about, as well as those ever-active hormones that contribute to increased vaginal lubrication. If your partner's passion matches your revved-up libido, enjoy!

But try not to be crushed if you find his lust waning just when you're raring to go again. As your belly blossoms, his fear of hurting you or the baby becomes that much more tangible. Unless your caregiver has told you other-

Just for Dad

How I Made Her Feel Beautiful

"I left a trail of paper hearts guiding her to our candlelit bedroom, where I gave her a massage and served her dinner. She loved it! She told me she was feeling sick until I did that." —*Travis*

"It's important to reassure her when she's not expecting it, not just when she brings it up. If you only respond when she's fishing for a compliment, it will come across as less sincere." —*Anonymous*

"I bought my wife some sexy maternity dresses and lingerie. Trying on new clothes always makes her feel good." —*Anonymous*

wise, reassure him that sex is perfectly safe and that you'll speak up if anything feels uncomfortable. If that doesn't allay his concerns, take him along to your next prenatal checkup so your provider can put his mind at ease.

Another hang-up for some men is the notion that a mother isn't an appropriate sex partner. Talk openly about his feelings without pressuring him. Let him know that you still want to see each other as lovers even though you're also going to become parents.

Then again, sometimes *you* may be the one who puts sex on the back burner, either from discomfort or from inhibitions about your changing body. Regardless of how much sex you're having and which partner is saying "Not tonight, dear," it's important to preserve the bond of intimacy. Continue to hold, caress, and kiss each other. Likewise, don't forget compliments, love notes, time together, and other ways of showing you care.

Positions for Pregnancy Sex: What to Do When Your Belly Comes Between You

The bad news: Once you're well into your second trimester, you'll find that your growing baby literally pushes you and your mate apart when you're trying to make love. The good news: This physical obstacle will force you to get creative. So go ahead—try some new moves! Time-tested positions and pointers for making love while you're pregnant:

Tilt sideways. Having your partner on top demands increasingly creative gymnastics as your tummy swells—he'll need to use his hands and

BabyCenter Buzz

I'm Worried That My Mate's Not Attracted to Me Anymore

"I feel like a walking hormone, and my husband is acting like a monk. He assures me that he still thinks I'm beautiful and desirable. I know he loves me; I just miss him *wanting* me, too." —*Anonymous*

"My husband has said that to him, a pregnant woman's body is doing an amazing thing in creating another life and that to have sex with her at that time would be a sort of violation of that. So yes, I masturbate—a lot." —*Paula*

"He says he's still attracted to me and that I'm beautiful because I'm going to be the mom of our baby. But I want him to *look* at me like he used to!" —*Tiffany*

"I'm worried that we're turning into friends instead of lovers. I'm some kind of motherly, sisterly, wholesome person to him now." —*Garita*

"I was feeling hurt because my husband was showing less interest in sex. But I asked myself, 'Is he still affectionate?' 'Does he still tell me he loves me?' When I answered 'yes' to those questions, I realized there's really not a problem." —*Amy*

"My husband was afraid to have sex with me because he thought it would hurt the baby. After we talked about it and he did a little reading himself, we never had that problem again." —*Anonymous*

"Speaking from a man's perspective, I find it hard to go from feeling our baby kick to thinking about having sex. It has nothing to do with my partner's physical appearance, though. She's just as beautiful to me as ever." —*Rick*

knees to hold his weight off you. But lying partly sideways while you're on your back (with a pillow wedged under one hip so you're not *flat* on your back) allows him to keep most of his weight off your belly without straining his muscles.

Use the bed as a prop. Your bump won't get in the way if you lie on your back (again, slightly tilted to one side) at the side or foot of the bed with your knees bent and your bottom and feet perched at the edge of the mattress. Your partner can then either kneel or stand in front of you.

Spoon. Lying side by side allows for only shallow penetration. Deep thrusts can become uncomfortable as the months pass.

Get on top. It puts less weight on your abdomen and allows you control over the depth of penetration.

Try sitting down. Having him enter you from a sitting position also

BabyCenter Buzz

My Family Is Driving Me Crazy!

"My well-meaning but cheap mother-in-law buys used baby furniture and toys for us. She never bothers to check whether the items have been recalled or pose safety hazards due to wear and tear."   —Susan

"My mom insists on staying with us after the birth, even though she knows my husband, baby, and I will be living in a tiny studio apartment. She has no idea how stressful this will be for us."   —Anonymous

"Our families have totally taken control of the pregnancy. They tell me what to eat and drink, which doctor and hospital I should go to, and even what we should name our baby."   —S.R.

"My husband's parents are so full of quacky advice that I dread their visits! A lot has changed since they had their kids, and some of their recommendations are not only bizarre—they're dangerous."   —Anonymous

"My mother-in-law wants to be in the room when I deliver! I've already given birth to one of her grandchildren without her present, and I didn't hear the end of it. I absolutely know I won't feel comfortable with her there."   —April

"My partner's family has never accepted my relationship with their daughter. They chose to ignore it completely. Now, at 17 weeks, they still refuse to talk about my pregnancy and our impending motherhood. At least *my* family is over the moon."   —Kelly

keeps his weight off your belly. Straddle your partner—either facing him or facing the other direction—as he sits on a sturdy chair or sofa.

Finally, have faith—where there's a will, there's a way. With a little experimenting, you'll find a technique that works for you.

Friends and Family
Your Friends

If you don't have a lot of friends with kids and if you feel yourself starting to drift away from your footloose-and-fancy-free childless buddies, now's the time to start reaching out to other women in the same boat as you. Not only do you need pals who can relate to what you're going through as your pregnancy progresses, but these women will become your lifeline in the exhausting, emotional weeks after your baby arrives.

BabyCenter Buzz

How I Respond to Rude Remarks

"To those who mention my size, I say, 'Yes, I *am* getting huge—and you're getting rude. I'll have something wonderful when this is over. You'll still be rude.' " —*Anonymous*

"My pet peeve is people touching my belly. I stopped that by turning and asking if they'd like to touch my ass, too." —*Anonymous*

"I'm a woman, but my female partner's mom asked me, 'Are you ready to be a daddy?' when we announced her pregnancy. I said, 'No, I'm ready to be a *mommy.*' " —*Leanne*

"I'm in a long-term relationship, but we're in no rush to tie the knot. When a married coworker learned about my pregnancy, he asked, 'So when are you going to make it legal?' I responded with 'Please, one mistake at a time!' " —*Anonymous*

"When I was pregnant with twins, people always asked if I'd had fertility treatments. My answer: 'No, all it took was my husband, God, and a couple of good swimmers.' " —*Anonymous*

Your Family (and Others Who May Get Too Close for Comfort)

A baby in the works has a way of inviting heretofore hands-off family members to get in your face. Do your best to grin and bear it (after all, annoying as the meddling may be, it's a sign that they care). Still, excited relatives eager to offer advice and assistance sometimes overstep their bounds. Try to remain civil—express your appreciation, but don't be shy about telling nosy grandmothers-to-be and know-it-all older sisters to back off when they've gone too far. After all, it's *your* pregnancy and *your* baby.

Your Older Child

Your baby's not even born yet—and already you may feel torn between the child-to-come and the one you already have. It's one thing to know that you need to rest and take care of yourself when you're pregnant—and quite another to figure out how to actually do it when you have a small child to look after.

BabyCenter Buzz

How I Juggle Pregnancy and Taking Care of My Toddler

It can be a challenge to give your child the attention he needs when you're not feeling yourself. A few ideas from other second-time moms:

"Whenever I need a break, I go over to my parents' house. No cooking, no cleaning-plus, someone *else* can play with my son." —*Anonymous*

"After I caught myself getting angry with my toddler because I was so frazzled, I hired a babysitter to come a few times a week and a housekeeper to clean. It's definitely worth the money—I have the energy to be a good mother again." —*Sheryl*

"I've become the 'quiet time' parent. I read books, do meals, bedtime, and so on. My husband does the diaper changes, baths, and the full-out playtime that I just can't handle right now." —*Dawn*

Caring for Yourself When You Have a Child at Home

Relax your standards. You can't do it all, so focus on what's important—your family—and let the small stuff slide. Skipping the vacuuming or serving a frozen dinner (or takeout) isn't a crime. Let your child help with chores. She'll love the one-on-one time with you, and who cares if the laundry isn't folded perfectly?

Use nap time wisely. Take a nap yourself, or enjoy a long soak in the tub. Don't worry about accomplishing anything. Remember: Having a healthy pregnancy and being rested enough to care for your older child's needs are worthwhile achievements in and of themselves.

Get help. Have a teenage neighbor or college student come in for a few hours to play with your toddler while you nap, shop, or go for a walk. Accept offers from relatives and friends to babysit or run errands—you'll get a break, and they'll feel good about helping you out.

Your Job

How to Break the News to Your Boss

Now that your first trimester is behind you, you're probably ready to let the cat out of the bag at work (unless you couldn't wait or early-pregnancy symptoms already made your announce-ment for you). This is an important discus-sion, and it's vital that you handle it professionally.

Do your homework. If you can, find out about your pregnancy and maternity leave options before talking to your supervisor. Review your employee hand-book, or discreetly contact a human re-sources or union representative who can clue you in about your employer's formal pregnancy and maternity policies. These reps will likely offer you informed and objective advice, since they've probably counseled many women in similar situations, and they won't be personally affected by your upcoming absence.

> **BY THE NUMBERS**
>
> **The Boss's Reaction**
>
> **83%** of moms-to-be said their boss was support-ive when they revealed their pregnancy.
>
> **17%** said their supervisor didn't take the news well.
>
> *Source: A BabyCenter.com poll of more than 54,000 women*

Seek out support. If you're lucky enough to be in a workplace where there are new mothers or—better yet—other pregnant women, seek out their support and counsel (make sure you can trust them with your secret, though, because your boss should hear the news from you before it travels through the office grapevine). Ask them what kind of response they got when they announced their pregnancies, which managers were helpful—and which weren't—when it came to accommodating any special needs they had, what their maternity leave proposals were like, and how much time they took off after their babies were born.

Make a plan. Though you won't need to finalize all the details of your maternity leave plan quite yet, it's good to start thinking about them now. Figure out how much time you'll want to take off once your baby arrives. If you're considering taking unpaid leave, carefully calculate how long you can reasonably afford to go without your salary. Also consider whether you'll want to take your maternity leave as one big block of time or you'd rather parcel it out (by coming back to work on a part-time schedule for the first few months, perhaps). As you start to discuss taking leave with your super-visor, be ready to offer solutions to potential problems and concerns she may raise. For instance, come prepared with ideas for how your workload could be handled while you're away and which colleagues are best suited for shoul-dering particular aspects of your job.

What to Do If Your Supervisor Isn't Supportive

Not every manager musters an appropriate and gracious response to the news of an employee's pregnancy. The sad truth is that being pregnant can affect how you're treated at work. Your boss and coworkers may worry or even assume that your work will suffer, that your responsibilities will be dumped on them when you're out on leave, and that you won't come back after the baby arrives. If you get a negative reaction when you break your baby news, respond professionally, positively, and firmly. Assure your employer that you'll do whatever it takes to ensure a smooth transition for all involved.

If you're demoted, laid off, or even fired after announcing your pregnancy, consult your human resources or union representative or call the National Association of Working Women at (800) 522-0925. Also be sure to look into your rights under the federal Pregnancy Discrimination Act, which prohibits job bias or discrimination against pregnant women. If you've been let go unjustly, consider hiring a lawyer to help you make your case.

Keep your options open. Your supervisor may ask you point-blank if you really plan to return to work after your baby is born. This is not a question that you have to answer, and in fact it's not a question that you can be expected to know the answer to before you actually become a mother. It's hard to predict how you'll feel once your baby is actually here or what your family needs will be in terms of time and income. If you tell your boss that you plan to resign after your baby is born, you may lose health insurance and other benefits the day you walk out the door. Technically, you have until the end of your maternity leave to decide whether you'll come back full-time, part-time, or not at all.

Deciphering Your Employer's Maternity Leave Policy

Do STD and FMLA sound like alphabet soup to you? Not sure what will happen to your benefits when you're out on leave? There's a lot to sort out when you're researching your maternity leave options. A look at the different types of leave, and how to figure out what you've got coming to you:

Maternity Leave

Maternity leave is the time you take off work after the birth of your child. Actual paid maternity leave is unusual in the United States, although some companies do offer new parents up to six weeks of paid time off. Most likely, though, you'll use a combination of short-term disability, sick leave, vacation, personal days, and unpaid family leave to cover your time away from the office. (Your employer's policy may dictate the order in which you can take different kinds of leave.)

BabyCenter Buzz

How I Found Support at Work

"I work in a predominantly male office, so I rely on the few other women there to keep me truckin'! The mothers love to tell stories about when they were pregnant, and they're great about coming around to see how I'm feeling." —*Lyn*

"There were several other pregnant women at my company. Unfortunately, we all worked in different departments and didn't have much regular contact. I asked if they were interested in setting up an e-mail exchange. They eagerly agreed, so we added a group list to our address books and kept in touch about things like getting together for lunchtime walks or checking out the prenatal yoga class at the local gym. Not only did I not feel so alone at work, but I found several new friends who were hiding right under my nose." —*Meredith*

"Surprisingly, I get most of my support from the older women at my workplace who've already had their kids—rather than from the women my age, since none of them are pregnant yet and they don't seem to be able to relate." —*Stacy*

Short-Term Disability

Short-term disability (STD) insurance will cover your salary (or a portion of it) while you're sidelined with pregnancy complications or recuperating from childbirth. Many large employers and unions offer it, as do several states. (It's generally provided automatically—not as an optional benefit that you have to sign up for.) If your *state* provides STD benefits, you may have a small amount deducted from each paycheck to cover your share. If your *employer or union* provides STD, they may cover the cost for you.

STD through your employer or a private provider generally pays 50 to 100 percent of your salary for a certain number of weeks, depending on how many years you've worked for your company. Six weeks is standard, but some plans allow more time if you've had a c-section or other labor or postpartum complications, and should also cover complications prior to birth when your doctor or midwife has certified that you can't work for health reasons.

State STD benefits typically cover half to two-thirds of your salary, and the maximum length of coverage for serious pregnancy complications varies from plan to plan. For the postpartum period, STD typically covers six weeks of recovery time for a vaginal delivery and eight weeks for a c-section.

If both your state and your employer offer STD, you may be required

Taxes and Disability Income

Whatever portion of your salary you get from your employer's short-term disability coverage is taxable, but no income taxes will be taken out of your checks. That means you'll have to cough it up to Uncle Sam come April 15, so don't forget to set aside a portion of this money for your tax bill. (That said, you'll be able to take an extra deduction for your new dependent, which may offset what you owe.) State disability benefits, on the other hand, generally aren't subject to federal or state income taxes. If you pay for private disability insurance yourself, your benefits are also tax-free.

to use the full state benefit and have your employer's coverage make up the rest. You'll still end up with the same amount of disability pay, but you'll get it in two checks—one from the state and one from your company's provider. Many disability programs require that you be out of work for several days before you can start to collect STD benefits, so you may have to use sick days or accrued vacation to cover this interim period.

If you decide to report back to work once your STD coverage runs out, you may be able to use saved up vacation, personal, or sick days to extend your leave beyond that point. Some companies will even let you take vacation or sick days that you haven't yet earned—though they'll probably make you reimburse them for those days if you decide to quit your job at the end of your leave.

You may also be eligible for unpaid disability leave once your paid leave ends. If you're still not physically ready to go back to work when your STD coverage runs out, some states will let you take a certain amount of unpaid disability leave after that. During that time, your employer must hold your job open until you're able to return (or until the leave period runs out). If you're physically able to go back to work but you want or need more time with your child, you may be eligible for state- or federally-mandated family leave. With either unpaid disability or family leave, though, your employer may require you to first use up any remaining vacation or sick days you have.

Family and Medical Leave

The federal Family and Medical Leave Act (FMLA) allows up to 12 weeks of unpaid family leave during pregnancy or following the birth of a child, after which you must be allowed to return to your job (or to a comparable one). It's the very minimum that's required; some states have more generous leave plans.

If you're planning to take leave under the FMLA, it's best to give your boss as much advance notice as you can. But if you need to go on leave sud-

Just the Facts

Who Can Take Family Leave

You're among the 60 percent of U.S. workers eligible for leave under the FMLA if you meet all of the following requirements: (Note, though, that eligibility for your state family policy may be less stringent.)

- You work for the federal, state, or local government or for any company with at least 50 employees within 75 miles of your workplace.

- You've worked for your employer for at least 12 months and logged at least 1,250 hours in the year before your leave starts (which comes out to about 24 hours a week).

- You're not among the highest-paid 10 percent of employees at your company, and you're not among those whose absence would cause "substantial economic harm" to the organization.

- You and your partner don't both work for the same company. In that case, you're entitled only to a combined 12 weeks of parental leave between the two of you.

denly due to unforeseen circumstances (such as preterm labor), you'll still be able to do so. Your employer will likely require that all the paid leave you're planning to take (STD, vacation, sick days) count toward the 12-week total. But some states and individual employers will let you take the full 12 weeks of unpaid leave in addition to whatever paid leave you're planning to use.

You can parcel out your unpaid leave any way you want during your pregnancy and the first year of your child's life. That means you can take it all at once (right after giving birth, say) or—provided your employer agrees—spread it out by taking time off in chunks and/or reducing your normal weekly or daily work schedule for a few months after your return to work. For instance, you may decide to take off two weeks before your due date, then six weeks after, and finally come back half-time for the first eight weeks. Or you may take off six weeks after your child is born, return to work for a period of time while your partner takes his family leave, and then take off your remaining six weeks after he returns to work.

If you're considering unpaid leave, think carefully about how much time you can reasonably afford to take. Also think about whether your partner can take off any time and when it would be best for him to do that. You both may decide to take leave right after your baby is born, but if you want to stretch out the time that at least one of you is home with your baby, consider overlapping your leaves, taking them consecutively, or spreading your time off over the year.

Your Employment Benefits during Maternity Leave

The FMLA requires that your company keep you on its health insurance plan while you're on leave, whether it's disability or family leave. Typically, your company will pay your health premiums for you but ask to be reim-

---

WORKSHEET: MATERNITY LEAVE CHECKLIST

If you're not sure what questions to ask or whom to turn to when trying to sort out your maternity leave options, use this checklist to keep it straight.

QUESTIONS TO ASK YOUR COWORKERS:

How much time did you take off, and how did you structure your leave?

What arrangements did you make to have your responsibilities covered while you were gone?

How did you transition back to work afterward?

Have you arranged any kind of flexible schedule since you returned?

QUESTIONS TO ASK YOUR HUMAN RESOURCES DEPARTMENT OR UNION REPRESENTATIVE:

Does the company or union offer paid maternity leave? How many days?

Am I entitled to short-term disability pay through the state, my union, or a company policy?

How many weeks are covered at what percentage?

Can I take additional time if I have practitioner-certified complications?

Can I buy additional STD coverage through the company's or union's provider?

Do I have to use state STD benefits first, if they're available?

bursed for your share—the amount that's normally taken out of your pay-check. (If your company normally picks up the entire amount, they're re-quired by law to continue to do so.) In rare cases, though, your employer may choose to put you on COBRA, a program in which you're covered under the same plan but must pay the entire premium yourself (at a cost of several hundred dollars a month).

If you decide during your leave that you won't be returning to work after all or if your job is eliminated while you're gone, your employer can stop

Can I take additional time if I have complications?

How and when do I apply for STD?

Is there a waiting period before I can collect benefits?

How many vacation, personal, or sick days will I have accrued by my due date?

Are there any limitations to how I can use these days?

Do I have to use vacation, personal, or sick days before any other kind of leave?

Can I take vacation days that I haven't yet accrued?

Am I eligible for 12 weeks of unpaid family leave under the FMLA?

Am I eligible for paid or unpaid family leave under my state's provisions or company or union policy? How much, and when can I take it?

Will I have to wait longer to be eligible for a raise, more annual vacation time, or other employee benefits if I take unpaid leave?

How will my health insurance premiums be handled while I'm on leave?

Will I still be covered by life insurance, and how will premiums for any extra cov-erage I may have be handled while I'm on leave?

Will any of my other employee benefits be affected?

Filing a Complaint against Your Employer

If you believe your employer is wrongly denying you pregnancy or maternity leave, contact your regional office of the Wage and Hour Division of the U.S. Department of Labor (www.dol.gov/esa/whd/) to file a complaint. A phone call from a Labor Department rep to your employer usually resolves most leave issues. If your problem persists, the Labor Department will investigate your complaint and may sue your employer on your behalf. If you don't get immediate results, consider hiring a labor lawyer to help you. If you can't afford to retain an attorney, find out whether there are legal aid groups or other advocacy groups in your community who can help.

paying your premiums and may even require you to pay back the money spent on premiums up to that point in your leave. (The exception to this rule is if you don't return to work due to circumstances beyond your control—if you develop a serious medical condition, say, or your spouse gets a job transfer that requires your family to relocate.)

Your company does not have to allow you to accrue other benefits when you're out on leave. That means the clock may stop on things like vacation days earned and your length of service when it comes to qualifying for:

• Raises based on seniority or time served

• Additional vacation days based on time served

• Participation in your company's 401(k) plan or vesting of your company's matching investment

• Vesting of stock options

Finally, you won't be able to contribute to your 401(k) or flexible spending account while you're taking unpaid leave because you won't be receiving a paycheck and thus can't contribute pretax dollars.

Your Money

Dollars and Sense: Sorting Through Your Family's Finances

Even if you're a whiz at juggling grocery bills, housing expenses, student loans, and credit card debt, factoring in new expenses such as hospital bills, baby gear, diapers, and child care will put your financial savvy to the test. Use the next few months to scrutinize your spending and tweak it as needed to ensure that your bank account can handle what lies ahead. And while no one wants to dwell on worst-case scenarios, now's also a good time to start thinking about what you can do to protect your child should anything happen to you or your mate.

Plan for the Future: Reevaluate Your Life Insurance and Write a Will

Thinking about death isn't easy—especially when a new life is in the making. But as difficult as it is, it's crucial to make time for a heart-to-heart with your partner about the possibility that one or both of you could pass away or become disabled before your child is grown. By planning for the unspeakable, you'll ensure that your family will still be able to make the mortgage, cover health expenses, pay for other debts, and write those college tuition checks when the time comes.

The Ins and Outs of Insurance

Though the typical advice is to buy six to ten times your annual salary in life insurance coverage, how much your family actually needs depends on a number of factors.

• How much you spend each year on items like housing, food, and clothing

• How much you'll need to cover large onetime expenses, such as your children's college educations

• How much your mate earns (hence how much of your family's expenses that covers)

• How much your investments and other assets are worth (hence how much of your family's expenses they'll cover)

When it comes to selecting life insurance, you have two basic choices: term or whole life. Term insurance works like car or homeowner's coverage:

If you die while the policy is active, your family gets the money for which you're covered. If you don't die, the policy expires and the insurance company keeps the money you've paid (still better than the alternative!). Some term policies give you the right to renew at the same rate, though they're generally a bit more expensive.

Term insurance makes sense for most young, middle-income families because it covers a set period, with affordable premiums. A typical premium for $250,000 in coverage might be $150 to $200 a year for a 30-year-old nonsmoker. Rates are fixed when you buy, and increase as you age.

Whole life insurance, also called cash-value insurance, offers both an insurance policy and an investment account. The premiums are significantly more expensive, but a portion of those funds go into a tax-deferred savings account. The rates are fixed: You'll pay the same premium at 30 as you will at 60. Upon your death, your spouse or family will collect the death benefit. But you can also choose to cash out the policy when you're older or retired and net the tax-deferred savings.

The Whys and Wherefores of Wills

Though you may assume that your assets will go to your partner if the unthinkable were to happen, he or she may inherit as little as a third of your property unless you specify otherwise in a will (and a will is absolutely *vital* if you and your mate aren't married). Likewise, though a relative or close friend may be your first choice to raise your child and manage your property if you and your partner both died, in actuality your lack of a will—and an appointed legal guardian for your baby-to-be—means that you're leaving these decisions in the court's hands. So steel yourself, and plot out what you'd want to happen if you and your mate passed away.

You don't necessarily need a lawyer to write a will. If you choose to do it yourself, you'll need to invest time, energy, and probably a little money to do it right. Many families have written legally valid wills with a self-help book or a will-writing software program. Here's a good rule: If the cost of hiring a lawyer is holding you back from writing a will, buy a book or software program and do it yourself—or ask your public librarian to guide you to the latest books on the subject.

On the other hand, if you have substantial assets or if the thought of plowing through pages of legalese is too daunting and you have some cash to spare, call a family lawyer or a lawyer who specializes in trusts and estates (ask for recommendations from family and friends). A lawyer will run you anywhere from a few hundred to a few thousand dollars, but that kind of cash buys you expertise and peace of mind. To save money, think through what you want to include in your will first and then contact a lawyer to go over the finer details.

Whichever option you choose, a few ideas to get you started:

• Choose a guardian for your children; then choose an alternate guardian in case your first choice is unwilling or unable to do the job.

• Make a list of all your assets, including bank accounts, investments, real estate, life insurance, pension plans or retirement accounts, and personal property.

• Decide exactly whom you want to inherit what—and when. For instance, you might want your daughter to inherit the gold bracelet your mother gave you when she turns 16.

• Decide if you want someone else to handle the assets you leave your children. If so, choose that person.

• Choose an executor to carry out your wishes and handle the necessary paperwork after you die.

• Decide if you want to include a letter stating how you'd like your children to be raised and educated, how you want your funeral arranged, and so on.

There are several requirements for making your will a legal document:

• It usually must be typed or computer-generated. Handwritten wills are legal in only some states.

• You must state somewhere in the document that it is your will.

• You must outline your decisions about property and guardianship of your children.

> ## QUICK TIP
>
> **Check Your Beneficiaries**
>
> Certain assets—such as life insurance policies, 401(k)s, and IRA accounts—have beneficiary forms that supersede wills. That means the funds in these accounts will be distributed to whomever you named as beneficiaries, no matter what you specify in your will. Be sure to check the beneficiaries on these accounts—and make any necessary changes—to match up with your will.

- You must date and sign your will.
- You must sign your will in the presence of at least two witnesses (three in some states), and your witnesses must also sign.

A legal will doesn't have to be notarized, nor does it have to be recorded or registered with any government agency. After your will has been signed, put it in a safe and fairly obvious place, like a locked metal file cabinet, and tell your spouse, partner, or executor where you put it. It's a good idea to have two signed copies (not photocopies) and to keep them in separate locations. Safe-deposit boxes aren't always a good place for a will because many banks restrict who can withdraw items from them. If a family member or executor can't open your safe deposit box, it could tie up your estate for some time. Make sure you understand your bank's rules about withdrawals from safe-deposit boxes before you lock your will inside one.

Staying Healthy and Comfortable on the Road

Now that you've passed the 13-week mark, a business or pleasure trip probably sounds more appealing. Morning sickness and bone-deep fatigue are likely becoming a thing of the past, and the risk of miscar-

BabyCenter Buzz

Taking a "Babymoon"

"We took a romantic hiking trip to get away from it all before the big arrival."
—*Anonymous*

"As soon as I found out I was pregnant, we booked a trip to Las Vegas. It was a blast! I had to get that out of my system." —*Kim*

"The two of us go away for a weekend every December to celebrate our anniversary. Last year our son was two months old, but that didn't stop us from going. And my being 18 weeks pregnant this year isn't stopping us either. Mom and Dad need time together, too, regardless of what else is going on." —*Anonymous*

riage is greatly diminished. It's a perfect time to take advantage of your newfound well being by visiting friends and family who want to share in the excitement of your pregnancy. Or how about a romantic getaway for you and your partner—a last chance for a pre-baby honeymoon?

As good as you may be feeling right now, it's important to remember that you are pregnant. Take these simple steps to take care of yourself and the precious cargo you're carrying, even when you're away from home.

Get medical clearance. Discuss your trip plans with your doctor or midwife ahead of time. If you're carrying twins or have certain complications—such as diabetes, high blood pressure, placental abnormalities, a history of blood clotting disorder, or a risk for preterm labor—your healthcare provider will probably advise you to stay close to home. (Well-controlled mild gestational diabetes shouldn't be a problem.) Also, get a referral to an obstetrician or midwife at your destination in case you need medical attention during your vacation.

Pack medical supplies. It never hurts to be prepared when you're on the road—so pack a basic first-aid kit. The items you'll need will depend on where you're going and how long you'll be there (travel to a major metropolitan area with 24-hour pharmacies is one thing—camping in a remote area or venturing overseas is quite another). You can buy a ready-made kit or put one together yourself. What to include:

- Your prescription medications
- Prenatal vitamins
- Acetaminophen
- Antacids
- Thermometer

BY THE NUMBERS

Travel Challenges

37% of expectant mothers say that constantly needing a restroom makes travel difficult.

21% cite dealing with fatigue as their big on-the-road battle.

14% worry about miscarriage.

11% are anxious about going into preterm labor away from home.

7% say swollen feet slowed them down.

Source: *A BabyCenter.com poll of more than 10,500 women*

- Liquid cleanser that doesn't require water, or moist towelettes
- Antiseptic wipes for cleaning cuts and scrapes
- Antibiotic ointment
- Tweezers for removing splinters or ticks
- Rubbing alcohol to clean thermometers, tweezers, and scissors
- Assorted bandages and sterile gauze (pads and roll)
- Adhesive tape and small scissors
- Broad-spectrum sunscreen and lip protection with SPF 15 or higher
- Calamine lotion to soothe insect bites and rashes
- Insect-sting kit (if you're allergic to bees or other insects)
- Topical anesthetic spray to cool sunburns
- Cold pack to reduce swelling from bumps, strains, bites, and minor burns (get the kind you simply squeeze to start the cooling reaction)
- Electrolyte replacement solution to prevent diarrhea-related dehydration

Schedule around prenatal tests. You'll need to fit your travel plans around upcoming prenatal tests, allowing time to get the results and plan any next steps in response. The following tests are ones you may need to keep in mind when making your travel plans.

- **Amniocentesis:** 15 to 20 weeks (it's usually done around 16 weeks)
- **Multiple marker screening:** 15 to 20 weeks (usually done between 16 and 18 weeks)
- **Ultrasound:** 16 to 20 weeks
- **Glucose screening test:** 24 to 28 weeks

Pack your health info and medications. Carry a copy of your medical history, which should include pregnancy risk factors, your due date, your blood type, any medications you're currently taking, and any that you're allergic to. See our emergency contact sheet (page 117) for pregnant travelers for a complete list of names, phone numbers, and information to have with you when you travel. Don't forget to take along any medications you'll need, including your prenatal vitamins.

Steer clear of risky activities. It's important to avoid sports or other activities where you risk collision or falling. That usually means no downhill skiing, water-skiing, surfing, horseback riding, or ice-skating. Scuba diving is also out because dangerous air bubbles can form in your (and your baby's) bloodstream as you surface. Waterslides and many amusement park rides are risky as well because a forceful landing and sudden starts and stops can harm your baby. Raising your internal temperature during pregnancy can increase the risk of birth defects, so avoid hot tubs and saunas, too.

Take care of your tummy. Part of the fun of travel is eating out—no grocery shopping, cooking, or dirty dishes to worry about. But overindulging—or indulging in the wrong things—can worsen already bothersome bloating, indigestion, heartburn, and constipation. (See page 116 for advice on eating and drinking wisely to keep your inner workings in good order.)

Get enough rest. As tempting as it is to try to see and do it all on vacation, schedule some downtime. Your body is working hard to create a new person, and deserves regular pampering. So plan for time to nap or just put your feet up a couple of times a day.

Dress for ease and comfort. To accommodate frequent trips to the bathroom, choose a dress or separates (skirt or pants with a top), rather than a jumpsuit or overalls. The fewer fasteners, the better. Layer your clothing to cope with sudden temperature changes, from the arctic blast of an air-conditioned airport to the stifling heat of a crowded bus. Choose breathable, wrinkle-resistant fabrics such as stretchy cotton knits in coordinating colors and patterns. And don't forget to pack a wide-brimmed hat for sun protection.

Choose comfortable, supportive footwear. The best shoes or sandals have a contoured foot bed to help prevent aches and a thick, skid-resistant sole for good traction and good support for walking. Sneakers built for high-impact aerobic sports fit the bill; strappy heels and mules do not. Elastic inserts, ties, or adjustable straps are perfect for when your feet swell. Maternity support panty hose, available at most maternity clothing stores, can help prevent circulation problems when you're sitting for long stretches in a car or on a plane.

Getting There by Plane

As long as you're healthy and your pregnancy is progressing normally, it's safe to fly during most of your pregnancy. Granted, a plane ride isn't always

BabyCenter Buzz

Plane Trip Tips

"It's easiest to just sleep through the plane rides. I booked a late-afternoon flight and skipped my regular nap—I was out like a light once the plane took off. The reverse trip was a red-eye, so it was even easier to sleep through it."
—*Katrina*

"My biggest issues were nausea, frequent bathroom trips, and jet lag/lack of sleep. My tips:

- Call the airline, explain that you're pregnant, and nicely ask for a bulkhead seat near a bathroom. Also mention it when you check in.

- Get an aisle seat—you won't feel as bad about inconveniencing your traveling companions by getting up ten times during the flight.

- Take lots of snacks that you like: crackers, oranges, celery sticks, nuts, and rice cakes worked for me.

- On night flights especially, wear a comfy pair of leggings or sweats.

- If you're a tea drinker, take caffeine-free herbal tea bags with you—most airlines don't have decaf on board, but they'll happily bring you hot water and lemon." —*SVDUB*

the most comfortable way to travel because you don't have as much freedom to stretch out and walk around, but it's mercifully quick compared with other forms of long-distance transportation.

Air-Travel Advice

• Request a seat in the middle of the plane over the wing for the smoothest ride, or a bulkhead seat for more legroom. (Don't bother asking for a seat by an emergency exit, though, because airlines prefer more "able-bodied" passengers in those seats.) In either case, reserve a seat on the aisle to facilitate bathroom runs and stretch breaks.

• Combat foot and ankle swelling by taking off your shoes and elevating your legs. Either rest your feet on your carry-on luggage under the seat in front of you or, if the seat next to you is empty, put your feet up there. If you're prone to varicose veins or swelling, wear maternity support panty hose to help quell these complaints.

• Keep your blood circulating by strolling the aisle every hour and doing some simple stretches every half-hour. Flex your feet to stretch your calf muscles, rotate your ankles, and wiggle your toes.

• When seated, keep your seat belt fastened under your belly and low on your hips.

• Drink plenty of fluids to stave off the dehydrating effects of dry cabin air. Caffeine acts as a diuretic, so pass on in-flight coffee, tea, and soft drinks in favor of water, juice, or milk.

• Beware of gas-producing meals or drinks before takeoff. The trapped gas from foods such as cabbage and beans expands at higher altitude, making for an uncomfortable trip.

• Dress comfortably, and bring a thick pair of socks to wear around the cabin if you take your shoes off.

Getting There by Train

The rhythmic rocking motion, steady clickety-clack of the wheels against the tracks, and the landscape unfolding outside your window make trains an especially appealing mode of travel for moms-to-be. In European and

Ask the Experts

Is It Safe to Use a Seat Belt When I'm Pregnant?

Ann Linden, certified nurse-midwife: Absolutely! It's dangerous *not* to. To avoid injuring your baby, though, the belt must be properly fastened. A lap belt should be secured *below* your belly and across your hips so that it lies snugly over your pelvis (one of the strongest bones in your body). Never wear the belt *across* your belly—during a crash, the sudden jolt could cause the placenta to tear away from your uterus. Always use a shoulder belt, too, if the vehicle you're riding in has one. It should fit snugly between your breasts. If the shoulder belt cuts across your neck, try repositioning the belt or your seat so the belt fits better.

Your body provides a cushion for your baby and helps keep her safe. That means the best way to protect your growing baby is to protect *yourself*—by wearing a properly positioned seat belt.

QUICK TIPS

Preparing for Road Emergencies

Carry a cell phone and sign up for roadside assistance to save yourself the potential aggravation and risk of changing a flat tire with a bulging belly. Also stock your car with these supplies in case you're stuck for a while:

- Warm clothes and a blanket
- A flashlight
- Drinking water and nonperishable snacks
- Toilet paper and a container to pee in
- Flares

other countries, trains are the transportation of choice—they're very convenient and often downright luxurious. Stateside train lines have no restrictions for pregnant travelers but as a general policy suggest that pregnant passengers check with their doctor or midwife before traveling (good advice for *any* type of trip).

Train travel can be one of the most comfortable means of transportation. You'll enjoy greater freedom of movement on a train than in a car, bus, or plane. It's easy to walk around and stretch your legs, provided you watch out for unexpected lurches and moving floor panels between cars. Since you don't have to worry about negotiating traffic, you can read a book, listen to music, or simply close your eyes and drift away. Restrooms tend to be numerous (usually one per car), if not always super clean or freshly stocked with supplies. Many trains have dining cars or snack bars, though prices can be steep and the quality and variety of the food limited. And sleeping compartments, however small, outshine the alternative on a plane or bus or in a car.

Train Travel Tips

Trains do have a few drawbacks: A cross-country trip takes several days, in contrast to a five-hour flight. And bench-style seating, still common on many short-distance runs, can be hard on your bottom and back. Some strategies for enhancing your journey:

- It's worth paying the higher fare to book a sleeping compartment if you're taking an overnight or extended train trip. Make sure you reserve a lower berth so you can get in and out easily, but avoid noisy compartments directly over the wheels.
- Ask for a compartment with separate bathroom facilities, instead of one with beds that must be raised to get to the toilet.

- Request a blanket and a pillow as soon as you board.
- Get up and walk around every hour that you're awake to keep your circulation moving.
- Bring along some of your own food (especially fresh fruits and veggies) because dining-car fare may amount to cellophane-wrapped sandwiches and snack food, often at exorbitant prices. But pack only what you can carry or fit in a suitcase on wheels because you may not be able to find a porter who can carry your bags.
- Dress in layers, since some cars can be hot and stuffy, while others are drafty and cold.
- If you know you're going to need help with your bags or with boarding the train, call a ticket agent at least 24 hours before you travel to ask about special services. You may be able to request special meals, too.

Getting There by Car

There's no reason to sit out a road trip just because you're pregnant—provided you allow extra time for bathroom and stretch breaks. If you

BabyCenter Buzz

How I Survived a Long Car Trip

"Make sure the air conditioner works! And if you can, take along a second driver. Although you'll still be sitting in the car just as long, it helps to be able to stretch out your legs on the passenger side." —*Veronica*

"We just took a nine-hour car trip. I was miserable with lower-back pain on the way up, but my mother-in-law loaned me a small, partially inflated air pillow to put behind my back for the ride home, and it made all the difference. I was actually comfortable for the entire drive back." —*Mary*

"Keep a thermos filled with boiled water and some herbal tea bags. Stop and take a tea break whenever you want to relax and refresh yourself." —*Tami*

"Bring a big bottle of water with you—and drink it. This forces you to take frequent pee breaks and stretch your legs. Plan on the trip taking longer than usual, too. Don't have an aggressive driving schedule because you won't want to push yourself." —*Chris*

Just the Facts

In the Event of an Accident

If you're in a car accident—whether it's a fender bender or something more serious—it's important to be examined as soon as possible. Even if you feel fine, call your doctor or midwife or head to an emergency room right away. While your womb does offer some protection for your baby and placenta during a sudden impact, a severe jolt can cause your placenta to partially or completely tear away from the wall of your uterus. Called a placental abruption, this can lead to serious problems such as hemorrhage, miscarriage, preterm delivery, or stillbirth. (In fact, anytime you receive a blow to the abdomen during pregnancy, you need to be evaluated.)

In the emergency room, you'll have a thorough obstetric exam and an ultrasound to check on your baby and placenta. Depending on how far along you are in your pregnancy and whether you have symptoms such as bleeding or contractions, you and your baby may be monitored for several hours or even admitted to the hospital for a thorough evaluation. If you're Rh negative, you may be given a shot of Rh immunoglobulin if there's any chance that your blood has mixed with your baby's.

After you're released, you'll need to be on high alert for any vaginal bleeding, leaking fluid, contractions or other abdominal pain, or a noticeable decline in the baby's movement. If you have any of these symptoms, call your doctor or midwife right away.

can, bring a companion so you don't have to do all the driving and will have a chance to nap and relax en route.

Car Comfort Tips

• Take a break from driving at least every 90 minutes. (You may need to stop more often than that for bathroom breaks anyway.) Pull over at a rest area to walk around and do some simple stretches.

• If you're riding shotgun, keep your seat reclined to a comfortable position (with your seat belt on), and try these simple exercises: Extend your leg, heel first, and gently flex your foot to stretch your calf muscles. Then rotate your ankles and wiggle your toes.

• Before you leave home, pack toilet paper (remove the inner card-

Just the Facts

All About Air Bags

Air bags are as safe during pregnancy as they are at any other time—as long as you buckle your seat belt correctly. In a crash, the seat belt helps restrain your upper body and keeps you as far as possible from the steering wheel or dashboard, and the air bag helps to distribute the impact of the crash. Because air bags open with tremendous force, there is some risk of injury associated with them, but safety experts believe the bags' protective benefits far outweigh any potential harm.

To minimize the risk, sit as far back from the air bag as possible. Move your seat back or recline it to allow at least 10 inches from the center of your breastbone to the air bag (located in either the steering wheel or the dashboard). Avoid leaning or reaching forward, and sit back against your seat with as little slack in your seat belt as possible—this minimizes your forward movement in a crash and allows the air bag to open without hitting you. If it's too hard to sit 10 inches from the air bag and comfortably reach the steering wheel or pedals, boost yourself up a bit by sitting on a cushion. If you're still too close to the wheel, check your vehicle owner's manual or visit your local authorized car dealer for advice about adjusting your position.

board tube and flatten the roll for compact carrying), disposable toilet seat covers, sanitary wipes, and antibacterial hand cleanser.

- You may also want to wear a sanitary pad to combat leaks and tuck a spare pair of undies into your purse in case you don't quite make it to the john.

Getting There by Boat

Cruising can make for a relaxing, romantic prebaby vacation. With bracing ocean breezes and countless ship and shore activities to try, your biggest problem may be how to avoid getting worn-out by all the excitement. You'll find a wide selection of full meals and snacks to satisfy almost any craving, 24 hours a day. Most cruise lines offer room service as well. Fortunately, you'll probably also find plenty of ways to work off those extra calories as you sail. Many ships offer both group and individual exercise programs, early-morning deck walks, swimming, stationary cycling, yoga, and even resistance training in the onboard gym.

Cruising Tips

Safeguard your health. Check with the cruise line about whether a doctor or nurse will be on board. Keep in mind that many smaller ships (those carrying fewer than 100 passengers) aren't required to have medical personnel on staff. And don't count on a shipboard pharmacy to stock your medications. Bring a supply to last the entire trip. Also find out if your health insurance policy covers any complications on board or at any of the ports of call. If not, you can buy additional travel medical coverage from most cruise lines or directly from insurance companies.

Check your dates. Most cruise operators don't allow women to sail after about week 26. Specific policies vary, though, so check with the cruise line before booking your trip. It's a good idea to carry a letter from your health-care provider stating your due date, medical condition, travel fitness, and any medications you're taking. That way, you can avoid unpleasant surprises at the boarding dock.

Get your sea legs. Pregnancy won't make you more likely to feel seasick, but ocean travel can upset your stomach whether you're pregnant or not. If you're prone to motion sickness, you're likely to feel queasy at sea. And if you're still suffering from morning sickness, the motion of the boat may make your nausea and vomiting worse.

When choosing a cruise, keep in mind that the larger ships tend to be the stablest on rough seas. Request a cabin in the middle of the ship, close to the waterline, for the smoothest ride. Before you sail, ask your health-care provider about seasickness medications and other remedies that are safe during pregnancy. Once you're on board, spend as much time on deck as possible. If you start to feel nauseated, fix your gaze on the horizon. Frequent light, nongreasy snacks, such as crackers, can also help soothe an unsettled stomach.

Sleep tight. When you book your cruise, ask for a cabin with a full- or queen-size bed, since shipboard bunks tend to be very narrow. Once you board, ask the cabin steward for extra blankets and pillows, too.

Try on your life preserver. Adult life preservers, also called personal flotation devices, are usually unisex, which translates to "huge." They usually fit easily over a pregnant belly. But the only way to know for sure is to try one on as soon as you arrive at your cabin. If yours is too small or if you need help adjusting it around your belly, ask the cabin steward for assistance.

PART III

THE THIRD TRIMESTER: 28 TO 41 WEEKS

At last, the end is near! These last few months may be marked by a mixture of impatience (I feel like I've been pregnant forever!), nervousness (How will I know when I'm really in labor?), and excitement (Our baby's almost here!). Fatigue is likely to return as your body makes one last push to grow that baby. Still, you may feel a surge of energy right before you give birth—the so-called "nesting" phenomenon. In this chapter, you'll discover how your baby's getting ready for his grand entrance—and how your body continues to change as delivery day draws near.

Third-Trimester Highlights

During this trimester, your baby will:

▶ Gain about 5 pounds and grow about 5 inches

▶ Develop smoother skin, fingernails and toenails, and bona fide hair

▶ Continue forming neurological pathways—the building blocks for learning—in the brain

▶ Complete all physical development

▶ Turn head down and drop into your pelvis

You will:

▶ Graduate from your childbirth class

▶ See your healthcare provider once a week starting around 36 weeks

▶ See your baby's tiny fists and feet punch and kick

▶ Feel more fatigue as your body grows ever larger and sleep becomes more difficult

▶ Gain about 11 pounds

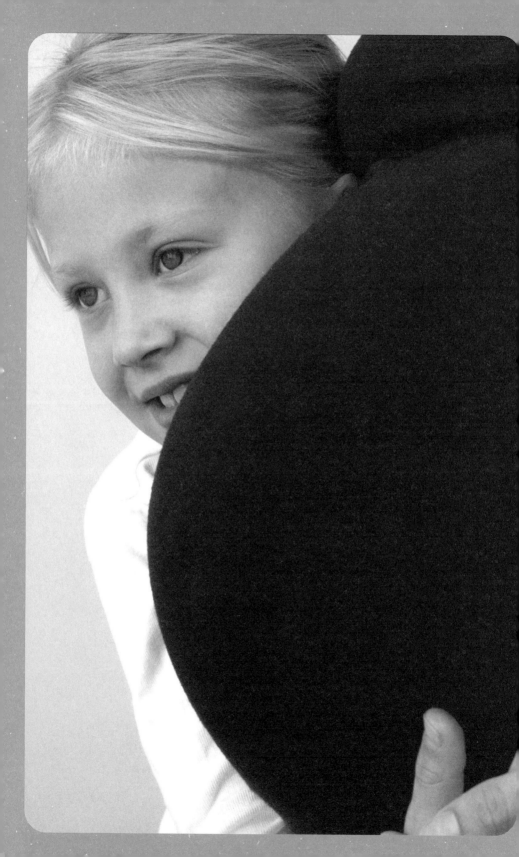

YOUR PREGNANCY WEEK BY WEEK

Your Pregnancy: 28 Weeks
Your Changing Body

At this point, you'll likely visit your doctor or midwife every two weeks; then, at 36 weeks, you'll switch to weekly visits. Depending on your risk factors, your practitioner may recommend repeating blood tests for HIV and syphilis now, as well as doing cultures for chlamydia and gonorrhea, to be certain of your status before delivery. Also, if your glucose screening test result was

HOT TOPICS

- Taking the glucose tolerance test (page 160)
- What to expect at your prenatal checkups (page 281)
- Common third-trimester complaints (page 293)
- Signs of preterm labor (page 297)
- Restless legs syndrome (page 317)

BabyCenter Buzz

What Other Women Say at 28 Weeks

"I can't believe how intrusive people are. Every stranger thinks it's okay to touch my stomach." —*Amy*

"It's great to really *look* pregnant now. I'm surprised at how differently I'm treated—in a good way!" —*Connilee*

"If I sleep on either side with a pillow tucked beneath my stomach, I can make it through the night—*just.*" —*Venece*

high and you haven't yet had follow-up testing, you'll soon be given the 3-hour glucose tolerance test. And if the blood work done at your first prenatal visit showed that you're Rh negative, you'll get an injection of Rh immunoglobulin to prevent your body from developing antibodies that could attack your baby's blood. (If your baby is indeed Rh positive and you're Rh negative, you'll receive another shot of Rh immunoglobulin after you give birth.)

Around this time, while trying to relax or sleep, some women feel a tingling in their lower legs and an irresistible urge to move them, a condition known as restless legs syndrome (RLS). No one knows what causes RLS, but it's relatively common among expectant mothers. Try cutting down on caffeine, which can make the symptoms worse, and massage your calves when they feel tense. If your iron stores are low, iron supplements may help ease the symptoms.

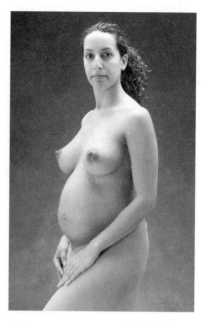

Your shape is undeniably pregnant. Your breasts are larger, your belly clearly announces your pregnancy, and your navel may go from an "innie" to an "outie." Loosening joints can make your larger body challenging to maneuver.

Your Growing Baby

By this week, your baby weighs a little over 2 pounds and measures almost 15 inches from head to heels. He can blink his eyes, which now sport lashes. With his eyesight maturing, your baby may actually be able to see the light that filters in through your womb.

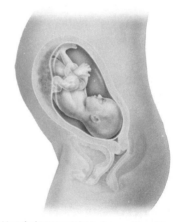

Your baby's eyesight is sharpening with each passing day. He's also developing billions of neurons in his brain and adding more body fat in preparation for life in the outside world.

Your Pregnancy: 29 Weeks

Your Changing Body

Some old friends—heartburn and constipation—may take center stage now. The pregnancy hormone progesterone relaxes smooth muscle tissue throughout your body, including your gastrointestinal tract. This relaxation, coupled with the crowding in your abdomen, slows digestion, which in turn can cause gas and heartburn—especially after a big meal—and contribute to constipation as well. Your growing uterus may also be contributing to hemorrhoids. These swollen blood vessels in your rectal area, which can cause pain, itching, and burning, are common during pregnancy—especially if you're constipated—and usually clear up in the weeks after giving birth.

> ### HOT TOPICS
>
> - Dealing with dizzy spells (page 168)
> - Good sources of calcium (page 193)
> - Warning signs you should never ignore (page 280)
> - How to do fetal kick counts (page 287)
> - Coping with constipation (page 298) and heartburn (page 301)

Some mothers-to-be develop a condition called "supine hypotensive syndrome." When you lie flat on your back, you get a change in heart rate and blood pressure that makes you feel dizzy until you change position. You might note that you feel lightheaded if you stand up too quickly, too. To avoid "the spins," lie on your side rather than your back, and move slowly as you go from lying down to sitting and then standing.

Your Growing Baby

Your baby now weighs about 2½ pounds and is a tad over 15 inches long from head to heel. Her muscles and lungs are continuing to mature, and her head is growing bigger to make room for her developing brain. To meet her increasing nutritional demands, you'll need plenty of protein, vitamin C, folic acid, and iron. And because her bones are soaking up lots of calcium, be sure to drink your milk (or find another good source of calcium, such as cheese, yogurt, or enriched orange juice). This trimester, about 250 milligrams of calcium are deposited in your baby's hardening skeleton each day.

Your baby's very active now. Pay attention to her kicks and nudges,

BabyCenter Buzz

What Other Women Say at 29 Weeks

"I've been in two modes for the past week: Slow and Stop! I want to go for a nice walk, and I can't even seem to get the energy to put my shoes on. It's pathetic!" —*Allison*

"I miss sleeping on my belly *so* much. I can't wait to lie on my stomach again. It's amazing how you miss small things like that." —*Kristen*

"I feel these weird pushing and rolling movements. I can feel the baby's body parts as they poke out and push across my belly, too. I had a dream about the baby's entire arm poking through—I could grab it!" —*Lindsey*

"I'm totally not interested in having sex right now. I feel so big and bulky, and my mind is preoccupied with labor and delivery—not making love." —*Anonymous*

"I had a couple of miscarriages before this pregnancy and was pretty anxious about carrying a baby to term. But now that I'm in the third trimester and my baby seems to be thriving, I've started to relax and am really trying to enjoy this time." —*Sherilyn*

and alert your practitioner if you notice them dropping off. She may ask you to do fetal kick counts to make sure everything's okay.

Your Pregnancy: 30 Weeks
Your Changing Body

You may be feeling a little tired these days, especially if you're having trouble sleeping at night. You might also feel clumsier than normal: Not only are you heavier (most women gain about 11 pounds this trimester), but the concentration of weight in your pregnant belly causes a shift in your center of gravity. Plus, thanks to pregnancy hormones, your ligaments are more lax, so your joints are looser, which

HOT TOPICS

- What—and when—to eat now (page 305)
- Understanding mood swings (page 328)
- Stashing away a "first-month" fund (page 358)
- Third-trimester travel tips (page 362)
- Too much or too little amniotic fluid (page 514)

may also contribute to your balance being a bit off. Finally, this relaxation of your ligaments can actually cause your feet to permanently spread, which means you may have to invest in some new shoes in a bigger size.

Remember the mood swings you had earlier in pregnancy? The combination of uncomfortable symptoms and pregnancy hormones can result in a return of those emotional ups and downs. It's normal to worry about what your labor will be like or whether you'll be a good parent. But if you can't shake the blues or feel increasingly anxious or irritable, talk to your doctor or midwife. You may be among the 1 in 10 expectant women who battle depression during pregnancy.

Your Growing Baby

Your baby's a bit more than 15½ inches long now, and he weighs almost 3 pounds. A pint and a half of amniotic fluid surrounds him, but that volume will decrease as he gets bigger and takes up more room in your uterus. His eyesight continues to develop, though it's not very keen; even after he's born, he'll keep his eyes closed for a good part of the day. When he does open them, he'll respond to changes in light but will have 20/400 vision—which means he can only make out objects a few inches from his face. (Normal adult vision is 20/20.)

BabyCenter Buzz

What Other Women Say at 30 Weeks

"It feels like I've been pregnant forever. Looking at my old clothes depresses me. Will I ever be that small again? My feet went from 7½ to a size 9—yikes! But I can't wait to meet my little man." —*Anna*

"I've gained 25 pounds so far. I was hoping for less, but I know a healthy baby is most important!" —*Anonymous*

"I feel as if my energy has been totally sapped this week. I just feel so drained. My iron levels are fine, but I'm not sleeping well because I'm up every few hours going to the bathroom." —*Jessi*

"I can't eat big meals like I used to. I find that I'm snacking more during the day and not really that hungry at dinnertime." —*Margot*

Your Pregnancy: 31 Weeks
Your Changing Body

HOT TOPICS

• Kegels (page 203)

• Braxton Hicks contractions (page 294)

• Getting a good night's sleep (page 314)

• Your labor pain-relief options (page 394)

• Big decisions: Circumcision (page 379) and breastfeeding (page 472)

Have you noticed the muscles in your uterus tightening now and then? Many women feel these random contractions—called Braxton Hicks—in the second half of pregnancy. Often lasting about 30 seconds (though sometimes up to 60 seconds), they're irregular, and at this point they should be infrequent and painless. Frequent contractions, on the other hand—even those that *don't* hurt—may be a sign of preterm labor. Call your practitioner immediately if you have more than four contractions an hour or if you have any other signs of preterm labor (page 297).

You may have noticed some colostrum, or "premilk," leaking from your breasts lately. If so, try tucking some nursing pads into your bra to protect your clothes. (And if not, it's certainly nothing to worry about; your breasts are making colostrum all the same, even if you don't see any.) If your current bra is too snug, you might want to pick up a nursing bra. (Choose a nursing bra at least one cup size bigger than you need now—when your milk comes in, you'll be grateful for that extra room!)

By now, you've likely started taking childbirth classes (if not, sign up for one as soon as possible) and been introduced to a lot of issues surrounding labor and birth. This is also a good time to start thinking about whether you might want some kind of pain relief for labor and delivery and to explore other things that you might want to include in your birth plan.

Your Growing Baby

This week, your baby measures about 16 inches long. She weighs a little over 3 pounds and is heading into a growth spurt. She can turn her head from side to side, and her arms, legs, and body are continuing to plump out as needed fat accumulates under her skin. She's probably moving a lot, too, so you may have trouble sleeping because your baby's kicks and somersaults

BabyCenter Buzz

What Other Women Say at 31 Weeks

"I absolutely love being pregnant! This has been the best time in my life. Yes, I'm getting uncomfortable, and I had a hard time sleeping last night, but I'm by no means complaining. It's such a blessing to be able to bring a life into this world." —*Kathy*

"It's painful if I sit for more than an hour with restricted legroom. It makes my hour-long commute to work a real drag." —*Shari*

"My back has really started to hurt. I'm wearing one of those maternity support belts to relieve some of the pressure." —*Karla*

"I work full-time and do a lot of errands at lunch, before I get too tired. When I get home, I have less to do and can relax or spend time with my toddler." —*Jodean*

"I'm back to being pooped. For the last week, I've been totally exhausted, but can't sleep at night. It's not fair—especially when I have to lie there and stare at my peaceful, snoozing husband!" —*Shelly*

keep you up. Take comfort: All this movement is a sign that your baby is active and healthy.

Your Pregnancy: 32 Weeks

Your Changing Body

To accommodate you and your baby's growing needs, your blood volume has increased 40 to 50 percent since you got pregnant. With your uterus pushing up near your diaphragm and crowding your stomach, the consequences may be shortness of breath and heartburn. To help relieve your discomfort, try sleeping propped up with pillows and eating smaller meals more often.

HOT TOPICS

- Strategies for soothing stomach upsets (page 54)
- Coping with lower-back pain (page 164)
- Breathlessness (page 296)
- Sleep inducers (page 314)
- When your baby is breech (page 517)

You may have increasing lower-back pain as your pregnancy advances. Both hormonal and other factors may be contributing to this discomfort: Hormones make your ligaments more lax, your abdominal muscles are stretched, your growing uterus may put pressure on some nerves, and the extra weight you're carrying up front changes your posture and further strains your back. You might feel some pain in your buttocks and thighs as well. Uncommonly, women get a condition called sciatica. With sciatica, you may feel pain below your knee, you're likely to feel more pain in your legs than in your back, and may feel numbness or a tingling "pins and needles" sensation in your legs. Using a heating pad or changing positions while you sit or sleep should provide some relief, and the problem is likely to abate after you give birth. If the discomfort is mild, some simple stretches (page 202) might help as well. If it's very uncomfortable or if you feel any numbness, be sure to let your healthcare provider know.

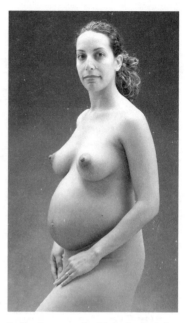

By the time you give birth, the capacity of your uterus will be up to a thousand times greater than normal. As your skin stretches over your growing belly now, you may start to feel itchy or notice stretch marks streaking across your taut skin. Don't despair: Most stretch marks fade considerably in the months following birth.

Your Growing Baby

By now, your baby is just shy of 4 pounds and is nearly 17 inches long, taking up a lot of space in your uterus. You're gaining about a pound a week, and roughly half of that goes right to your baby. In fact, he'll gain a third to half of his birthweight during the next 7 weeks as he fattens up for survival outside the womb.

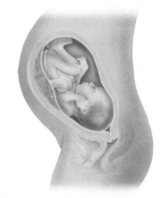

Your baby will put on more than a pound this month. He now has toenails, fingernails, and real hair (or at least respectable peach fuzz). His skin is becoming soft and smooth as he plumps up in preparation for birth.

BabyCenter Buzz

What Other Women Say at 32 Weeks

"I'm *still* suffering from morning sickness. I just can't wait to feel normal again!" —*Amber*

"Sleeping is getting unbearable. The only way I can get any rest is to lie with my back to my husband as he cradles my body. The support from him and a pillow between my legs is the best help." —*Anonymous*

"I'm getting really nervous about labor. I'm not sure I'll be able to handle the pain, so it's nice to know that I have pain-relief options if I need them." —*Virginia*

Your Pregnancy: 33 Weeks
Your Changing Body

As your baby fills out even more of your belly, lots of things might start to change: Whereas before you were sashaying, you may now find yourself waddling. Finding an easy position to sit in—let alone sleep—is becoming more of a challenge. And bumping into chairs and counters is par for the course.

You may be feeling some achiness and even numbness in your fingers, wrists and hands. Like many other tissues in your body, those in your wrist can retain fluid, which increases pressure in the carpal tunnel, a bony canal in your wrist. Nerves that run through this "tunnel" may end up pinched, causing numbness; tingling, shooting or burning pain; or a dull ache. Try wearing a splint to stabilize your wrist or propping your arm up with a pillow when you sleep. If your work requires repetitive hand movements (at a keyboard or on an assembly line, for instance), remember to stretch your hands when you take breaks (which should be frequently).

Many women are still feeling sexy at this stage—and their partners often agree. You'll need to make some adjustments, but for most women sex is fine right up until their water breaks.

HOT TOPICS

- Relief for carpal tunnel syndrome (page 167)
- Coping with stress urinary incontinence (page 300)
- Managing your weight gain (page 307)
- Making peace with the "pregnancy blahs" (page 328)
- Sex in the third trimester (page 335)

BabyCenter Buzz

What Other Women Say at 33 Weeks

"I've gained about 20 pounds so far. I'm terrified of never getting back in shape, though I know I will once I start exercising again."   —Shannon

"Sleeplessness has set in. I know this is all to prepare us for life with a newborn, but I would've been okay with getting prepared around 38 or 39 weeks!"   —Jo

"I've started to make some food to put in the freezer in case the baby comes early. This way, I won't have to worry about meals once the baby's here."   —Maureen

"I feel like I could star in one of those 'overactive bladder' commercials. I have to bring spare panties everywhere, just in case."   —Anonymous

"Every time I start to get bored with my pregnancy, I lie down and rub my belly. Sure enough, my baby starts to kick, and I think about how wonderful it will be when I'm able to hold him."   —Barbara

Your Growing Baby

This week, your baby weighs a little over 4 pounds and has passed the 17-inch mark. She's rapidly losing that wrinkled, alien look, and her skeleton is hardening. The bones in her skull aren't fused together, which allows them to move and slightly overlap, thus making it easier for her to fit through the birth canal. (These bones don't entirely fuse until early adulthood, so they can grow as her brain and other tissue expands during infancy and childhood.)

Your Pregnancy: 34 Weeks

Your Changing Body

By this week, fatigue has probably set in again, though maybe not with the same coma-like intensity of your first trimester. Your tiredness is perfectly understandable, given the physical strain you're under and the restless nights of frequent pee breaks and tossing and turning to get

HOT TOPICS

- Warning signs of preeclampsia (page 177)
- Itchy skin and rashes (page 302)
- Making the most of your prebaby time (page 328)
- Packing for the hospital or birth center (page 376)
- Perineal massage (page 419)

comfortable. Now's the time to slow down: Save up your energy for labor day (and beyond). If you've been sitting or lying down for a long time, don't jump up too quickly. Blood can pool in your feet and legs; the temporary drop in your blood pressure when you get up may make you feel dizzy.

Many midwives recommend massaging the perineum (the tissue between your vagina and rectum) to help prevent tearing during childbirth. If you want to try this technique, now's a good time to start, though not every woman (or practitioner) is comfortable with it, and it may not help in every case.

Now is also when you may notice itchy red bumps or welts on your belly—and possibly your thighs and buttocks as well. Most likely, this is a harmless condition called pruritic urticarial papules and plaques of pregnancy (PUPPP for short, page 303), but let your practitioner make the diagnosis. Also be sure to call her if you feel itchy all over, even if you don't have a rash. It could signal a liver problem.

BabyCenter Buzz

What Other Women Say at 34 Weeks

"This baby is so low that I have to waddle around (and yes, I *have* been quacked at). When I sit or lie down, my hips feel like they'll split apart—ouch!"   —*Kelly*

"I try to see my legs and feet when I'm standing, but all I see is this huge round mass with my belly button sticking out like those pop-up thermometers in a Thanksgiving turkey."   —*Tina*

"With my big belly in the way, getting in and out of the car is starting to be a real challenge. And there's no way I can pick up my 3-year-old anymore."   —*Peggy*

"My car seat is in. I was thinking of packing my hospital bag this weekend. I'll probably go past my due date just because I'm all ready to go. But if I did nothing, I just know that she'd come early!"   —*Katie*

"I'm trying to enjoy my last months of freedom, doing all the things I may not have time for—movies, facials, romantic dinners—once my baby is here."   —*Bethany*

Your Growing Baby

Your baby now weighs about 4¾ pounds and is almost 18 inches long. His fat layers—which he'll need to regulate his body temperature once he's born—are filling out, making him rounder; his skin is also smoother than ever. His central nervous system is maturing, and his lungs are continuing to mature as well. If you've been nervous about preterm labor, you'll be happy to know that 99 percent of babies born at this age can survive outside the womb. Though most may require a little help in the short term, they usually have no major long-term health problems.

Your Pregnancy: 35 Weeks

Your Changing Body

Your uterus—which was tucked away inside your pelvis when you conceived—is now nestled under your rib cage. If you could peek inside your womb, you'd see that there's more baby than amniotic fluid in there now. Your ballooning uterus is crowding your internal organs, too, which is why you probably have to pee more often and may be dealing with heartburn and other gastrointestinal distress. If you're not grappling with these annoyances, you're one of the lucky few.

HOT TOPICS

- Group B strep (page 285)
- Fatigue busters (page 299)
- Third-trimester dream themes (page 319)
- Preparing for your departure at work (page 350)
- Creating a birth plan (page 378)

From here on out, you'll start seeing your practitioner every week. Sometime between this week and week 37, she'll also do a vaginal and rectal culture to check for bacteria called Group B streptococci (GBS). (Don't worry: The swab is the size of a Q-tip, and it won't hurt at all.) GBS is usually harmless in adults, but if you pass it to your baby during birth, it can cause serious complications such as pneumonia, meningitis, or a blood infection. Because 10 to 30 percent of pregnant women carry the bacteria and don't know it, it's vital to be screened. (The bacteria come and go on their own—that's why you weren't screened earlier in pregnancy.) If you're a GBS carrier, you'll get IV

BabyCenter Buzz

What Other Women Say at 35 Weeks

"Tomorrow is my last day at work. It was my intention to work until I delivered. But I realize now that I can't do it anymore. Even though I have a desk job, I'm just too tired." —*Karen*

"I had postpartum depression after giving birth to my first child. Now that the due date for baby number two is approaching, I'm worried that it will happen again. Fortunately, my OB knows my history, and we'll keep an eye on how I'm feeling from here on out." —*Anonymous*

"I sleep in our recliner. That way I'm not sleeping on my side (making my hips hurt) and I'm not sleeping flat on my back (not good for the baby). This does the trick, and I wake up in the morning feeling semi-decent." —*Nicki*

antibiotics during labor, which will greatly reduce your baby's risk of infection.

This is also a good time to create your birth plan. Check out our sample form (page 382) to help you get specific: who'll be there, what pain-management techniques you want to try, and where you want your baby to stay after you deliver. Childbirth is unpredictable, and chances are you won't follow your plan to the letter, but thinking about your choices ahead of time—and sharing your preferences with your caregiver—should take some of the anxiety out of the process.

Your Growing Baby

Your baby doesn't have much room to maneuver now that she's over 18 inches long and tips the scales at 5 pounds plus. Because it's so snug in your womb, she isn't likely to be doing somersaults anymore, but the number of times she kicks should remain about the same. Her kidneys are fully developed now, and her liver can process some waste products. Most of her basic physical development is now complete, and she'll spend the next few weeks putting on weight.

Your Pregnancy: 36 Weeks

Your Changing Body

HOT TOPICS

- Preparing your child for a sibling (page 344)
- Baby basics checklist (page 348)
- What it means when your baby "drops" (page 387)
- Stages of labor (page 407)
- Turning a breech baby (page 517)

Now that your baby is taking up so much room, you may have trouble eating a normal-size meal; smaller, more frequent meals are often easier to handle at this point. On the other hand, you may have less heartburn and have an easier time breathing once your baby starts to "drop" into your pelvis. This phenomenon—called lightening—often happens a few weeks before labor if this is your first baby. If you've given birth before, it probably won't happen until labor kicks in. If your baby drops, you may also feel increased pressure in your lower abdomen and bladder, which will make walking increasingly uncomfortable. And if your baby is very low, you may feel lots of vaginal pressure and discomfort as well—some women say that they feel as though they're carrying a bowling ball between their legs!

You might also notice that Braxton Hicks contractions are more frequent now. Be sure to review with your practitioner exactly when and where to call her if you think your labor has started. As a general rule, call when you start having painful contractions every five minutes for an hour, if your water breaks, or if you think you're leaking amniotic fluid. Of course, you'll want to call right away if you have signs of labor before 37 weeks. Also call without delay if you notice a decrease in your baby's activity or if you have vaginal bleeding, fever, swelling in your hands or face, a severe or persistent headache, abdominal pain, or vision changes.

Even if you're enjoying an uncomplicated pregnancy, it's best to avoid flying (or

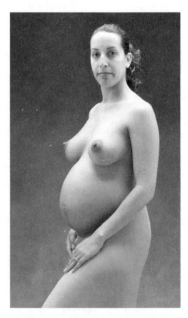

You're likely feeling some discomfort from all the extra weight you're carrying, but you may get a little relief if your baby "drops" into your pelvis sometime this month. That will make it easier to catch your breath.

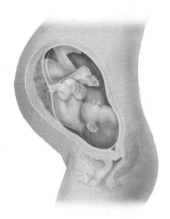

Your baby's in the home stretch, too. All he has left to do now is get into position (if he hasn't already) and plump up to his birthweight. He looks like a newborn as well—he may even sport a full head of hair.

any travel far from home by *any* mode of transportation) during your final month because you can go into labor at any time. In fact, some airlines won't even let women on board who are due to deliver within 30 days of the flight.

Your Growing Baby

Your baby is still packing on the pounds—at the rate of about an ounce a day. He now weighs almost 6 pounds and is a little under 19 inches long. He's shedding most of the downy hair that covered his body, as well as the vernix caseosa, the waxy substance that has coated and protected his skin during his nine-month amniotic bath. He swallows both of these substances, along with other secretions, resulting in a blackish mixture called meconium that will form the contents of his first bowel movement.

At the end of this week, your baby will be considered full-term. (Full-term is 37 to 42 weeks; babies born before 37 weeks are "preterm," and

BabyCenter Buzz

What Other Women Say at 36 Weeks

"Swimming is the only exercise that eases all my aches and pains. I love feeling weightless!" —*Paula*

"I can barely type, my hands hurt so much. They're swollen, and my joints are aching. I feel like I have arthritis or something." —*Jen*

"I have gestational diabetes, and my sugar levels have been mostly okay. I'm *so* ready to have this baby so I can eat normally again!" —*Jessie*

"I felt some fluid leak out of me one morning, and my underwear was damp. It ended up being amniotic fluid, so my doctor induced labor. I had a healthy baby girl 3½ weeks early!" —*Michelle*

"I've started collecting take-out and delivery menus from local restaurants because I know I won't have time to cook in the early weeks after giving birth." —*Kristina*

those born after 42 are "postterm.") Most likely, he's in a head-down position. But if he isn't, your provider may suggest scheduling an "external cephalic version," which is a fancy way of saying she'll try to coax your baby into a head-down position by manipulating him on the outside of your belly.

Your Pregnancy: 37 Weeks

Your Changing Body

Congratulations—your baby is full-term! This means that you could deliver any day now, and your baby's lungs should be fully mature and ready to adjust to life outside the womb. Braxton Hicks contractions may be coming more frequently now and may last longer and be more uncomfortable. You might also notice an increase in vaginal discharge. If you see some "bloody show" (mucus tinged with a tiny amount of blood) in the toilet or your undies, labor is probably a few days away—or less. (If you have heavier spotting or bleeding, call your doctor or midwife immediately.) Also, be sure to ask your caregiver about the results of your Group B strep culture. That way, if the result isn't yet on your chart when you get to the hospital or birth center, you'll be able to give the staff there a timely heads-up if you need antibiotics.

> **HOT TOPICS**
>
> - When to start your maternity leave (page 231)
> - The nesting instinct (page 344)
> - Do you need a postpartum doula? (page 376)
> - False versus true labor (page 388)
> - What "bloody show" signals (page 388)

For most women, the next couple of weeks are a waiting game. Use this time to prepare your baby's nursery and take care of necessary tasks or indulgences (naps, reading time, dates with your partner) that you may not get around to for a while after your baby's born.

During those luxurious naps, you're likely to have some intense dreams. Anxiety both about labor and about becoming a parent can fuel a lot of strange flights of unconscious fancy. If you're so inclined, jot them down while they're fresh in your mind so you can analyze them later.

Your Growing Baby

Your baby weighs a little over 6 pounds and measures between 19 and 20 inches head to heel. Many babies have a full head of hair at birth, with locks from ½ to 1½ inches long. But don't be surprised if your baby's hair isn't the same color

BabyCenter Buzz

What Other Women Say at 37 Weeks

"My hips get numb when I sit for even short periods. I spend a lot of time in front of a computer, so it's making it hard to work." —*Laura*

"I'm planning to work as long as I can to get the most out of my salary and maternity benefits. I'm feeling great now, but we'll see how things go." —*Anonymous*

"I never thought I'd say it, but I'm just plain bored waiting around for this baby to come! My hospital bag is packed, the nursery is ready, and I've seen all the movies and read all the books that I want to. My girlfriends are the only ones who understand!" —*Mary*

"This has not been an easy pregnancy for me, and I'm just so grateful that we've made it this far. I've been on bedrest and can't wait to finally meet my baby girl!" —*Chelle*

"I was induced this week because I had preeclampsia. I started having pretty strong contractions immediately. After just an hour of pushing, my daughter was born!" —*Amanda*

as yours. Dark-haired couples are sometimes thrown for a loop when their children come out as blonds or redheads, and fair-haired couples have been surprised by Elvis look-alikes. (Note, though, that this newborn hair often falls out after a few months and bears little resemblance to the permanent locks that will grow in its place.) And then, of course, some newborns sport only peach fuzz.

Your Pregnancy: 38 Weeks
Your Changing Body

It may be harder than ever to get comfortable enough to sleep well at night—you may have trouble falling asleep, and when you finally do, you may experience frequent nighttime awakenings. If you can, take it easy during the day—this may be your last chance to do so for a while! Keep monitoring your baby's movements, too. Though his quarters are getting cozy, he should still be as active as before.

HOT TOPICS

- Strategies for soothing swollen feet (page 167)
- How to handle hemorrhoids (page 301)
- Common worries about labor and delivery (page 322)
- What to expect at the hospital (page 390)
- When a breech baby won't turn (page 425)

Swelling in your feet and ankles is normal during these weeks, but if you notice any swelling in your hands or face, sudden weight gain, persistent or severe headaches, blurred vision or spots before your eyes, or severe upper-abdominal pain, call your practitioner right away; these are symptoms of a serious condition called preeclampsia (page 531).

Your Growing Baby

Your baby has really plumped up. He weighs between 6 and 7½ pounds (boys tend to be slightly heavier than girls), and he's nearly 20 inches long. He has a firm grasp, which you'll soon be able to test when you hold his hand for the first time! His organs have matured and are ready for life outside the womb.

Wondering what color his peepers will be? You may not be able to tell right away. If he's born with brown eyes, they'll likely stay brown. If he's born with steel gray or dark blue eyes, they may stay gray or blue or turn green, hazel, or brown by the time he's nine months old. That's because a child's irises (the colored part of the eye) may gain more pigment in the months after he's born, but they won't get "lighter" or bluer. (Green, hazel, and brown eyes have more pigment than gray or blue eyes.)

BabyCenter Buzz

What Other Women Say at 38 Weeks

"I'm having trouble distinguishing between painful baby movement and contractions. How will I know if I'm really in labor?" —*Joanna*

"I had no foot swelling until a few days ago—then *bam*! I'm trying to drink extra amounts of water and am elevating my feet when I can, but I'm pretty miserable. I can only fit into flip-flops!" —*Jen*

"I love my unborn daughter already and I can't wait to be her mommy, but I fear becoming a goofy mother—one of those people in the grocery store who babble baby talk to their infants, oblivious to how annoying it is to others!" —*Anonymous*

"I know that most women don't have their water break before going into labor, but I keep a plastic bag and a towel in my car just in case it does break when I'm away from home." —*Becky*

"All that people want to talk to me about is my pregnancy. Sometimes I want to yell that I'm more than a pregnant woman! Ask me about some other aspect of my life. When I have this baby, are people only going to be interested in the baby and not me?" —*Anonymous*

Your Pregnancy: 39 Weeks
Your Changing Body

At each of your now-weekly visits, your caregiver will do an abdominal exam to check your baby's growth and position. She might also do an internal exam to see whether you cervix has started ripening: softening, effacing (thinning out), and dilating (opening). Only 1 in 20 infants is actually born on his due date. Some have already arrived and others come later, so if the week passes and your baby stays put, don't worry.

> **HOT TOPICS**
>
> - Dealing with rude comments about your size (page 333)
> - Should you go back to work after the baby? (page 351)
> - What to do when your water breaks (page 389)
> - What your partner will do in the delivery room (page 414)
> - What to expect during a c-section (page 426)

While you're waiting, try not to worry too much about your water breaking before you go into labor. Membranes rupture before the beginning of labor in fewer than 15 percent of pregnancies. If your water does break (whether you have a large gush or a small stream, or you suspect you might have a small leak), call your doctor or midwife, but stay calm. It may be hours before your first contraction. (If you tested positive for Group B strep

BabyCenter Buzz

What Other Women Say at 39 Weeks

"I'm 2 centimeters dilated and 80 percent effaced and have had a few contractions off and on, but nothing consistent or too painful. But at least my body has started to prepare for the big day!" —*Anonymous*

"I'm pretty anxious about how my labor is going to go: Will I know when it starts? Will we get stuck in traffic on the way to the hospital? Will my husband be able to get home from work when I go into labor? What if I can't handle the pain?" —*Cece*

"I'm having lower back pain and cramping in my lower abdomen. I would love to have this baby now, but I know it's out of my control." —*Dara*

"My water broke at 1:30 this morning! It felt like the baby kicked really hard, and then there was a gush. I actually soaked through four pads in 15 minutes. It's now 4:30 in the afternoon, and I'm heading to the hospital!" —*Meaghan*

"This baby must be taking his time. My cervix hasn't even started softening yet, according to my doc." —*Susan*

on your recent culture, you will need to get to the hospital soon so you can start receiving IV antibiotics, and will likely be induced before too long if you don't start contracting on your own. You'll also need to get there right away if you have any signs of a herpes outbreak when your water breaks or your labor starts.) Also call your practitioner immediately if you notice that your baby's movements have slowed, whether or not you're leaking fluid.

Your Growing Baby

Your baby's waiting to greet the world! She continues to build a layer of fat to help control her body temperature after birth, but it's likely she already measures about 20 inches and weighs a tad over 7 pounds. The outer layers of her skin are shedding as new skin forms underneath.

Your Pregnancy: 40 Weeks
Your Changing Body

After months of anticipation, your due date finally rolls around, and . . . you're still pregnant. It's a frustrating, but common, situation in which to find yourself. You may not be as late as you think, especially if your baby wasn't conceived exactly when you thought. Even with reliable dating, some women have prolonged pregnancies for no apparent reason.

> ### HOT TOPICS
> - Fetal kick counts (page 287)
> - Biophysical profile (page 290) and nonstress testing (page 289)
> - False labor (page 388)
> - Inducing labor (page 436)
> - Recovering from childbirth (page 447)

You still have a week or two before you'll be considered "late." (Remember, full-term is anywhere from 37 to 42 weeks.) That said, the rate of complications begins to rise at about 41 weeks, so to be sure your baby is still thriving, your practitioner may schedule you for special testing to keep an eye on her (page 286). (If you have any pregnancy complications, you've likely started this testing already, but if everything's been going well, you probably won't start testing until the end of this week.) A biophysical profile (BPP) consists of an ultrasound to check your baby's overall movements, breathing movements, and muscle tone (whether she opens and closes her hand or extends and then flexes her limbs), as well as the amount of amniotic fluid that surrounds her (important because it's a reflection of how well the placenta is supporting your baby). Fetal heart rate monitoring (called a nonstress test, or

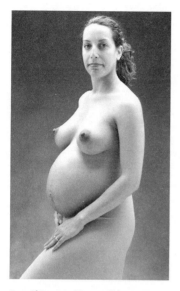

Even if it seems like you'll be pregnant forever, your baby will be here soon—though your practitioner may eventually have to give nature a little nudge. Take a picture of yourself and your glorious belly now to put in your baby's memory book.

NST) will generally be done as well—by itself or as part of the BPP. Whether you've started testing or not, it's important for you to keep track of your baby's movements and report any decrease in activity to your caregiver without delay.

Use caution if you're tempted to try some techniques at home to get labor started. Having sex won't actually *start* labor, but it may help to get the ball rolling because having an orgasm and the prostaglandins in semen can stimulate contractions and help soften your cervix. You may have heard that nipple stimulation can trigger contractions, but you shouldn't try it at home because it can bring on some long, strong contractions that could stress your baby. Castor oil is a powerful laxative that can stimulate your bowels and, at times, some contractions as

BabyCenter Buzz

What Other Women Say at 40 Weeks

"Either I'm in labor or I have the world's worst intestinal bug! I've been having what feels like contractions all night long and a bit of diarrhea. The contractions started around noon yesterday, but I haven't bothered to time them until this morning—30 minutes apart and manageable, just annoying." —*Anonymous*

"I am so huge and so uncomfortable. Something's gotta give! I've been having mild contractions off and on for the last two days, so I'm keeping my fingers crossed that my body's getting ready for delivery." —*Sandy*

"I just started maternity leave after a very busy last few weeks at work, so I'm really hoping, for another week or two, just to rest and get my head together before the baby makes her appearance!" —*Leah*

"My cervix is still closed and high, even though I've been having irregular contractions. My doctor said to walk, but every two blocks, I have to pee. If nothing happens soon, we have to talk about an induction." —*Nhaylene*

"No one told me that pregnancy is really *10* months!" —*Anonymous*

well. Still, there's no good proof that it actually helps induce labor, though plenty of women can attest to its other unpleasant effects! Though many people think a spicy meal can help, it will probably only result in heartburn. Finally, the safety and effectiveness of herbal remedies to induce labor are largely unknown, and a few are downright dangerous. So ask your doctor or midwife before doing or taking *anything* to kick-start contractions.

Your Growing Baby

It's hard to say for sure how big your baby will be, but the average newborn weighs in at a little over 7 pounds and measures about 20 inches long. Her skull bones are not yet fused, which allows them to overlap a bit if it's a snug fit in the birth canal. This so-called "molding" is the reason that your baby's noggin may look a little conehead-ish after birth. Rest assured, it's normal—and temporary.

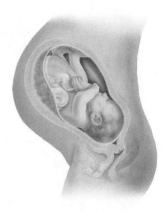

Your baby will keep getting bigger—and his nails and hair will continue to grow—every day that he's in your womb. His skull plates remain unfused to ease his passage through your birth canal.

Your Pregnancy: 41 Weeks
Your Changing Body

Just when you start to worry that you'll be pregnant forever, a light appears at the end of the tunnel. There's a good chance you'll go into labor on your own in the next several days, and if you don't, you'll be induced this week or the start of next.

The method your practitioner will use to get labor going will depend on what condition your cervix is in. If it hasn't yet started to soften, efface (thin out), or dilate (open), it's "unripe"—in other words, not yet ready for labor. In that case, she'll try either "mechanical" methods or hormonelike sub-

HOT TOPICS

- What to do while you're playing the waiting game (page 369)

- Dealing with last-minute anxiety (page 394)

- Labor complications (page 423)

- All about emergency c-sections (page 429)

- How to stay comfortable during an induction (page 436)

stances called prostaglandins to ripen your cervix before the induction. Sometimes these will end up jump-starting labor as well. Depending on your situation, these techniques can include "stripping" or rupturing your amniotic membranes, inserting a flexible catheter all the way into your cervix and inflating a small balloon on the end to put pressure on it from above, and applying prostaglandin gel to your cervix. Finally, if contractions haven't started, you'll get intravenous oxytocin (Pitocin) to get them going.

In the meantime, tell your doctor or midwife right away if your baby's movements slow down or if you're leaking amniotic fluid.

Your Growing Baby

A bit over 20 inches long, your baby has continued to grow and may now weigh 8 pounds or more. As cozy as he is, he can't stay inside you much longer. Most practitioners won't let you go more than two weeks past your due date because it puts you and your baby at increased risk for complications. Your placenta may be starting to peter out, for instance, thus reducing the amount of oxygen and nutrients your baby receives. And babies born after 42 weeks are often overweight and can have dry, parchmentlike skin from their too-long amniotic bath. What's more, your labor is more likely to be prolonged or stalled, both you and your baby have an increased risk of injury during a vaginal delivery, and you double your chances of needing a c-section.

BabyCenter Buzz

What Other Women Say at 41 Weeks

"So far, no progress. Seems like my cervix is not cooperating. My doctor will wait one more week and then induce me if my daughter doesn't come naturally." —*Emel*

"I'm actually happy for the extra time. I worked right up to 40 weeks and am enjoying some time to myself!" —*Jody*

"I'm so tired of everyone calling to find out if I've had the baby yet. I don't even pick up the phone anymore. I'm definitely pretty cranky these days." —*Sarah*

"It's really hard for my 3-year-old right now. I can't pick him up, I don't have any energy to play, and I'm really short-tempered because I ache all over. But he seems genuinely excited about having a baby sister." —*Hilary*

"My doctor's going to induce me tonight because they don't want my baby to get any bigger. I'm scared—this is my first—but so excited!" —*Candice*

Symptoms You Should Never Ignore in the Third Trimester

If you have any of the following complaints, call your doctor or midwife immediately:

Before you reach 37 weeks:

- Pelvic pressure, low back pain, abdominal pain, cramping, or more than four contractions in an hour (even if they don't hurt)
- An increase in vaginal discharge or a change in the type of discharge—if it becomes watery, mucous-like, or bloody (even if it's only pink or blood-tinged)

At any time:

- A decrease in your baby's movements
- Vaginal bleeding or spotting, or watery or foul-smellling discharge
- A severe or persistent headache
- Blurred or double vision, or seeing spots or "floaters"
- Severe or persistent abdominal pain or tenderness
- Severe or persistent vomiting, or any vomiting accompanied by pain or fever
- Any swelling in your face or puffiness around your eyes, anything more than mild swelling in your fingers or hands, or severe or sudden swelling in your legs, feet, or ankles
- Rapid weight gain (more than 4 pounds in a week)
- Pain or burning when you urinate, or little or no urination
- Severe or persistent leg or calf pain that doesn't ease up when you flex your ankle and point your toes toward your nose, or one leg that's much more swollen than the other
- Chills or a fever over 100 degrees F
- Fainting, frequent dizziness, rapid heartbeat or palpitations
- Difficulty breathing, coughing up blood
- Persistent itching all over
- Trauma to your abdomen
- Any health problem that you'd ordinarily call your practitioner about

Note: If you're near your due date, check out the signs of labor (page 388).

YOUR HEALTH

You've come a long way, baby! And though the big event is just around the corner, the final months of your pregnancy will hopefully be just the opposite: uneventful. In this chapter, you'll learn what tests may be due, which new physical complaints will likely pop up now (and what to do about them), and finally, how to chase those increasingly elusive ZZZs. And, of course, don't forget that the most exciting thing of all—your baby's birth—is still ahead.

What to Expect at Prenatal Checkups in the Third Trimester

You'll probably start having checkups every two weeks beginning in week 28 and going up to week 36, then switch to once-a-week visits. As you and your practitioner get to know each other better and as your due date draws nearer, you can expect a mix of regular physical exams, late-pregnancy screening tests, and discussions about the coming birth. Some of the things your caregiver will do at these appointments:

Ask how you're feeling. As before, your caregiver will probably start your visit by asking how you're doing and follow up on any issues raised at your last appointment. Before proceeding to the physical exam, she'll ask you about contractions, swelling, headaches, and any other complaints you might have. Fatigue, moodiness, aches and pains—they're all fair game for discussion and could provide valuable medical information to boot. (That's why, even if she *doesn't* ask, you should still share this information. Don't be put off by a too-busy-to-talk vibe: Your practitioner may see dozens of patients a day, but your pregnancy is still the most important thing in the world to *you*.)

Question you about fetal movement. She'll also want to know what your baby's been up to—and how *often* he's been up to it—and remind you to call at any time if you sense a decrease in activity compared with his usual pattern. She may even ask you to start counting the baby's movements for a set period of time each day.

Check you out and run routine tests. Your practitioner will weigh you; take urine samples to check for signs of preeclampsia, urinary tract infection, and other problems; track your blood pressure to make sure it isn't high; and check your ankles, hands, and face for swelling.

Do an abdominal exam. Just as she did in the second trimester, your caregiver will feel your belly at every visit in order to estimate your baby's size. She'll also measure the distance between your pubic bone and the top of your uterus and compare it with the number from your previous visit to see if your baby's growth rate seems normal. If he seems either too big or too small, you'll get an ultrasound to measure him more precisely and to check your amniotic fluid levels. Your practitioner will probably be able to tell whether your baby is in the head-down position or is breech. If she thinks he's still breech (or simply can't tell for sure) at week 36 or so, she'll order an ultrasound to confirm her findings, and you'll likely be offered the option of undergoing a procedure called an external cephalic version to try to turn the baby. Finally, she'll check your baby's heartbeat—which, for most women, is the highlight of the appointment.

Possibly do a pelvic exam. Don't expect routine pelvic exams at your prenatal visits, even in the third trimester. Many midwives and doctors don't do them unless they have a specific concern, such as preterm labor, because the exams can be uncomfortable and don't offer any actionable information. But if you're past your due date, your provider will check your cervix to see if it's softening, effacing (thinning out), and dilating (opening)—because this may help her decide whether and when to induce labor. She may also do a pelvic exam to double-check your baby's position, particularly if you're nearing your due date and it's not clear from the abdominal exam. (If your baby has dropped and his head is quite low, it can be hard to feel abdominally but may be easy to do with a vaginal exam.) All that said, if your caregiver doesn't routinely do vaginal exams, but you're near your due date and just curious as to whether anything much is happening, you can request one.

BY THE NUMBERS

Giving Nature a Nudge

Labors induced in 1989: **9%**

Labors induced in 2002: **20%**

Source: *National Center for Health Statistics*

Ask the Experts

I've Lost Faith in My Pregnancy Care Provider—Is It Too Late to Switch?

Dr. Meredith Goodwin, family practitioner: Absolutely not. *You* call the shots in this relationship. Just make sure to take a copy of your medical records with you when you go (yes, you do have a right to them). Your new doctor or midwife will need to be aware of your medical history and your pregnancy's progress. Switching providers might be awkward—but it won't be a risk to your health care.

Provide pregnancy counseling. If your provider hasn't already done so, she'll talk to you early this trimester about the signs of preterm labor and preeclampsia and review other warning signs that should prompt a call to her. As you near your due date, she'll discuss the signs of labor and let you know when you should get in touch with her. And at the end of each prenatal visit, your caregiver will let you know if she has any concerns. She should also clue you in about what to look for between now and your next visit and explain any tests you may need.

Answer labor and delivery questions. If you haven't done so already, it's time to resolve any lingering concerns you have about the way your labor and delivery will be handled. Common questions include "Will you be there throughout my labor?" "Are the nurses a constant presence, or does each one take care of a lot of patients at once?" "What happens if I go into labor in the middle of the night?" Some of these issues will be addressed in your childbirth preparation class, but it's always a good idea to ask your provider to clarify things, especially if you took a childbirth class somewhere other than where you plan to deliver your baby. Make your concerns and preferences known, too; a birth plan can help with this.

Discuss postpartum considerations. Because you may not be in any shape to make decisions right after giving birth, now's the time to talk about whether you want your baby boy circumcised, whether you plan to breastfeed, and what you'd like to do for contraception after giving birth. (Though you may see your midwife or doctor make a note of your preferences in your chart, you can change your mind later!) And if you haven't found a doctor for your baby yet, your practitioner can give you some names.

Tell you how a latecomer is doing. If you're a week past your due date

BabyCenter Buzz

Why I Decided to Find a New Caregiver

"My doctor hardly spoke to me. I felt like I was just another pregnant woman he had to deal with. I ended up with another doctor in the same practice. He's been so helpful, and I feel totally at ease with him." —*Paris*

"My first doctor made me wait more than an hour to see her, and then only spent three minutes with me. I often found myself chasing her into the hallway to get my questions answered. It made me realize that I wanted a smaller practice and a more personal touch. I interviewed a couple of doctors, and found my new doctor through a friend's recommendation. I'm very happy so far." —*Anonymous*

"I switched from an OB to a midwife in week 32. I'm planning an unmedicated birth, and my OB thought that was funny. So I switched to a great midwife who works with an OB, and I've been so glad I did it. She treats me like a person, not just another patient. And she's supportive of my decisions, which helps a lot." —*Karilee*

"I had to switch doctors in week 33 because mine left my HMO. I was really disappointed to have to find someone new at that point, but it may have been a blessing in disguise. My new doctor does everything to avoid episiotomies and seems very invested in his patients' welfare." —*Anonymous*

(or maybe even less), your caregiver will order tests to make sure your baby's thriving. You may get a full biophysical profile or a modified one, which includes a nonstress test (page 289) to assess your baby's heart rate and an ultrasound to check your amniotic fluid level. These tests are usually performed twice a week. Even if everything looks normal, if you don't have your baby by the start of week 42, your practitioner will probably induce labor (page 436) because after that point, the health risks for both you and your baby rise dramatically. (And if your cervix is ripe, you may be induced even sooner.)

Third-Trimester Prenatal Tests

Some late-pregnancy tests are routine, and others are done on an as-needed basis. Here's a look at what's in store for you on the testing front this trimester.

Blood Tests and Cultures

Gestational diabetes screening. If you had a normal glucose challenge test late in your second trimester, consider yourself done. But if you haven't taken it yet, or if the results were abnormal and you haven't yet done the glucose tolerance test, you'll be tested for diabetes now.

Hematocrit/hemoglobin. This test for anemia was done at your first prenatal visit and will likely be repeated sometime during this trimester. That's because your blood volume continues to increase during pregnancy, putting you at higher risk for anemia.

Rh antibody screening. Your blood was tested for Rh factor at your first prenatal visit. If you're Rh negative, an antibody screen will be repeated now (to save you a needle prick, it's usually done at the same time as your glucose challenge test), and you'll get an injection of Rh immunoglobulin in week 28 (unless the baby's father is also Rh negative). This will protect you from developing antibodies—which could pose a risk to future babies, or even this one—in the unlikely event that some of your baby's blood gets into your bloodstream during this trimester. (And because the effects of the Rh immunoglobulin wear off after a few months, if your baby is Rh positive, you'll get another injection after he's born to ensure that you won't have any problem carrying an Rh-positive baby in future pregnancies.)

Testing for sexually transmitted infections. You were likely tested for STIs at your first prenatal appointment, but if you're at high risk for infection you'll be retested now. Your caregiver will do cervical cultures to check for chlamydia and gonorrhea, and your blood will be tested for syphilis. It's a wise idea to be retested for HIV as well if there's any chance that you may have contracted it since your original test. If you are HIV positive, you will receive treatments that dramatically reduce your risk of transmitting HIV to your baby.

Group B strep testing. Sometime between weeks 35 and 37, you'll be checked for the presence of Group B streptococci (GBS) in your vagina and rectum—this is a painless test done by swabbing the lower end of your vagina and your rectum. Your practitioner

> **QUICK TIP**
>
> **Spread the News about Your GBS Status**
>
> If you test positive for GBS, it will be noted on your chart so that you can get antibiotic treatment during labor. But just in case that important piece of news falls through the cracks, be sure to remind your caregiver of your status when your water breaks or when you're in labor— whichever happens first. And don't be shy about informing your nurses or the on-call practitioner attending your birth as well. Penicillin is the antibiotic most commonly used to treat GBS carriers—if you're allergic to this medication, make sure that's known as well, and you'll be treated with a different antibiotic.

Ask the Experts

What Is Group B Strep?

Dr. Russell Turk, obstetrician: Group B streptococcus (GBS) is a common bacterium associated with a relatively rare but very serious infection in newborns. GBS is found in the genital tract, urinary tract, and bowels of 20 to 25 percent of pregnant women. (Group B is not the same as Group A strep, the bacterium that causes strep throat.)

Though about one in four pregnant women harbors the bacteria, because of screening and treatment, only one newborn in 2,000 contracts GBS and gets sick during the first week of life.

Of those babies who do become infected, though, "early-onset GBS" is a major cause of life-threatening conditions, including blood infection, pneumonia, and brain inflammation. And for a small percentage of them, GBS proves fatal. Many others are left with permanent disabilities, such as brain or lung damage, blindness, or hearing loss. Group B strep can also cause urinary tract and uterine infections in women and, very rarely, lead to stillbirth.

The good news is that most cases of early-onset GBS and maternal uterine infections are easily prevented through timely testing and antibiotics.

will get the results in two or three days and give them to you at your next visit.

Unless you have symptoms of preterm labor, this test isn't done before week 35 because the bacteria can come and go; testing early won't predict whether you're likely to be carrying GBS when you finally do go into labor. (If you have preterm labor, you'll be tested then, and treatment will be started while your caregiver is waiting for results, just in case you're infected.)

If your vaginal/rectal cultures are positive, you won't be treated right away because early treatment is no guarantee that the bacteria won't return. But if you get a urinary tract infection from GBS, that *will* be treated right away because untreated UTIs of any kind increase your risk for kidney infection and premature labor.

Testing for Your Baby's Well-Being

If everything's going well and you deliver by your due date, having your routine prenatal checkups and learning how to count fetal kicks are likely all you'll need to do to monitor your baby's health. But if you've been high risk from the start, if you develop problems along the way, or if you don't deliver soon after your due date, your caregiver will schedule some tests to see how your baby's doing. This information can help reassure both of you that every-thing's on track or, alternatively, alert her that your baby needs to be delivered.

Fetal Movements/Kick Counts

WHAT: Though all practitioners advise pregnant women to pay close attention to fetal movement, some midwives and doctors recommend that women actually count their baby's kicks, punches, and other movements once or twice a day.

WHO: Many pregnant women will be asked to do daily kick counts—and *all* pregnant women should be alert for decreases in their baby's move-ment, even if they aren't actually counting.

WHEN: From week 28 until delivery.

WHY: An absence or slowdown of fetal movement can signal a problem. If you notice less movement, let your practitioner know right away—you'll need a nonstress test or a biophysical profile to check on your baby's condition.

HOW: There are many ways of counting fetal kicks, so ask your doctor or midwife how she'd like you to do it. One common approach is this: Time how long it takes you to feel ten distinct movements (kicks, punches, and rolls all count). Ideally, you want to feel at least ten movements within one or two hours. (In reality, it probably won't take that long.) Sit or lie on your left side while you count your baby's movements; don't try to count while you're busy doing something else because you're likely to be distracted and miss some movements. It's also a good idea to try to do your counts at roughly the same time every day. If you don't feel enough movement, call your caregiver.

Ultrasound

WHAT: A noninvasive diagnostic test that uses sound waves to create a visual image of your uterus, baby, and placenta. Ultrasound can also be used to estimate the amount of your amniotic fluid and assess the length of your cervix.

WHO: Women whose practitioner has questions about their baby's weight, position, or general health.

WHEN: The timing will depend on the reason for the testing.

WHY: Your practitioner may order an ultrasound now to:

Determine the cause of vaginal bleeding. Bleeding this late in the game can signal problems with your placenta. If an ultrasound shows you have a condition called placenta previa, you'll need to deliver by c-section.

Check your baby's growth. If your doctor or midwife is concerned that your baby isn't growing properly, she'll schedule an ultrasound (or a series of them) to measure certain parts of his body—including his head, the length of his thighbone, and the distance around his midsection. The rest of his body may be evaluated as well. If your baby isn't growing the way he should, your practitioner will follow him closely in the coming weeks, or you may be induced. (The decision will depend on a variety of factors, including how far along you are and how serious the problem is.) Ultrasound may also be used to check on your baby if he seems too big, though the closer you are to term, the less precise ultrasound may be. If he's especially large (particularly if you have diabetes), your caregiver may talk to you about delivering by c-section.

Check your amniotic fluid level. If your practitioner suspects that you have too much or too little fluid, she'll order an ultrasound to check the amount. Depending on the results and your stage of pregnancy, she may request further tests, or you may be induced.

See if your baby is thriving. If you have high blood pressure or diabetes, if you're overdue, if you've previously had a stillbirth, or if you have a host of other complications, your practitioner may order a biophysical profile (BPP) in addition to a nonstress test, which uses ultrasound to evaluate your baby's body movements, muscle tone, and breathing movements and to measure the amount of amniotic fluid in your uterus.

Check your baby's position. After week 36, if your caregiver suspects that your baby isn't in the usual head-down position (or if she simply can't tell for sure), she'll order an ultrasound to confirm your baby's position. If your baby is breech or lying horizontally, you can opt for an external cephalic version to try to get him to turn. (Ultrasound is used during the procedure itself, too.)

Doppler Sonography

WHAT: This noninvasive test can be done at the same time as an ultrasound and uses the same equipment to measure blood flow in different parts of your baby's body, such as the umbilical cord, brain, liver, and heart. Depending on the direction of the flow and its intensity, different colored signals appear on the ultrasound screen and can help your caregiver assess your baby's health.

WHO: Women with high-risk pregnancies, including those who have low amniotic fluid levels, who have Rh sensitization, who have twins sharing the same placenta, or whose babies aren't growing like they should be.

WHEN: Between week 28 and delivery.

WHY: In certain situations, such as when your practitioner has a question about whether your placenta is running out of steam (thus delivering less oxygen- and nutrient-rich blood to your baby) and whether your baby is growing enough, she can use Doppler sonography to evaluate the flow of blood in the umbilical cord or in your baby's body itself. This information will help her decide whether your baby needs to be delivered early or other medical measures are needed to protect her health.

HOW: Most modern ultrasound machines have a Doppler function that allows your sonographer to simply locate a specific blood vessel that she wants to evaluate (one of the arteries in your umbilical cord, for instance) and then turn on a button. Blue or red highlights on the screen will signal the characteristics of the blood flow, which the machine will then analyze. All of this will just take a few minutes during the course of your ultrasound.

Nonstress Test

WHAT: A simple, painless procedure in which your baby's heartbeat is continuously monitored and recorded for at least 20 minutes in order to evaluate his condition. Just as *your* heart beats faster when you're active, your baby's heart rate should go up while he's moving or kicking.

WHO: Women who have preexisting medical conditions that complicate their pregnancy or who develop problems that make it high risk. Some of the most common reasons for ordering a nonstress test are:

• You have diabetes treated with insulin, have high blood pressure, or have other medical conditions that may affect your pregnancy.
• You develop pregnancy-induced hypertension.
• Your baby seems small or isn't growing properly.
• Your baby is less active than normal.
• You have either too much or too little amniotic fluid.
• You've had a procedure such as an external cephalic version or third-trimester amniocentesis. Afterward, your practitioner will order a nonstress test to make sure your baby's doing well.
• You're past your due date and your practitioner wants to see how your baby's holding up during his extended stay in the womb.
• You've previously lost a baby in the second half of pregnancy (due either to an unknown reason or to a problem that might recur in this pregnancy).

WHEN: The timing will depend on the reason for the testing.

WHY: To evaluate how your baby's doing in the womb. If his heart beats faster (at least 15 beats a minute over his resting rate) while he's moving and this acceleration lasts at least 15 seconds on two separate occasions during a 20-minute span, the result is normal, or "reactive." A normal result means that your baby is likely doing fine for now. If the reason that your practitioner ordered the testing in the first place persists, she'll want you to undergo testing every week (or more often) until your baby is born.

If your baby's heart isn't reactive during the first few minutes of testing, it may just be that he's sleeping, so the monitoring will be continued. If after another hour or so there still aren't at least two accelerations, the result is "nonreactive." A nonreactive result doesn't necessarily mean that something's wrong—it merely means that the test didn't yield enough information, so the testing may be extended or you may need to move on to more comprehensive tests, such as a biophysical profile or a contraction stress test. (*Note:* If you haven't yet hit week 32, you might get a nonreactive result simply because of your baby's age—reactivity requires a certain amount of fetal maturity.) If your practitioner feels that your baby is no longer doing well in the womb, she'll likely decide to induce labor.

HOW: You may have heard that you should eat before the test because it will spur your baby to move. While there's no hard evidence for this suggestion, it can't hurt. Plus, it's a good idea to have a snack (and to pee!) before a nonstress test because you may be lying strapped to a monitor for up to an hour. For the procedure itself, the technician or nurse will ask you to lie on your left side or put a wedge under your back so you're slightly tilted to the left. Then she'll strap two electronic devices to your belly. One, an ultrasound transducer, monitors your baby's heartbeat; the other records any uterine contractions you may be having. If your baby isn't moving, the technician may try to wake him up with a buzzer. In some cases, you may be asked to press a button when you feel the baby move. The test usually takes 20 minutes to an hour.

Biophysical Profile (BPP)

WHAT: This noninvasive test gauges your baby's well-being with a combination of the nonstress test and an ultrasound to measure his body and limb movements, muscle tone (flexing of his arms and legs), breathing (his ability to move his chest muscles), and the amount of amniotic fluid surrounding him.

WHO: Women who have preexisting medical conditions that may complicate their pregnancy, and those who develop problems that make pregnancy high risk. These conditions include:

- Diabetes treated with insulin, high blood pressure, or other medical problems
- Pregnancy-induced hypertension
- A baby who seems too small or who isn't growing properly
- A baby who's less active than normal
- Either too much or too little amniotic fluid
- Pregnancy that goes beyond 40 weeks
- The previous loss of a baby in the second half of pregnancy (due to unknown reasons or to a problem that might recur now)
- A nonreactive nonstress test result

WHEN: The timing will depend on the reason for the testing.

WHY: This test indicates—indirectly—whether your baby's getting enough oxygen in the womb. Each of its five components—nonstress test, body movements, muscle tone, breathing movements, and amniotic fluid level—is assigned a score of either 0 (abnormal) or 2 (normal). These scores are added up for a score ranging from 0 to 10. In general, a score of 8 or 10 is normal, 6 is considered borderline, and below 6 is worrisome. If all the ultrasound scores are normal, your practitioner may forgo the heart-rate evaluation. But if the amount of amniotic fluid scores a 0, your baby will need more testing or you may be induced right away (particularly if you're near term)—even if the other components seem fine.

Depending on your baby's score and other factors (such as how far along you are and whether you have other complicating conditions), your practitioner may advise further testing. Or, if she decides that your baby isn't doing well and needs to be delivered, she'll recommend inducing labor or—if your baby is in imminent danger—perform a c-section.

HOW: The test consists of a detailed ultrasound plus a nonstress test. The entire test can take up to an hour, so you may want to have something to eat (and stop for a bathroom break!) beforehand. Your practitioner may repeat the test once or twice a week or more, depending on your situation.

Contraction Stress Test

WHAT: A contraction stress test—also called an oxytocin challenge test—involves deliberately stimulating uterine contractions and then measuring your baby's heart rate to make sure that your placenta is still healthy and that your baby can tolerate the stress of labor. When you have a contraction, the flow of blood and oxygen to your placenta temporarily slows. If the placenta has extra stores of blood ready to provide your baby with the oxygen she needs, her heart rate will be fine during contractions. But if your placenta isn't working the way it should, your baby won't get enough oxygen and her heart rate will slow in response to contractions.

WHO: Though biophysical profiles have largely replaced cumbersome, time-consuming, and expensive stress tests as a way of evaluating high-risk pregnancies, your practitioner may still recommend one. Because this test involves stimulating uterine contractions (which could in rare cases start true labor), it isn't recommended if you have risk factors for preterm labor, if you have a placenta previa, or if you've had a previous "classical" (up-and-down) c-section incision.

WHEN: The timing will depend on the particulars of your situation.

WHY: If your baby's heartbeat reacts normally in response to contractions, she's probably doing fine. This is called a "normal," or "negative," result. In this case, you may wait to go into labor naturally, but you will continue to be followed closely in the meantime. If your baby's heart *does* slow after more than half of your contractions, the test result is "positive," signaling that your baby may be under stress. In this case, your practitioner may recommend delivery right away, either by c-section if your baby couldn't tolerate any contractions or appears to be in imminent danger or by induction of labor if your cervix is soft or starting to dilate.

As alarming as this may sound, try not to worry too much. "Negative" results (meaning everything's okay for now) are very reliable, but "positive" results (signaling a possible problem) are false alarms in about one out of three cases.

HOW: You'll be asked to fast for six to eight hours beforehand, on the slim chance that the results will call for an emergency c-section. (Peeing prior to the test is still a good idea.) Just as with the nonstress test, you'll need to lie on your left side while the technician straps two electric devices to your belly. One, an ultrasound transducer, monitors the baby's heartbeat; the other measures your uterine contractions. A machine records your contractions and your baby's heartbeat as two separate lines on graph paper.

First, you'll be monitored for 15 minutes or so. If you're not having contractions on your own, your practitioner may ask you to stimulate your nipples (which releases natural oxytocin) or she'll give you intravenous synthetic oxytocin (Pitocin). You may barely feel these contractions or they may feel a bit like menstrual cramps, and they shouldn't be strong enough to bring on labor. The test lasts until you've had three contractions, each lasting 40 to 60 seconds, within a ten-minute span. This may take up to two hours. Afterward, you'll need to stick around until your contractions cease or go back to their pretest level.

Symptoms and Complaints

After the relative bliss of mid-pregnancy, hitting your third trimester can be a rude shock. The size of your belly may make you feel like the proverbial bull in a china shop, especially as you near your due date. You'll likely find it harder to get comfortable at night and fall (or stay) asleep, thanks to a variety of woes such as frequent urination and back pain. You may also be plagued by worsening digestive problems, and if you're suffering from hemorrhoids or varicose veins, they'll probably get more uncomfortable as well. And if your physical transformation wasn't already complex enough, when you're within a few weeks of your due date, Braxton Hicks contractions may become fairly frequent and even painful; this can make it difficult to know if labor has really started or if you're just having a bout of "false labor."

If you're feeling more than your share of aches and pains, try to remember that you won't be pregnant forever. A look at what your body may have in store for you this trimester:

Allover Aches and Pains

Around this time, you may start feeling a hard-to-pin-down full-body discomfort. For most women, this hits in the morning and toward the end of the day, and no wonder: After a night of lying on your side or tossing and turning, and a day of lugging your body around or trying to find a good position at your desk or workstation, your poor aching muscles have had enough. Your baby's increased heft can strain your body, making even simple sitting or standing uncomfortable on your back, your hips . . . well, all over. Your legs may ache, and you may also feel increasing pain deep in your but-

BabyCenter Buzz

Oh, My Aching . . .

"It feels like my entire body aches *all the time*—hips, wrists, pelvis, you name it! I'm miserable."   —*Anonymous*

"It helps to get on all fours on my bed. I make use of gravity and let the baby hang away from my back. I look dumb, but it works."   —*Anonymous*

"I've had headaches for almost two weeks. Only one side of my face hurts. My OB recommended acetaminophen, and boy, does it help!   —*Summer*

tocks as your hip joints relax so that your pelvis can better accommodate your baby during childbirth.

Braxton Hicks Contractions

Your uterus actually started contracting sporadically at about week 6, though you probably only noticed this tightening sometime after mid-pregnancy. Until you get to the last few weeks of pregnancy, these contractions—called Braxton Hicks—should be infrequent, irregular, and essentially painless. As your pregnancy advances, Braxton Hicks tend to come more often and sometimes are hard to tell apart from early signs of preterm labor. Don't try to make the diagnosis yourself: If you haven't yet hit week 37 and you're having four or more contractions in an hour or have any other signs of preterm labor, call your caregiver immediately.

By the time you get within a couple of weeks of your due date, these contractions may increase in intensity and frequency and can even become a bit painful. Unlike the earlier, painless, and very sporadic Braxton Hicks, which caused no obvious cervical change, these may actually help your cervix "ripen"—that is, soften, thin (efface), and maybe even begin to open (dilate) a bit. (When that happens, this period is sometimes referred to as "prelabor.") As your due date draws near, Braxton Hicks contractions may even become somewhat rhythmic and relatively close together, at times fooling you into thinking you're in labor. But unlike true labor contractions, they don't grow consistently longer, stronger, and closer together, nor do they cause major cervical dilation.

BabyCenter Buzz

Braxton Hicks Contractions

"I've been getting Braxton Hicks every day since week 20. Believe me, drinking water and sitting down to relax for a minute really helps. I noticed that I got a lot more of them at work (when I was more active), and that they were quite uncomfortable. Now that I'm home, I only get them a few times a day, and they're not as bothersome." —*Sheryl*

"I only have two weeks to go, and I've been feeling mild, painless contractions. But this morning I've had two painful contractions. The last one nearly knocked me off my feet." —*Anonymous*

"I went into the hospital with painful contractions that I've been having for a few days. My doctor told me that I was only 1 centimeter dilated and not even effaced yet. I'm really hating these pains." —*Anonymous*

If you're within a few weeks of your due date and your Braxton Hicks contractions start getting frequent and uncomfortable (if it's earlier in pregnancy, call your doctor or midwife right away), try these measures:

• Change your activity or position. Sometimes walking may provide you with relief, and other times resting may ease your contractions. (Real labor contractions, on the other hand, will persist and progress regardless of what you do.)
• Take a warm bath to help your body relax.
• Try drinking a couple of glasses of water, since these contractions can sometimes be brought on by dehydration.
• Try relaxation exercises or slow, deep breathing. This won't stop the Braxton Hicks, but it may help you cope with the discomfort. (Use this opportunity to practice some of the pain-management strategies you learned in your childbirth preparation class, page 394.)

Breast Changes

Though your mammary glands have been secreting a small amount of thick, yellowish premilk, called colostrum, for many months now, only some women leak before the last few months of pregnancy. By now, though, your breasts are filled with colostrum—so don't be surprised if you look down

Just for Dad

How to Help Her Get Comfy

Be her chair. Have her sit on the bed, in any position that feels good to her. Then spoon your body around hers and invite her to rest back on you. Your arms, chest, and soft murmurs in her ear can support her better than any chair—no matter how ergonomically correct it may be.

Give her a massage. Put a pillow on a chair and ask her to straddle it with her chest facing the chair back, the pillow cushioning her front, and her head resting on some combination of her arms and the pillow. Then sit or stand behind her and, using an open palm, gently circle your hands on her lower back and shoulders. Think in terms of warming these areas, as opposed to doing any sort of "deep" massage. Run your thumbs along her spine, and lightly squeeze her shoulders. Make sure to ask how each motion feels and what she'd like you to do differently, if anything.

Lend a hand. If she's comfortable where she is, or just dreads having to get up, help her out. Offer her a hand if she's getting from one awkward position into another, and try not to laugh if she looks foolish. (If *she* thinks it's funny, you can laugh—a little.) Having to get up in the middle of the night to fetch a glass of water, tuck pillows around her, or pick up something she's dropped is your chance to be a prince among men. She'll definitely appreciate it (especially if you don't complain about it).

---

one day and see two damp blotches on the front of your shirt. Some women also leak colostrum when they're sexually aroused. On the other hand, don't worry if your breasts stay dry—they're producing colostrum and are ready for breastfeeding just the same.

Breathlessness

With your uterus on a continuing quest up and out, you may find yourself feeling like you've just run a 100-meter dash when all you've really done is lumber from the couch to the fridge. The newest culprit: your baby, who's poking up against your diaphragm and limiting your lungs' ability to fully expand. Though you may feel like the Little Engine That Could as you huff and puff, don't worry—the feeling that breathing is a little more difficult is normal and harmless and has zero effect on you or your baby. In fact, the amount of air you inhale with each breath actually *increases* as your pregnancy advances so that you're sure to get all the oxygen you need. (It's only the *volume* of air that remains in your lungs after you exhale that's affected when your growing uterus exerts pressure on your diaphragm.) If this is

Preterm Labor Warning Signs

Call your caregiver if you've yet to reach week 37 and your contractions are becoming more frequent, rhythmic, or painful, or if you have any of the following:

- Abdominal pain, menstrual-like cramping, or more than four contractions in an hour (even if they don't hurt)
- Any vaginal bleeding or spotting
- An increase in vaginal discharge or a change in the type of discharge—if it becomes watery, mucous-like, or bloody (even if it's only pink or blood-tinged)
- Increased pelvic pressure (a feeling that your baby's pushing down)
- Lower-back pain, especially if it's a new problem for you

. . . .

your first pregnancy, this sensation might ease up as your baby "drops" into your pelvis a few weeks before you're due. (If you're not a first-timer, your baby generally won't settle down into your pelvis until labor is under way.)

To breathe a little easier:

Take it slow. Be realistic about what you can and can't do, and listen to your body. If an activity *seems* too taxing, then it is.

Watch your posture. By holding your shoulders back and avoiding slumping over, your lungs will have more room to expand.

Focus on your breath. Concentrate on taking deep, satisfying breaths, channeling them down your throat, and imagining them making it all the way down to your baby.

Prop yourself up. You may find that you're able to breathe more deeply at night if you elevate your head and chest with extra pillows when you're in bed.

Clumsiness

Let's face it: Grace and dexterity aren't part of the late-pregnancy package. In fact, feeling like a klutz is par for the course, especially as you enter these final, fumbling months. And that's no surprise: You're carrying more weight, your center of gravity has shifted along with your uterus,

BabyCenter Buzz

I've Turned into a Total Klutz

"I've started dropping glasses. If there's a glass in the house, I manage to drop or crack it nine times out of ten. My husband finally bought me a set of plastic tumblers. He says that if I keep using real glasses, we won't have any left by the time I deliver!" —*Anonymous*

"For some reason, I've lost all sense of spatial relationships—as well as the ability to parallel park! After bumping into the cars behind *and* in front of me, inadvertently honking my car horn in the process, I decided I'd rather pay to park in the lot." —*Erica*

and your hips and other joints may be looser due to hormones. You're also likely to be distracted by thoughts of what's to come, and therefore more prone to clumsiness. Aside from looking silly, you might be worried about tripping or banging into things. If you do, your baby will most likely be fine—he's well-cushioned by your belly, uterus, and amniotic fluid.

Don't expect yourself to have the same agility you used to: Situations that carry a high risk of falling, like climbing stadium steps or negotiating icy sidewalks, are best done slowly and while holding handrails. And don't even think about getting on a ladder or standing on a chair to change a light-bulb—this is your time to take advantage of the helping hands around you, not to try to do it all on your own.

Constipation, Gas, and Bloating

Earlier in pregnancy, you might have experienced constipation, gas, and bloating due to the hormone progesterone (which slows digestion) and iron (particularly if you've been taking a high-dose supplement). But now another factor comes into play: the increasing pressure of your growing uterus on your rectum, stomach, and intestines, which can exacerbate your digestive troubles.

Diarrhea

Just as when you're *not* pregnant, a stomach virus, food poisoning, or sensitivity to certain foods or medications can cause this unpleasant ailment. Diarrhea might also hit when you go into labor, as part of your body's "clearing-out" process.

If you've come down with a stomach virus or a mild case of food poisoning, you should improve within 24 hours. In the meantime, drink plenty of fluids, and stick to bland foods like bananas, rice, and toast.

Dropping/Lightening

Just when you've really had it with breathlessness and feeling stuffed to the gills after only a few bites of food, your baby may descend into your pelvic cavity and give you some relief. This process is sometimes called "lightening" because once your baby drops, you'll probably have a lighter feeling. If this is your first baby, "dropping" is likely to happen sometime during the last few weeks (for subsequent births, probably not until labor is under way). The downside: Once he's dropped, your baby will take up more room in your pelvis and increase pressure on your bladder, making trips to the bathroom a near constant in your final weeks. And if he's particularly low, you may get an uncomfortable feeling of pressure deep in your pelvis—not to mention developing that trademark late-pregnancy waddle.

Fatigue

Feeling groggy? Weariness often returns now. But in contrast to the total, full-body, falling-into-a-coma brand of exhaustion you felt at the beginning of your pregnancy, third-trimester fatigue often feels more like you stayed up late the night before-which, thanks to the sleep stealers that are so common now, you probably did! What's more, transporting your growing girth can take a toll on your muscles and energy level. That's why it's important to build rest into your schedule as much as you can, be realistic about what your body can handle right now, and continue to make adjustments as your pregnancy advances.

Fetal Movements

The charming flutters and nudges you were enjoying when you first started to notice your baby moving will feel more like full-fledged pokes, prods, and (yes) kicks now that he's bigger. Chances are, you'll feel your little boxer most while you're at rest because babies at this stage tend to be more active at night and you're more likely to notice your baby's movements when you're lying still.

Ask the Experts

**My Baby Sometimes Makes Funny, Rhythmic Movements—
Could He Be Hiccuping?**

Ann Linden, certified nurse-midwife: Yes. Fetal hiccuping is a normal phenomenon that's been observed on many an ultrasound. In fact, your baby may have started hiccuping intermittently beginning in the late first or early second trimester (though you wouldn't have been able to feel them at that early stage). And he'll have occasional bouts of hiccups after he's born, too.

And you soon may experience one of the strangest sensations of the third trimester: feeling a specific part of your baby's body—her heel, for instance—rubbing up against a specific part of yours. Some women swear they can tell their baby's foot is lodged under their ribs; others complain of feeling fingers or toes poking their nether regions. And while your baby may no longer be doing frequent somersaults, he's still making full-body movements—rolling, stretching, and moving his head—and now that he's bigger, they may be more visible than ever before. Watching your baby's gyrations across your belly is one of the more surreal activities you'll probably ever partake in. Enjoy it while you can!

If you compare notes with a pregnant friend or if you've been pregnant before, you'll find that all babies have different patterns and amounts of activity. It's key to pay attention to your baby's movements so you get a good sense of his usual level of activity and to be alert to any changes. Fetal movement is an important indicator of his well-being.

Call your caregiver if you experience either of the following:

• You notice a decrease in activity compared with what you've come to expect from your baby.

• You're counting movements and you don't feel at least ten in one to two hours. (*Note:* There are different acceptable methods of performing kick counts, so your practitioner may give you somewhat different guidelines.)

Frequent Urination and Stress Urinary Incontinence

Your ever-heavier uterus means that during this trimester you'll probably have to pee even more than before. And once your baby drops, you'll have the added pressure of her head on your bladder. Plus, if you have swelling in your lower limbs, you may find that your *pattern* of urination changes, too, with an increased need to pee during the night. (This happens because when you lie on your side to sleep, some of the fluid you've retained during the day makes its way back into your bloodstream and eventually ends up in your bladder.)

Your advancing pregnancy affects not only your bladder but your pelvic floor muscles as well. Many women develop stress urinary incontinence in the later stages of pregnancy, meaning that exercise or activities like coughing, laughing, sneezing, or lifting may cause them to leak some urine.

Heartburn

This unpleasant burning sensation may occur more often now. In addition to the effect of progesterone (which has already made your digestion sluggish and has relaxed the valve between your stomach and esophagus), in later pregnancy your growing baby crowds your abdominal cavity, slowing elimination even *more* and pushing stomach acids upward. This annoyance will probably come and go until you give birth.

Hemorrhoids

Hemorrhoids are essentially varicose veins in your rectal area. There are a number of reasons why pregnancy makes you more prone to these pesky, often itchy eruptions: Your growing uterus puts pressure on your pelvic veins and vena cava, which slows the return of blood from your lower body to your heart and increases pressure on the veins below your uterus, sometimes causing them to dilate and swell. Constipation, another common pregnancy problem, can also bring on or aggravate hemorrhoids because you tend to strain when you're having a hard bowel movement. Finally, an increase in progesterone causes the walls of your veins to relax, allowing them to swell more easily.

Sometimes these enlarged rectal veins actually protrude through your anus. If so, you'll be able to feel a soft, swollen mass—ranging from the size of a raisin to the size of a grape—near your rectum. Though hemorrhoids don't pose a risk to your baby, they can be itchy or painful for you and can cause rectal bleeding, especially during a bowel movement. (Call your caregiver if you have any rectal bleeding.)

To help alleviate or avoid hemorrhoids:

• **Stay regular.** Eat a high-fiber diet, drink plenty of water (at least eight glasses a day), and try to get regular exercise, even if you only have time for a short, brisk walk. If you're constipated, ask your caregiver about using a fiber supplement or a stool softener.

• **Don't "hold it."** Go as soon as you have the urge, try not to strain when moving your bowels, and don't linger on the toilet (sorry, that means no reading!)—all of which put pressure on your rectal area.

• **Do your Kegels** (page 203). They'll increase circulation in your rectal area and strengthen the muscles around your anus (thereby decreasing the chance of hemorrhoids).

• **Avoid sitting or standing for long stretches.** If your job involves sitting, get up and move around for a few minutes every hour or so. At home, lie on your left side when you're sleeping, reading, or watching TV, to take the pressure off your rectal veins and help increase blood return from the lower half of your body.

• **Take a sitz bath.** Soak your bottom for 10 to 20 minutes several times a day (or whenever you can). You don't have to run a bath in the tub—most drugstores sell small plastic tubs that you can fill with warm water and position over your toilet, allowing you to submerge only your bottom and your genitals.

• **Try cold or warm treatments.** Some women find comfort from ice packs or cold compresses medicated with witch hazel, while others swear by a soak in warm water. Try alternating treatments; start with an ice pack followed by a warm sitz bath.

• **Wipe with care.** Use soft, unscented white toilet tissue, which is less irritating than colored, scented brands. Moistening the tissue can help, too. Many women find wiping with medicated moist towelettes designed just for hemorrhoid sufferers more comfortable than using regular toilet paper.

• **Ask your practitioner to recommend safe topical anesthetics or medicated suppositories.** There are many hemorrhoid-relief products on the market, but get your doctor or midwife's okay before trying one on your own. Most of these products are meant for short-term use only (a week or less) because continued use can cause even more inflammation.

Rashes

Now that your belly's in full bloom, you may start itching (and not just for the baby to be born!). While eczema, psoriasis, and other chronic skin disorders can cause itching or rashes—pregnant or not—a few conditions are unique to pregnancy and the postpartum period.

In the last few months of pregnancy, about 1 in 200 women develops a skin disorder called pruritic urticarial papules and plaques of pregnancy (PUPPP). It's characterized by itchy red bumps and larger patches of a hives-like rash that usually show up on your abdomen first. Often the initial bumps are within stretch marks you may have developed, and then, over the next few days, the rash spreads to your thighs, buttocks, and sometimes arms. While PUPPP is harmless to your baby, these itchy eruptions can drive even the calmest woman crazy. The good news is that PUPPP can be safely treated with antihistamines, topical corticosteroid creams, or oral steroids and will disappear after delivery, usually in a matter of days.

Less frequently, women get a skin condition called prurigo of pregnancy (or prurigo gestationis), characterized by tiny, discrete bumps that may resemble bug bites. These eruptions can occur anywhere on your body, but you're most apt to get them on your arms and legs. Though they can be itchy and annoying, they pose no risk to your baby. Prurigo of pregnancy can develop in any trimester, but it's more common in the second half of pregnancy.

If you just have some mild, run-of-the-mill itchiness on your expanding belly, try these comfort measures:

- Avoid hot showers and baths—they'll just dry out your skin and make itching worse.
- Use mild soaps, rinse well, and towel off lightly.
- Slather on a nonscented moisturizer (some scents can worsen irritation).
- Try an oatmeal-bath preparation (available in most drugstores).
- Wear loose cotton clothing and avoid going out in the heat of the day, since heat can intensify the itching.

Call your caregiver if you experience either of the following:

- You have *any* itchy rash—so she can evaluate it, make a diagnosis, and recommend appropriate treatment (or perhaps give you a referral to a dermatologist).
- You feel itchy everywhere. This can be a sign of a liver problem, called intrahepatic cholestasis of pregnancy, that affects about 1 to 2 percent of pregnant women. It generally develops in late pregnancy and happens

when bile doesn't flow normally in the small ducts in your liver, causing bile salts to accumulate in your skin. This can make you itch all over, and the itching can be quite intense. The disorder itself doesn't cause a rash, but you may end up with irritated and reddened skin with little cuts in areas where you're scratching a lot. Call your doctor or midwife immediately if you think you have cholestasis because it carries some risk for your baby. You'll get blood tests to help make the diagnosis and to check your liver function, and an ultrasound to check on your baby. Depending on your situation, you may need to have labor induced.

Swelling (Edema)

Swelling of your ankles and feet tends to strike with full force this trimester and can be especially bad at the end of the day or in hot weather. You may also develop some mild swelling of your hands. (*Hint:* If you haven't yet removed your wedding ring and other snug jewelry, now's the time.)

Vaginal Discharge

The flow of vaginal discharge may increase as you approach your due date. In very early pregnancy, cervical secretions filled your cervical canal and created a protective barrier—the so-called mucus plug. As you approach labor and your cervix begins to thin out, you may notice a dramatic uptick in the amount of mucous discharge over a couple of days. It may look like egg white or mucus from a stuffy nose. Or you might expel the plug in one gelatinous glob. The plug is usually tinged with a bit of blood—so is also referred to as "bloody show" and is a sign that you'll likely be going into labor within the next few days. That said, some women don't have any show at all until labor is under way, and bloody show right after a pelvic exam isn't a sign of impending labor because the exam itself can dislodge the mucus plug.

YOUR NUTRITION
AND FITNESS

Eating Well
What to Eat (and Drink) Now

This is no time to skimp. Your baby is growing rapidly, and his nutritional and caloric needs are reaching their peak. His skeleton is hardening, his brain is developing billions of neurons, his muscles and lungs are maturing, and he's adding a much-needed layer of fat to buffer him once he's out in the world. Plus, your body is working extra hard to facilitate all of that growth. To keep both of you well-nourished and -hydrated, these nutrients are especially important now:

Calcium and vitamin D. As his skeleton is developing, your baby is using up about 200 milligrams of calcium a day, so make sure you get 1,000 milligrams total. (And because vitamin D helps your body absorb the calcium you eat, make sure you get enough sunshine—about 15 minutes a day—to make your own vitamin D, or eat foods with vitamin D, such as fatty fish, milk, and fortified cereal.)

Iron. You'll need plenty of this important mineral for your growing baby and the placenta that nourishes him. You also need iron to produce extra red blood cells to keep up with your expanding blood volume and to give you extra protection if you lose a lot of blood during childbirth. You'll need 27 milligrams a day of elemental iron, and many practitioners recommend a supplement to make sure you get enough. (If you're taking prenatal vitamins, they likely contain at least this amount.) If you have iron deficiency anemia, your doctor or midwife will recommend iron supplements so your daily intake is about 60 to 120 milligrams of iron.

BabyCenter Buzz

How I Feel about the Weight I've Gained

"I'm nearly due and have gained only 26 pounds. I know it's not a whole lot, but to me it seems like a ton. I can't wait to have this baby just so I can feel normal again!" —Amber

"I know my weight should be the least important thing to me right now—after all, I'm growing this little person inside me and my first priority should be (and is) keeping him or her safe and healthy. But I'm worried about my weight and my body, too!" —Anonymous

"It's hard to reconcile having tried to stay slim for so many years with the fact that it's now okay to gain weight. I think I'm going to put the scale away and try not to worry so much." —Angie

"I just eat well for myself and my baby. I think some people gain a little more or a little less, depending on how their body works." —Anonymous

Fat. Your baby's brain and vision will undergo a big developmental spurt this trimester—a process that depends on adequate dietary fat. Pay particular attention to the kind of fat you eat now: Essential fatty acids are critical, and you need 1.4 milligrams of omega-3 fatty acids a day (Good food sources include fish, walnuts, flaxseed, canola oil, and dark leafy greens such as kale). But while some fat is good, be sure to take it easy on saturated and trans fats.

Protein. Your baby's growth and development depend on getting enough of this nutrient. Be sure you're eating at least 71 grams a day.

Water. Keep chugging at least eight 8-ounce glasses of water a day. You can't function without it, and your body uses extra water during pregnancy. You need H_2O to—among other things—supply fluid for your rising blood volume and to form the amniotic fluid that bathes and protects your baby.

Vitamin C. This nutrient is vital for tissue repair and can aid your recovery after giving birth. Shoot for 85 milligrams a day.

Folic acid. This important B vitamin is essential not only before conception and during the first trimester, to decrease the risk of neural tube defects, but throughout pregnancy as well. Your body and your baby need folic acid to produce and repair DNA and allow it to function. Folic acid is also

Just the Facts

The Spicy Food—Labor Link

It's a common piece of folk wisdom: If you're close to your due date and want to give nature a nudge, try a fiery Mexican meal or an eye-watering Indian dish. Is there any truth to the old wives' tale? There's certainly no definitive research that confirms the link, but if you enjoy a good spicy meal, then go ahead and chow down. But be forewarned: It may cause (or exacerbate) uncomfortable heartburn.

vital for the production of red blood cells. Aim for 600 micrograms of folic acid a day.

For more specific information about these nutrients and examples of good sources, see page 74.

Healthy Weight Gain
How Much You'll Gain This Trimester

Most women gain about a pound a week this trimester—though you may put on a little more or a little less, depending on your diet, lifestyle, and individual metabolism. Weight gain now is critical for your baby's development. As in early pregnancy, as long as you're trying to stick to a healthy diet and getting some regular exercise, you're probably right where you should be.

Staying Fit
Why You Should Keep Exercising

Now that you're truly "living large," exercise becomes more of a challenge—but it also offers some welcome rewards. A moderate, gentle exercise routine can be a great way to help keep common pregnancy discomforts at bay, improve your body image, and calm the anxiety that's likely to mount as your due date approaches. Plus, anything you can do to fight inertia and keep your body toned and flexible is bound to help as you head into labor. We can't say

Just the Facts

Dropping That Baby Weight

If you find your current scale reading distressing, remind yourself that you'll lose a substantial amount of weight immediately after giving birth—namely, the 16 to 20 pounds that make up your baby, amniotic fluid, placenta, and blood and bodily fluids. For the average mother-to-be, that leaves only about 10 pounds of extra weight to contend with after the baby's born. And though most of this sum is usually lost in the first three months after you give birth, it may take up to six months (or more) to melt away completely, particularly if you've gained more than the recommended amount. But with a healthy diet and regular exercise, it will eventually come off.

whether exercise will truly shorten your labor and decrease the likelihood of medical interventions, but it's certain to increase your endurance and confidence in your body and make you better prepared for whatever birth scenario you may face—as well as for getting your body back afterward.

The Best Exercises for Your Third Trimester

At this stage of your pregnancy, the size of your belly and the safety of its lively inhabitant will obviously limit your choice of workout routines. And, of course, general guidelines about who shouldn't exercise, which activities to avoid, and other prenatal exercise considerations (page 81) still apply. For the most part, you'll need to stick with familiar routines rather than trying something new, and focus on exercises that are gentle and low impact. Swimming, walking, and yoga are ideal third-trimester workouts, as are the simple labor-preparation exercises described here.

Swimming

As your pregnancy enters its final phase, there's no better way to get in an aerobic workout than through swimming. Besides making you feel better overall, aerobic exercise stimulates breathing and circulation-not to mention burning calories, strengthening muscles, building endurance, reducing stress, and improving your mood. What's more, simply climbing (avoid jumping or diving) into a pool and releasing your body from the aching pull of gravity feels wonderful. The water's buoyancy frees you to exercise safely: It supports your joints and ligaments, prevents injury, and protects you from overheating (as long as you swim in pools under 85°F). If bobbing up and down for air makes the muscles around your neck ache, try using a snorkel.

Walking

Like swimming, walking is a good way to get aerobic exercise well into your third trimester. And if you don't have much time to work out, walking can easily be built into your daily routine. (Plus, it's good preparation for walking up and down your hallway or the hospital corridor once you're in labor!) Keep up your walking regimen as long as you can, but avoid paths or hiking trails with uneven terrain that could throw you off balance. As you get closer to your due date, you may also want to consider walking on a track. The cushioned walking surface will be easier on your body—and you may feel safer staying close to home or your car in case of an emergency.

Yoga

If yoga has been part of your prenatal fitness routine so far, you'll appreciate its benefits now more than ever. Poses that gently open and expand your pelvic region—such as *Baddha Konasana* (similar to the tailor or cobbler sitting exercise described in the next section)—feel especially good at this stage for most women. Focus on keeping your breathing deep and relaxed as you stretch slowly into each pose, creating a sense of calmness that stays with you no matter how your body is positioned. Trust us: You'll be glad you practiced this when you're in the final stages of labor!

As in your second trimester, be cautious about stretching your loosening joints too far and about risking injury. (The extent of ligament and joint relaxation varies from woman to woman—even if the rest of your prenatal yoga class is comfortably doing a pose that you find

BY THE NUMBERS

Working Out in the Homestretch

46% of expectant moms ease up a bit on exercise in late pregnancy

20% keep up the same prenatal exercise pace in their third trimester as they did earlier

18% stop working out altogether once their pregnancy reaches its final months

5% worked out *more* now

Source: *A BabyCenter.com poll of more than 3,600 women*

uncomfortable, listen to your body and stop.) Standing poses will help your lower body stay toned in preparation for the big day, but you should steady your heel against the wall or use a supporting chair to keep from losing your balance. You may also want to use blocks or straps to increase your stability in various poses. Finally, remember to modify poses as needed to avoid lying flat on your back (for example, opt for a side-lying version of *Savasana* for relaxation).

Sport-Specific Safety Strategies

If you've been following a more strenuous routine and you want to keep going with it, be sure to run it by your practitioner first—and to take these late-pregnancy precautions:

Dancing. Avoid movements that can result in dizziness and shortness of breath. Jumps, lifts, dips, and fast spins are also off-limits now.

Low-impact aerobics. Pay attention to which types of movements aren't compatible with your pregnant belly. If a move feels too tricky or uncomfortable, march in place instead. This simple trick lets you keep your heart rate up while giving your body a bit of a break. Avoid bending over, spinning, or turning, too—these movements can make you dizzy and perhaps even lead to a fall. And consider taking a prenatal water aerobics class if one is available in your community. Not only will it be gentler on your joints, but exercise while standing in water may help lessen swelling in your legs.

Running or jogging. As always, be careful and listen to your body. If you feel too fatigued to go for a run, it's perfectly okay to take a break. And if you begin to find that running or jogging is making your hips or other joints ache, it's time to switch to a gentler activity. While being sedentary isn't healthy, pushing yourself too hard can be harmful, too; find a balance between these extremes. Even avid runners find that their pace slows considerably during their third trimester—a fast waddle or shuffle may be the best you can do.

Fit for Labor: Four Simple Exercises to Prepare Your Body for Delivery Day

If you don't have time for a half-hour walk, swim, or yoga session every day, don't beat yourself up about it. By spending a little time on one or more of the following exercises whenever you get a chance, you'll help tone the parts

BabyCenter Buzz

My Exercise Routine in the Third Trimester

"I'm at week 28 and still running three miles, four times a week. I bought a belly belt to help with the bounce and so far have had no problems. I'm much slower now than I used to be, but that's okay." —Amy

"I'm still running in week 35. I definitely don't run as far as I used to, though. Some days I just walk. I feel like a big whale running down the street, and I get *lots* of funny looks. Most people smile or cheer, but some look mortified—I think they're afraid I'll lie down on their front lawn and give birth!" —Cheryl

"I did regular, nonprenatal yoga for the first seven months, but my belly has finally taken over and some of the poses have become cumbersome. So lately I've been doing a 'baby and mom yoga' video at home. The exercises provide a lot of stretching and movement of my pelvic region." —Anonymous

"I'm going into my week 36, and I've never been more miserable! My only relief is swimming, which eases the pain in my varicose veins. I'm ready to try sleeping in the pool!" —Libby

"When my third trimester started, I made a commitment to work my heart and muscles more—and because walking was getting cumbersome and painful for my back, I took up swimming. I go three times a week for an hour, and I love it! I'm sleeping much better, and the back pain has really improved." —Anonymous

"I'm taking prenatal yoga and walking almost every night. This pregnancy has gone a lot smoother than my first, and I attribute that to staying in shape!" —Anonymous

"I'm at week 37 and still working out, but the heat and humidity have hit and I find breathing more difficult now. My baby's still very high, and she's pressing on my diaphragm quite a bit. Now I just take it one workout at a time." —S.P.

of your body that work the hardest during labor and delivery. And remember that you can do some of these exercises while you're doing some other enjoyable activity—like watching TV or listening to music. Ease into each exercise at your own pace, and repeat it as many times as it's comfortable for you—never strain or force a position.

Kegels. These discreet, do-anywhere motions will strengthen your pelvic-floor muscles and thus help prevent stress urinary incontinence now and aid postpartum recovery later. They help prevent postpartum urine leaks, too. Good pelvic-floor muscle tone makes sex more pleasurable, and some research suggests that pelvic-floor exercises may help shorten the pushing stage of labor for some women. (See page 203 for instructions on how to do Kegels.)

Angry cat. This variation of the pelvic tilt is done on all fours. It strengthens your abdominal muscles and eases back pain during pregnancy and labor. To do it, get down on your hands and knees with your arms held straight and spaced shoulder-width apart and with your knees spaced hip-width apart. Next, take a breath in, and exhale as you tighten your abdominal muscles, round your back, and tuck your butt under. Then inhale and relax your back into a neutral—but not a swayback—position. Repeat three times. Work up to ten repetitions as you get stronger.

Squatting. It may not look elegant, but squatting is a time-honored way of preparing for (and giving!) birth. Since your pelvic opening is widest when you're squatting, it can be a good position to use during the pushing stage of labor. Doing squats now strengthens your legs so you'll have the ability and stamina to use this position if need be when the big day arrives. To practice the position: Hold on to the back of a sturdy chair for support. Stand with your feet spread slightly wider than hip-width and your toes pointed outward. Bend your knees and slowly lower your bottom toward the floor as if you were going to sit in a chair. As you lower yourself, contract your abdominal muscles, lift your chest, and relax your shoulders. Most of your weight should be resting on your heels. Slowly return to standing. Repeat

Just the Facts

The Exercise-and-Labor Connection

As your due date approaches, well-meaning friends and relatives are sure to regale you with stories about their own labor starting after a particularly challenging hike, or about contractions kicking in the day they decided to move all the living room furniture around. But while such anecdotes are common, medical research has yet to bear out a connection between working out and going into labor.

You may have also heard that one form of "exercise"—sex—can induce labor. And though orgasm *can* trigger the release of oxytocin (the hormone that causes uterine contractions), and semen *does* contain prostaglandins (substances responsible for cervical ripening), the jury is still out on whether sexual intercourse actually helps kick-start labor in women near term. Whatever the final verdict, though, you can certainly have fun trying!

Just the Facts

When to Stop Exercising

Even if you've been active throughout your pregnancy without problems, it's wise to take a break from exercising and contact your doctor or midwife if you develop any of the following symptoms:

- Trouble breathing
- Calf pain or sudden swelling
- Chest pain or an irregular heartbeat
- Decreased fetal movement
- Feeling faint or dizzy
- Headache
- Leaking amniotic fluid
- Muscle weakness or significant pain
- Pelvic or abdominal pain or contractions (or any other signs of preterm labor)
- Vaginal spotting or bleeding

five times—or as many as you can manage comfortably. If you experience any discomfort—such as pelvic or knee pain—during this exercise, ease up; the other exercises in this section are better choices for you.

Tailor or cobbler sitting. Sitting on the floor in one of these positions helps condition and increase the flexibility of your inner-thigh muscles in preparation for birth, and eases lower-back tension as well: Sit either with your legs crossed or with the soles of your feet touching each other and your knees out to the side (you may want to put a folded blanket under each knee to prevent overstretching), and be sure to maintain good posture. If you like, you can sit with your back resting against a wall. Stay in this position for as long as you're comfortable.

BY THE NUMBERS

Sex to Start Labor

38% of mothers-to-be definitely plan to have sex in an effort to get labor going

31% might try it

31% are skeptical about intercourse as labor inducer

Of the mothers who tried this method:

14% say it worked

39% admit they aren't sure

47% say that a roll in the hay did little to nudge nature along

Source: *A BabyCenter.com poll of more than 2,300 women*

Getting Enough Sleep

Remember the so-called honeymoon stage of your pregnancy, just a few weeks ago? With the discomfort, awkwardness, and insomnia that typify late-pregnancy sleep—or lack thereof—those nights of leisurely slumber may soon seem like a distant dream. While the term "good night's sleep" is relative at this point, there *are* creative ways to get the rest you so desperately need.

Third Trimester Sleep: So Long, Slumber

You're not dreaming. Research proves that the quality of sleep in the third trimester is worse than ever before. You'll have fewer periods of deep sleep and wake up more often during the night. As your belly grows, it'll become increasingly more difficult to get comfortable at night. If sleeping on your side with pillows wedged between your legs and behind your back doesn't help, head for a comfy recliner instead—as your belly reaches watermelon proportions, you may sleep better propped up. And don't be surprised if heartburn, back pain, leg cramps, restless legs syndrome, and the frequent need to pee—not to mention your baby's in-utero acrobatics—keep you awake at night.

BY THE NUMBERS

Chasing the Sandman

29%	of moms-to-be read in an effort to lull themselves to sleep
26%	take a warm shower or bath
22%	have sex as a sleep inducer
9%	try a relaxation technique such as yoga or deep breathing
8%	have a glass of warm milk
5%	eat a high-carb snack

Source: *A BabyCenter.com poll of more than 10,800 women*

Third Trimester Sleep Problems— and Solutions

To be honest, there's only so much you can do to counteract the inevitable. Still, there *are* some simple strategies that may help you get a little more rest during the homestretch of your pregnancy. Common third-trimester sleep stealers, and how best to handle them:

FREQUENT URINATION

As your uterus continues to enlarge and put pressure on your bladder, you'll likely have to pee even more frequently than before. Limit your nighttime bathroom

BabyCenter Buzz

What I Do to Get to Sleep at Night

"I practice deep breathing and relaxation exercises; I fall right to sleep when I do them." —*Christina*

"Doing crossword puzzles right before bed relaxes me. I never finish the puzzles, but I do drop off after about 15 minutes!" —*Melissa*

"Sleeping in a lounge chair in our bedroom helps. I miss sleeping with the hubby, but at least I'm *sleeping*!" —*Kim*

"Lavender works wonders for soothing anxieties. Taking a warm bath with three to five drops of lavender oil or putting a drop on your pillowcase is great!" —*Adria*

"I bought a long body pillow, and it's a lifesaver. I put it under my head, chest, and stomach and between my legs. I couldn't—and wouldn't—sleep without it." —*Kelly*

breaks by cutting back on fluids in the late afternoon and evening and by completely emptying your bladder during every trip to the toilet. (*Hint:* Leaning forward when you pee will help.)

INSOMNIA

With such a litany of physical sleep disturbances—not to mention run-of-the-mill preparental jitters—it's no surprise that three out of four mothers-to-be have insomnia and other sleep problems. Although misery may love company, knowing that other women are tossing and turning won't provide much solace when you're watching the numbers on your clock radio change in the middle of the night. Some of the following advice, however, may:

* Keep to a regular bedtime and morning wake-up time. And try not to nap too late in the day.
* Cut down on caffeine consumption, and avoid it altogether in the late afternoon and evening. And completely avoid alcohol and tobacco; they not only are harmful to your baby but can disrupt your sleep as well.
* Avoid heavy, spicy meals before bedtime, and drink more fluids during the day and less in the late afternoon and evening.
* Use your bed only for sleep and sex.

Just for Dad

How to Help Your Partner Get a Good Night's Rest

Let's face it: It's no fun for you when your partner wakes up in the middle of the night, shifts around in bed, sighs in frustration, or turns on the light to flip through pages of a magazine—loudly. Luckily for you, this is one of the areas where your efforts might yield a quick payoff, or at least a lot of appreciation. Some things to try:

Take over the post-dinner cleanup. Your partner will be better off if she takes time to wind down before she gets in bed, and your tidying up the kitchen and fielding phone calls will help ease her way. Encourage her to read, listen to music, or just relax.

Give her a massage before she falls asleep. Concentrate on her neck, feet, and hands. Use her favorite body oil or lotion to make your motions smoother.

In bed, help her arrange the pillows to support her back and belly. Give her a hand getting out of bed, too.

Make the move. If snoring (yours or hers) is keeping one of you up, offer to be the one to relocate to the guest room.

Be patient with her different sleeping schedule. If she turns in an hour before you do, or doesn't need to leave for work until an hour after you depart, try to be quiet as you move around the bedroom. Remember: Her insomnia is a temporary situation. Soon you'll *both* be sleep-deprived!

- Establish a regular, relaxing bedtime routine. You may want to start winding down by taking a warm bath or—if you're in the mood and your partner is willing—asking for a massage.

- Try a prebed relaxation technique, such as progressive muscle relaxation or guided imagery (page 186).

- Don't tackle any anxiety-producing tasks or chores (like paying bills) close to your bedtime.

- Other than gentle stretching, don't exercise late in the day—that includes housework. Finish your workout at least three to four hours before bedtime. (But do get in the habit of exercising during the day—it's a stress reducer and can help you sleep.)

- Make sure your bedroom is conducive to sleep. Adjust the temperature so that it's comfortable (if your partner's cold, ask him to get another blanket rather than turn up the heat). Is the room dark and quiet enough? Heavy or dark-colored curtains can block out unwanted light, and white-noise sound machines (or using a fan) can help mask the drone of traffic.

- Stop watching the clock—you'll just get increasingly anxious as the sleepless moments creep by, and worrying about your lack of sleep will only compound the problem. (You may even want to turn your clock around so you can't see it.)
- If you aren't asleep 20 minutes after climbing into bed, get up and go to another room. Read a magazine or listen to music until you feel drowsy; then go back to bed.

RESTLESS LEGS SYNDROME

An overwhelming urge to move your legs is a hallmark of restless legs syndrome (RLS), a disorder that's relatively common in pregnancy. This urge begins (or worsens) while you're inactive, is worse during the evening or at night, and is at least partly (though temporarily) relieved by movement or rubbing your legs. Most people with RLS describe uncomfortable sensations in their limbs as well, such as a crawling, creeping, tingling, burning, or painful feeling. (Some women also notice symptoms in their arms as well.)

Since RLS is usually triggered by inactivity, it's no surprise that it can wreak havoc on your ability to fall asleep. And since women with RLS are also likely to experience involuntary leg movements while they sleep, it can affect your ability to *stay* asleep, too.

No one knows for sure what causes RLS, but one theory is that—at

Ask the Experts

Will My Lack of Sleep Harm My Baby?

Dr. Mary O'Malley, sleep medicine specialist: It's natural to assume that if you aren't sleeping well, your baby isn't, either. But relax—your baby can sleep even when you're wide-awake. No one knows for sure why your baby sleeps independently of you, though experts do know that the need to sleep is one our strongest physiological drives. We also know that a baby isn't bothered by the same sounds that keep you awake. Layers of skin and muscle, as well as amniotic fluid, insulate him from outside noise and movement. But your baby's not completely cut off from what's going on around him. A sharp noise or sudden movement can wake him, and you may feel a kick or punch as a result.

Your baby's health *is* at risk if your lack of sleep affects your ability to function—for instance, if you fall asleep while you're driving, or exhaustion leads you to stumble or fall.

Ask the Experts

Do Sleep Patterns before Birth Affect Patterns after Birth?

Dr. Mary O'Malley, sleep medicine expert: You've probably heard that if your baby is most active in the womb at night, he'll be a night owl once he's born. Some moms—as well as a few sleep experts—swear this old wives' tale is true, but no scientific evidence bears it out.

That doesn't contradict the fact that your baby *is* developing a sleep-wake cycle before he's born. At about 6 or 7 months gestation, he started having active or REM (rapid eye movement) sleep, the phase of sleep in which we dream. He'll add non-REM sleep—also known as quiet sleep—between his 7th and 8th months in the womb. Just like newborns, babies in utero don't have our typical day-night schedule; they rest for a few hours and then are awake for a few hours. So don't worry about disturbing his sleep routine—you'll have to wait until a month or two after he's born for him to even *have* one!

least in some cases—it's related to another common pregnancy condition: iron deficiency anemia, which tends to happen around the same time. Another theory is that a folate deficiency may play a role. There also appears to be a genetic component to RLS; if one of your immediate family members suffers from the disorder, you're more likely to as well.

DEALING WITH RLS

Though RLS itself isn't medically serious, its effects can range from mildly irritating to downright disturbing. Strategies for easing symptoms:

• Several kinds of drugs effectively treat RLS, but most are discouraged during pregnancy. Instead, ask your caregiver for simple blood tests to determine whether you're suffering from iron-deficiency anemia; if so, iron supplements may be all you need to banish RLS.

• Though getting up and moving around offers only temporary relief, simple stretching exercises for your legs—and your arms if they've been bothering you, too—every night before going to bed may give you more sustained relief.

• Try doing mild to moderate exercise daily to help keep your symptoms at bay.

• See if a warm bath gives you some relief. If that doesn't help, try a cool bath or alternating the two.

• Steer clear of caffeine, tobacco, and alcohol, all of which worsen RLS symptoms.

• Don't take antihistamines or cold and sinus medications with antihistamines, which can exacerbate your symptoms.

• Avoid reading or watching TV in bed—because the longer you lie still, the worse your symptoms will become. Go to bed only when you're actually ready to sleep.

SNORING AND CONGESTION

As you enter your third trimester, you may find yourself more congested than usual and possibly even snoring for the first time in your life. While you—and your partner—may be less than thrilled about this new development, take heart: There's a good chance you'll stop snoring after your baby is born.

One explanation behind your midnight melodies is congested or swollen nasal passages. An increase in pregnancy hormones may cause the soft tissues of your nasal passages to swell and partially block your airways. Also, pregnancy weight gain can lead to a bulkier neck and more tissue in your throat—making snoring even likelier. If your snoring is severe, it may be a sign that you have sleep apnea.

What's in a Dream? Third Trimester Dream Themes—And What They Might Mean

Your unconscious will continue to reflect your waking concerns—which now means getting ready for childbirth and motherhood. Vivid dreams continue, and nightmares are common. If you're like most expectant mothers, you're running through an ever-changing mental checklist of parental prep issues: How will I handle labor? Will I be a good mother? Who *is* this baby, anyway? Here, BabyCenter dream expert, clinical psychologist, and *Women's Bodies, Women's Dreams* author Patricia Garfield takes a look at some common third trimester dreams and offers possible interpretations.

You dream about your baby's sex. From their dreams alone, some mothers-to-be are quite certain of their baby's gender. One mom, for instance, was convinced she was carrying a girl because her dreams were filled with images of a field of flowers, quite unlike the visions of hard, jagged rocks that filled her dreams when she was expecting her firstborn, a son. And later she did indeed give birth to a daughter. But like most of the gender guesswork we do, it's not a hard science: Only half of expectant mothers accurately dream of their baby's sex—and since the chance of having a child of either gender is also 50–50, these dreamers' unconscious forecasts were no better at predicting their baby's sex than flipping a coin would be.

You see your baby. Many pregnant women report having some dreams where they "see" their babies. Instead of assuming that what you're seeing is a perfect vision of your child, it's probably more useful to look at these dreams as a key to understanding what you're hoping for or worrying about. What do you notice about the baby in your dreams, and how do you react to her? Does she have your father's strong jaw and your mother-in-law's gorgeous eyes? Or is she the spitting image of that great-aunt you can't stand? No matter what the subject of your dreams happens to be, remember that they're best at telling you what's going on inside your *own* mind.

You hear your baby's name. You may have a dream where your baby announces, requests, or even demands his name. Traditionally, some Native American tribes regard names given in a dream as having special power. If you haven't already come up with a name, this can be a great way to explore other, more creative options.

You take a trip. You board a plane to a country you've never visited before, or you pack your bags for a journey but you don't know where you're going. Travel dreams—especially for first-time moms—may signal that you're embarking on an adventure. Since you've never given birth before, you don't know what to expect, much as you wouldn't if you took off for the Seven Seas. Some expectant moms dream of moving through tunnels and corridors, which could also represent birth—either your baby's experience of the birth canal or your own feeling of being "reborn" as a mother.

You wait (and *wait* . . .). Train stations, baseball games, checkout lines . . . you may find yourself dreaming of situations that involve waiting for an expected or unexpected outcome. Just like what you're doing now—waiting, patiently or not, for your little one to arrive.

YOUR EMOTIONS

Before long, you'll be holding that wished-for baby in your arms—and chances are good that until then you'll spend a significant portion of your time daydreaming about your little one, fretting aimlessly, or crying over reality-TV baby shows. Yes, you may find yourself weeping—joyfully, miserably, or even somewhat vaguely—over just about anything these days because, as you're surely beginning to realize, third-trimester emotions are not for the faint of heart. Don't be surprised if you ride out your last weeks on a wave of *feelings*: worry and vulnerability, impatience, grief over your present life ending, boredom, mounting discomfort, and, above all, excitement.

The Highest High

As you enter your final trimester, your baby belly is unmistakable to the world, and so is your excitement. Everyone—friends, relatives, and strangers at the supermarket—wants to know when you're due, whether you know if it's a boy or girl, and if they can touch your belly. ("No" is always a perfectly appropriate response.)

There's only so much belly admiring you can do yourself, and so you're probably channeling your own enthusiasm into baby-readying tasks: You decorate the nursery; you pore over baby-name books; you attend childbirth classes and enroll in infant CPR classes; you clean the house in eager anticipation of your pending arrival; and you may even attempt to knit a baby bootie or two.

Your main agenda for the months ahead is to eat well, get plenty of sleep, avoid stress as best you can, and spend time with your partner, enjoying your last few months as a twosome. As your due date approaches, though, it can become a challenge simply to get through the day—you're

Just the Facts

When Worrying Gets out of Hand

Although a mix of strong emotions is common in the third trimester, it's important to seek help if your anxiety is really getting out of hand or if you're down and the feeling won't lift. Your midwife or doctor can help you find a therapist, and you—and your baby—will benefit. Remember, prenatal anxiety and depression often lead to postpartum problems, so the best time to seek help is now.

physically uncomfortable and emotionally volatile. But try to remember to cherish this time instead of merely *enduring* it—when you look back, it will seem like the prelude to the greatest love affair of your life.

What You May Be Worrying about Now

Whether this baby was a total surprise or long-planned, and whether your pregnancy so far has been rocky or smooth, it's normal to be nervous about what lies ahead. Common worries include:

Going into labor early. While some women are at greater risk for preterm labor than others, remind yourself that the vast majority of women carry their pregnancies to term. Still, if you haven't yet hit week 37, it's a good idea to familiarize yourself with the signs of preterm labor (page 297) and to ask your practitioner what to do if you start having contractions early, just in case. A plan of action will help ease your fears.

Recognizing real labor. You probably don't find it very helpful when your friends tell you, "Don't worry—you'll *know* when you're in labor!" But it's true that as your labor progresses, you'll be able to figure it out. If this is your first baby, you'll have plenty of time to tell whether your contractions are the real thing or just stronger Braxton Hicks contractions. Fortunately, you're not expected to be the professional here. Call your caregiver if your contractions have you baffled, and find out now when she wants you to get in touch once contractions start in earnest.

Having a difficult labor or delivery. Maybe you've spent too much time listening to the gory details of your sister-in-law's marathon labor, or perhaps your last birth experience wasn't what you'd hoped for. Whatever the reason, most women experience some anxiety about the birth process.

BabyCenter Buzz

What I Fear Most about Labor

"I'm afraid I won't be able to tell when it's time to go to the hospital. I've been having so many contractions off and on that I wonder if I'll know what a 'real' one feels like." —Kara

"I had a rough experience with my first and am worried that this time around won't be any different. Even though my doctor says there's no reason to expect the same problems, I can't help losing sleep over this." —Bette

Obvious as it is, the idea that the baby—the ever-larger baby—has to get out *somehow* may dawn on you with a new and sudden horror. Talking to your practitioner (and attending childbirth classes) may alleviate some of your fears, especially when you learn about the steps that will be taken should problems arise. In the meantime, try to maintain a positive attitude about your upcoming delivery—but don't get too locked in to specific expectations.

Test results or other complications. Toward the end of this trimester, your doctor or midwife will screen you for Group B strep, an infection that can be passed to your baby during delivery. Don't worry if you test positive; many women do, and antibiotics in labor will protect your baby from infection. If you develop any pregnancy complications, your caregiver will keep an extra-close eye on you and will likely order regular testing—such as biophysical profiles—to keep tabs on your baby, too. Some women are reassured by extra testing, while it makes others more anxious. Finding out what to expect ahead of time (and when you'll get the results) will help take the edge off. Keep going to all your prenatal appointments right up to the end; many late-pregnancy complications can be quickly and safely addressed if they're caught in time.

Getting your body back. If you're preoccupied with worry over your changing shape, take a look around at women who have older kids. You'll find that many of them have regained their "old" bodies and are just as active as they were before getting pregnant. With the right combination of regular exercise and good nutrition, you'll gradually lose most, if not all, of your pregnancy weight. That's not to say your body will be *exactly* the same as it was before. But most changes, such as a softer belly or breasts, aren't very obvious—and your love for your baby may even leave you with a warm spot for those souvenirs of this amazing time.

Being a good parent. The fact that you're worried about being a good parent is a strong indication that you already *are* one because you care about your baby's well-being. But if you're concerned that something from your past will directly affect your baby or your feelings about yourself as a mother, you're right to address it. Start by discussing your concerns with your caregiver; she can refer you to a counselor, if need be.

Overcoming an Unhappy Childhood

If you suspect that your past may impact your baby's future, it's important to take steps to protect both yourself and your baby.

Consider seeking therapy. This is an effective way to handle what may become an overwhelming time in your life—and beginning therapy *before* you have your baby will give you a head start. That way, your support system will already be in place if you run into emotional trouble spots after the birth. Plus, your counselor can coach you on positive parenting skills—both now and after your baby arrives.

Share your worries. Talk to someone you trust, be it your mate, a close friend, or a relative. Verbalizing your emotions helps you begin dealing with them. If you keep your feelings locked up inside, they can grow stronger and eventually overwhelm you. Instead, let them out, little by little, by sharing them with someone who cares.

Keep yourself strong and healthy. Eat well, rest as much as possible, sleep when you can, exercise moderately, and for your sake—and your baby's—avoid alcohol, tobacco, and drugs. When your mind and body are strong, you're in better shape to cope with negative emotions.

Think positively. If you've had a particularly good day, remind yourself how sweet life can be. Tell yourself that you have many more good days ahead of you. Think about the positive things you've done and the kind things that others have done for you. See yourself as sharing the best of yourself with your child.

Know that your past isn't your future. Vow to be conscious in the parenting choices you make—and remember that you're starting fresh with your own children. Read books on the subject, take a parenting class, write down your

Just for Dad

What *You* May Be Worried about Now

Many fathers-to-be fear that they won't hold up during labor and delivery. You may worry about getting queasy, throwing up, or even passing out in the presence of all those bodily fluids. Or you may simply find yourself dreading your partner's pain and worrying that you won't be a strong enough support person for her. But while these are real and daunting emotional hurdles, most fathers navigate them just fine. Still, acknowledge your fears and anticipate your own limitations. Talking to other guys who've been there will give you some ideas about what you'll need to do to get through.

You might also want to come up with some strategies for staying strong during your partner's labor and birth. Plan to step out of the labor room when you need a breath of fresh air, for instance. Or talk to her about asking another relative or friend to offer backup support. The two of you might even consider hiring a doula (professional birth coach) if you worry that you won't be in top form when the time comes.

In terms of being prepared, the best defense is a good offense. Develop a birth plan, and define your role long before her contractions begin. And above all, read all you can about labor and delivery. Maybe the pregnancy was a surprise, but you sure don't want the birth to be one! (Still, if plans change once you're in the delivery room or if you're having trouble with your assigned tasks, stay flexible and ask for backup. Your most important job is to let your partner know you're there for her. If you can't help her with her breathing exercises, hold her hand, bring her a cool washcloth, feed her ice chips, or call the nurse.)

If you and your partner haven't signed up for a childbirth class, make arrangements to do so right away. Not only will this show her that you're in this together, but you'll likely get the opportunity to watch several birth videos—a preview that can function as a real shock tamer when your own time comes. That said, there's no way to prepare yourself for the profound joy of your baby's birth. You'll just have to feel it yourself.

hopes and fears, and let yourself imagine what a happy childhood might be like. *That's* the one you can help create for your baby.

Reclaim your relationship with your partner once your baby is born. Many couples fear that their relationship is on the rocks during the last few months of pregnancy, when sex often becomes burdensome and an expectant mother's libido commonly loses oomph. Stress about the upcoming changes in your lives also may lead to bickering, quick tempers, and other heightened emotions. Once the baby is born, and after the initial shock of parenting has worn off (give yourselves at least six months to recuperate), the old flames usually still burn bright. *Note:* If your relationship has become physically or emotionally abusive—page 98—seek help immediately.

"Pregnancy Brain": Why You're So Scattered Now

With the distraction of this pending sea change in your life, it can be difficult to focus on the more mundane events of daily existence. This is even more true if you're used to juggling several projects at once or working at a job that requires intense concentration. Instead of getting that report out by noon, you may find yourself daydreaming about your baby—her little toes, the beautiful new bassinette, yourself as a radiant mother. What exactly was that report supposed to be about, anyway? And how did it get to be half past 3?

To make matters worse, many pregnant women believe that their short-term memory isn't up to par during pregnancy. And in many ways, it makes sense. You may be preoccupied with worries about your baby's well-being, and you're fatigued and uncomfortable from the changes overwhelming your body. Plus, given that the hormonal free-for-all of pregnancy has had so many effects on you, it's not unreasonable to wonder if it's affecting your memory as well.

In fact, the research on pregnancy and memory hasn't produced a clear answer on what's really going on up there. While some studies have found evidence of verbal and memory deficits in pregnant women, others show that mothers-to-be actually function just as well in cognitive tests as their non-pregnant counterparts. Interestingly, one small study found that the main difference between the two groups was that pregnant women rated *themselves* as performing worse than they would have before pregnancy—even though they tested just as well as the nonpregnant group. So if you think you're flakier than usual while you're pregnant, it may be real or it may just be your perception.

Try these simple strategies to cope with forgetfulness:

• Stay calm. The more flustered you get, the harder it is to remember things.

• Carry a small notebook (or PDA) to jot down reminders about appointments and other details of daily life.

• Place a detailed daily calendar in a spot where you'll see it several times a day.

BabyCenter Buzz

My Brain Is Like Swiss Cheese

"My personal theory is that the baby's brain develops by stealing part of the mom's. I'm pregnant with my fifth child, and I'm reaching critical mass now!" —*Nancy*

"The last time I was pregnant, I got into the shower with my socks and underwear still on! Hoping that doesn't happen again . . ." —*T.*

"I take my calendar everywhere I go to remind me of appointments, school activities, etc. My husband bought me a PalmPilot for Christmas. . . . If only I could remember where I put it!" —*Lisa*

"I keep a dry-erase board on the fridge and write everything there, from the grocery list to chores and errands. I just erase them when they're done and start over." —*Lynn*

"During my last pregnancy, I forgot to go to my ultrasound, so now I use the alarm on my cell phone to remember important appointments." —*Anonymous*

"I forget to do laundry, set my alarm, run errands, and I even left my car running with the keys locked inside for an entire hour before I realized what I'd done." —*Anonymous*

"It's the hormones! With my first pregnancy, I arrived at work one day wearing two different shoes. (Talk about embarrassing!) I advise cutting back on what you're trying to do. Remind yourself that you're building a baby. That's the number one job you have right now. Say 'no' to everything you possibly can." —*Lynn*

• If you spend a lot of time in front of a computer, use its calendar feature (often part of your e-mail program) to keep track of appointments and to-dos. You can even set it to send you on-screen reminders.

• Keep lists of what you hope to accomplish before you take off on maternity leave or go into labor. (Still, don't let it get out of control. Remember to pencil in time for yourself and your mate in addition to all the tasks you want to check off.)

• Keep items you use often, such as your keys or credit cards, in one place.

• Simplify your life. Cut back on activities so you have more time in the day to relax and reflect. Savor these prebaby moments while you can.

BabyCenter Buzz

What I Do When I'm Feeling Irritable

"I can't always swing it, but I try to take a long bath or shower whenever I start feeling irritable. It's the only thing that helps me relax." —*Veronica*

"I call up my best friend and vent about how miserable I feel. She just had a baby a few months ago and really understands. Other people can be so judgmental if you don't act as though you're completely thrilled about being pregnant." —*Kylie*

Why You May Feel Cranky Now

Does the way your mate chews his food make you want to scream? Are you ready to tear the elastic panel out of your maternity jeans? Don't worry; it's normal for little things to start driving you crazy this trimester. Even the most even-keeled women lose their cool every now and then. You're likely to feel especially irritable if your third trimester coincides with summer, when high temperatures can make you more miserable than usual (though trying to zip a down parka over your bulging belly likely won't do much for your mood, either). Toss in the requisite worries, lack of sleep, hormonal changes, and late-pregnancy aches and pains for good measure, and it's no *wonder* you're on edge.

Coping with the "Pregnancy Blahs"

Yes, your body is undergoing some amazing changes—but it's normal for the novelty to wear off toward the end of pregnancy (especially if this isn't your first). The added 30 or so pounds you're toting around, combined with restricted motion and the endless questions from friends and coworkers about your condition—"Has the baby dropped?" or "How past due *are* you?"—can make the whole experience particularly tiresome. And if you end up on bed rest, passing the time can be an even bigger challenge.

Making the Most of the Final Weeks

To get through these last weeks and months, accept that it's okay not to be excited about your pregnancy every minute of every day. Instead, enjoy the anticipation of holding that newborn in your arms. Many women get through the doldrums by nesting—preparing for the baby's arrival by doing everything from buying supplies to mapping out the details of maternity leave and day care to obsessively cleaning every nook and cranny in the nursery.

But take advantage of this waning prebaby time to indulge *yourself*, too: You may not have this kind of freedom again until you send your last child off to college! (And don't worry—you may not miss it as much as you imagine you will.)

Book a prenatal massage. A licensed massage therapist trained in prenatal massage can help alleviate the aches and pains in your lower back, joints, and everywhere else, giving your body—and your mind—a much-needed lift.

Investigate new-mom support groups *now*. Once the baby arrives, you'll need the companionship of other women going through the same thing, so research your options while you have the time and mental energy. If the idea of a group appeals to you but you can't find one in your community, consider organizing one yourself, or at least contacting a few other pregnant women or new moms and promising to be available to one another. A good place to start: See if any of the women you hit it off with in childbirth class are interested in staying in touch.

Take a baby-care class with your partner. Not only will you both learn valuable skills, boosting your parenting confidence, but these classes serve as good start-off points for important conversations about parenting styles and expectations. Plus, you'll get to meet other parents-to-be—future support for you and your mate (and the parents of future friends for your baby!).

Take a "babymoon." Like a honeymoon, a short weekend away with your partner (and perhaps your firstborn, too, if this is round two), gives you a chance to relax and enjoy yourselves before the new baby comes. Plus, time away gives you a break from the nesting cycle and your predelivery jitters, which can be hard to break when you're at home (and really, the onesies have been laundered enough already).

The Big Emotional Preview

Pregnancy in general, and the third trimester in particular, offers a sneak peek at the emotions to come. After all, you're in the process of becoming a parent, and some of the feelings you have now are ones that will stick with you, in one form or another, for a lifetime. You may feel:

Out of control. And, in truth, you are. For many women, especially those who are accustomed to having everything in their lives just so, pregnancy can inaugurate a feeling of disorder and helplessness. Suddenly, the most important things in your life—the well-being and safe arrival of your baby—are ones you can't totally control.

Fear of the unknown. Life may have been predictable for you so far—and now it's not. You can't know in advance what your labor will be like, who your baby will be, how you'll feel about parenting, or, in the big picture, what the future might hold for your family. Like loss of control, this may be an unfamiliar feeling. But just because you don't know exactly how things will go doesn't mean they'll turn out badly. Keep a positive outlook. You've made it this far—you'll learn to roll with the changes ahead, too.

Reluctant to give yourself over. Pregnancy—and parenting—demands that you put the needs of your children first. Chances are good that you already feel like you've been taken over by a giant, beloved parasite—and this is a feeling that's likely to intensify after the birth. Nursing, the disruption to your sleep schedule, taking time off from work, adjusting your relationship with your partner—you'll continue to give more of yourself than you ever imagined, but you'll learn over time how to balance your own needs as a person with those of your growing family.

Chapter 15

THE REST OF YOUR LIFE

Making the Most of Your Changing Look

It used to be that pregnant women tried to draw attention *away* from their bountiful bellies. These days, it's perfectly acceptable to show off your baby belly and to take pride in your luscious, rounded figure. And while you may be dismayed by some less fashionable late-pregnancy physical changes—like swollen ankles and extra padding on your thighs and behind—bear in mind that these changes are happening for a reason and are mostly temporary. And whether you're loving your new look or counting the days until you can toss your maternity jeans in the trash, we have a few tips and tricks for enhancing your appearance as your pregnancy peaks.

Hairstyling Tips and Tricks

Many women feel an urge to cut their hair during pregnancy—but don't make any dramatic changes right now. Your hair will likely thin out in the months after giving birth, so you may want to wait about six months after your baby's born to overhaul your look, though quick trims before then are fine. (Bonus: You'll get an hour to yourself!). In the meantime, try these simple tricks to keep your mane looking great.

• If you have long hair that seems too thick and unruly and you're tempted to cut it all off, try keeping it at least shoulder-length. Too dramatic a length change could leave you in tears. Switching styling products might help, or using a bit more than you think you should. Today's hair-care products are lighter and more sophisticated than in years past, and stylists say not using enough is a common mistake women make.

• Straight, blown-out hair can bring out your cheekbones and create the illusion of slimness in a round face. Use a flat brush, and if you end up with a wave where you want sleek, continue blow-drying that section in the opposite direction of the wave.

• You may want to avoid harsh bangs or a multilayered style, since these tend to accentuate a heavy face.

• Think low maintenance. Whatever your hair-care routine, try to settle on one that's easy and ideally doesn't involve anything that needs to be plugged into the wall! Wash-and-go styles or ponytails are timesavers now—and later, when you won't have the time or energy to do your hair.

What to Wear in Your Waning Months

By now, the novelty of maternity clothes has worn off. If you're staring into your closet and moaning, "I have *nothing* to wear!" try these tips to make it through the next few months.

Check your partner's closet . . . again. Even though you've been through there before, your new size might mean you gravitate toward items you hadn't considered earlier in your pregnancy: A vest worn over a white dress shirt and slim black pants is one classic late-pregnancy look.

Hit your friends up . . . again. Mention your fashion paralysis to the formerly pregnant women in your lives, and they may come up with something they hadn't thought of before.

BabyCenter Buzz

I Can't Live Without My . . .

"I love men's button-fly jeans. They can be worn from the beginning of pregnancy all the way through postpartum. Just button them up as far as you comfortably can and tuck in the flaps." —*Anonymous*

"I'm in health care and have found that scrub pants are great. I have them in white, black, khaki, and pale yellow. They're cheap, too—some are under $10 at uniform and medical-supply stores! I've even made capri pants out of them just by hemming the bottoms." —*Anonymous*

"The best pants aren't even maternity pants—believe it or not, they're yoga pants! They're the first thing I pull out, whether I'm going to work or on a long car ride. They're so comfortable, and still look very stylish." —*Anonymous*

BabyCenter Buzz

My Favorite Comeback to Clueless Comments about My Size

"To those who mention my size, I say, 'Yes, I *am* getting huge—and you're getting rude. I'll have something wonderful when this is over. You'll still be rude.'"
—*Anonymous*

"I think my pregnant body is beautiful, and my boyfriend seems to love it, too. When someone says something negative to me, I simply say, 'I'm still sexy.'"
—*Anonymous*

"It works to say something like 'If it's off-limits to discuss a person's weight when they're not pregnant, it's especially off-limits when they *are* pregnant.'"   —*Kimber*

"In response to 'Wow—you're getting big,' I say, 'So are you!' Shuts 'em up every time." —*Anonymous*

Splurge on one or two new pieces. Choose things you can wear in those first postpartum weeks, too, such as a shirt that drapes nicely and lifts easily (for nursing), a jacket that curves close in the right places and flows smoothly in the wrong places, or stretchy pants that will retain their shape as you regain yours.

Loving Your Larger-Than-Normal Body

Women are their own harshest critics, and pregnancy is a time when we may feel particularly sensitive about our body image. Remember: *You* may see extra pounds on your thighs or arms, but practically everyone else sees a miracle—a woman's body lush with new life.

You and Your Partner

You're into the homestretch! And you may *feel* the stretch—in more places than just your elastic maternity panel. As you become increasingly preoccupied with the baby—and increasingly weary of hauling around your growing bulk—expect that your relationship may strain a little, too. Now's a good time to practice asking your family and friends for help—with preparations, with child or pet care, and with a little *TLC* just for you.

Just for Dad

Paternal Pressures

While your partner is busy counting microscopic socks, you may start to wonder exactly what *you* should be doing. Should you take up woodworking and spend your weekends in the garage, building an heirloom grandfather clock for your child-to-be? Should you practice saying "son" in a deep baritone?

Well, no—not unless you want to. Maybe you prefer baking apple pies or singing lullabies or folding all of the baby's little things. There are a million wonderful ways to be a father, and with a little patience and a lot of love, you will surely find your own. You don't need to earn a ton of money, you don't need to own a baseball glove, and you don't need to look the part. Just be your best self, and the rest will come naturally.

Once the baby comes, you'll be glad to know you can count on them for support.

Dealing with Last-Minute Jitters about Becoming Parents

If your focus up until now has been on your pregnancy or the birth, it may suddenly start to sink in that there's actually a *baby* on the way—a baby who will be yours to care for even when the pregnancy and labor are just happy (or nauseating) memories. Parenting can feel like an awesome responsibility—and it is!—so clear the lines of communication with your mate now, before the baby arrives.

Talk about your concerns. It can be a tremendous relief to air your worries. If you're not already doing so, now's a good time to begin responding to your partner with honesty and humor—two qualities that will go far once you become parents.

Reassure each other about how capable you are. You've done hard things together before (remember the first trimester?). Remind each other of your strengths and successes—patience or discipline, a great laugh, or a job well-done—and the fact that these skills will offer you direction and sustenance on your parenting journey.

Read parenting books together. Besides offering helpful advice and food for thought, reading can give you something to do together in these final expectant months.

Discuss your postpartum plans. Talk about how you'll divide baby care and household responsibilities, and figure out which friends and relatives you can call on for help. Stay flexible (a colicky baby or round-the-clock nurser may render moot your plans to split everything 50-50, but start talking about these important issues *now*.)

Consider your own childhoods. If you and your partner are first-timers, most of your experience with parenting has probably come from being somebody *else's* child. Talk with your mate about the aspects of your own childhood you might want to re-create for your kids—and those aspects you'd more happily leave behind.

Sex in Your Third Trimester: Time to Get Creative

With one person growing inside of you, the thought of yet another person trying to get in there may make you feel like spending the rest of your pregnancy in a convent! Indeed, between the ever-bigger baby taking over your body, the various aches and indignities of late pregnancy, and your own pre-occupation with the upcoming birth, a roll in the hay might start to feel more like an acrobatic feat than an act of love. Plus, while those feisty baby kicks inevitably inflame your parenting excitement, they might quickly snuff out your more conjugal passions.

Not to worry. With a sense of humor, a sense of adventure, and a little creativity, you and your partner can enjoy each other to the end. And if your libido feels a little lackluster right now, rest assured that it *will* return—just don't expect it to right after the baby's born. During the early months with a newborn, fatigue, hormonal changes (particularly if you're breastfeeding), time constraints, a changing body, a sore vagina, and the adjustment to motherhood aren't likely to trigger your great sexual reawakening.

Starting now, make the most of any sensual contact with your mate—massages, showering together, sleeping in the nude, mutual masturbation—even if it doesn't always end in intercourse. And even when you're not in the mood for fooling around, be generous with the hugs, kisses, and "I love yous." Finally, make sure your partner knows that it's common

BY THE NUMBERS

Straying Thoughts During Sex

80% of mothers-to-be admit that thoughts of their baby distract them during sex

70% of dads have the same problem

Source: *A BabyCenter.com poll of more than 800 people*

BabyCenter Buzz

The Last-Name Game

"I believe that babies need to have their fathers' last names. My baby's dad and I aren't married, but she has his last name. That's the traditional thing to do, even if it's not a traditional relationship." —*Anonymous*

"My boyfriend of five years suddenly decided he needed to 'take a break' from our relationship. Because he's not here to support me through the pregnancy, our child will have my last name. If a woman is going to carry a baby with no emotional support from the father, why should her child get his last name?" —*Nicole*

"We've chosen to hyphenate our last names—they're not difficult names, and we feel strongly about both of our names being represented for our daughter. I'd originally thought about using just my partner's name (I'm the pregnant one), but she felt that we should use both, and I agree now. We like the idea that at school, doctors' offices, etc., we'll have the obvious last-name match." —*Lorraine*

"We've decided that the baby will take both of our last names (and that's what will be on the birth certificate), but that she'll just use her father's last name in day-to-day life." —*Aimee*

"I think that *what* you decide is less important than *how* you decide it. It's a partnership, right? It should be a decision that you make together, and with respect for each other and your child." —*Anonymous*

for women to be less interested in sex late in pregnancy, and reassure him that this doesn't mean you love him any less.

Third Trimester Sexual Roadblocks

The third trimester can bring with it all of the erotic challenges of earlier pregnancy—along with some added discomforts as your proportions change dramatically.

Fatigue, crankiness, and feeling unattractive. You're tired, you're sore, your stretch marks have stretch marks of their own, and it's been weeks since you could bend down to shave your legs. While some lucky pregnant women experience this as a time of energetic, glowing self-confidence, many others feel more toadlike than foxy. Be kind to yourself. You're doing a beautiful thing—growing a baby.

Difficulty maneuvering. When the mood does strike, your body might seem uncooperative at best. Something has come between you and your

BabyCenter Buzz

How We Stayed Close Without Intercourse

"My husband touches my belly. As I grow, he caresses it and looks at it like it's the most beautiful thing he's ever seen. I can think of nothing else that makes more of an impression on me. A lack of sex during pregnancy is something you get through just fine." —*Anonymous*

"Patience, romance, massage, patience, understanding, patience." —*Chris*

"I get full-body massages—which is about as close to sexual excitement as it gets for me these days. We kiss, cuddle, and snuggle all the time and, most importantly, *talk* about our feelings. My husband still misses sex, but the point is, we maintain the intimacy in our relationship. At this point, we're joking about how the first time we make love after the baby is born will be like 'the first time' all over again." —*Anonymous*

partner—literally. While you figure out the hydraulics of intercourse—Where do we put *this*?—use your imagination, and be prepared to laugh a lot.

Swollen vulva. Just when you thought it couldn't get any worse, your hemorrhoids suddenly have an unwelcome twin sister: vulvar varicosities. Like varicose veins, these painful swellings result from the weight of your growing uterus partially obstructing blood return, which increases pressure in the veins in the lower half of your body and causes blood to pool. But while vulvar varicosities may take the edge off your sexual appetite now, they usually recede rapidly after you give birth. In the meantime, avoid standing for long periods, and try waist-high support hose,

Ask the Experts

Is It Still Safe to Have Sex?

Dr. Gina Brown, obstetrician: Yes, with a few exceptions. It's *not* safe, for instance, if you're bleeding or have placenta previa (page 529). Also abstain from having sex after your membranes rupture because then your baby is no longer protected against infection. It's also risky to have sex early in your third trimester if you're having premature labor or if you have a short cervix. In those cases an orgasm can stimulate dangerous contractions. But if you're having a healthy, normal pregnancy, there's no risk at all in having sex.

Just the Facts

When to Avoid Sex (and Orgasm)

Because orgasm can cause mild uterine contractions (as can the prostaglandins in semen and, in some cases, nipple stimulation), most doctors and midwives advise against intercourse and/or orgasm if you have any of the following conditions:

- Placenta previa
- A history of preterm birth or preterm labor in this pregnancy
- Unexplained vaginal bleeding or discharge
- Abdominal cramping
- Cervical insufficiency
- Cervical dilation
- Ruptured membranes
- An unhealed genital herpes lesion in either you or your partner (*Note:* You should also abstain if you've never had herpes but your partner has—even if he hasn't had an outbreak in years.)
- Any other sexually transmitted infection

Avoid oral sex if your partner has an oral herpes (cold sore) outbreak.

walks, soaks in a warm tub, and lying down on your left side or with your legs up.

Cramping after orgasm. Your uterus contracts after orgasm even when you're *not* pregnant—but now you'll really feel these contractions. This is normal—but let your doctor or midwife know if the contractions or pain continue for more than a few minutes.

Family and Friends

As your own feelings of expectation heighten, you can probably expect some complicated interactions with relatives and friends as well. Your attempts to set boundaries, your worries about becoming needy or dependent, your feelings of privacy or isolation—any and all of these can strain even the strongest relationship. Remember that as troublesome as your loved ones may seem, they likely mean well—but do be clear about what *you* need now, even if it means keeping a little of their zealous attention at bay.

There's nothing quite like a coming baby to generate excitement—and to create (or unearth) family tension. The stakes are high, and everybody has an opinion: about baby names, child rearing, who should be at the birth, and how long a visit should last. Chances are good that you're already receiving advice by the bassinetful—especially if you're making choices that are different from the ones your own parents made. As you become a mother yourself, you may find it a little awkward to navigate your ongoing role as somebody else's child—to say nothing of your status as daughter-in-law! But now that you're expecting a baby of your own, your first responsibility is to yourself and your new family.

How to Respond to Unwanted Advice from Your Family

Screen your calls. Sure, avoidance may seem cowardly—but if constant phone calls are stressing you out during these final weeks, take a break. Try leaving a lighthearted answering machine message: "Sorry, we're not able to take your call right now. We're enjoying our last moments of freedom!"

Set clear limits. Whether you're hoping that your mom comes for the birth and stays forever or praying that your in-laws will settle for sending a congratulatory postcard, be clear about what you can live with as relatives plan their visits. Those first weeks with a new baby—to say nothing of the birth itself—will be highly emotional. If you want to curtail or postpone visits, do so now—or you may come to regret biting your tongue. Plan to spend more time alone with your mate and new baby than you think you'll need—you can always adjust your plans if you feel ready for company sooner.

Stick to your guns. As advice pours in—about breastfeeding and sleeping arrangements, names and nursery decor, staying home versus returning to work—keep a respectful attitude and an open mind, but stay in touch with your own instincts. Times have changed since your parents had their kids—and you'll know what's best for yours. "That sounds like it would be another good way to do things!" is a useful, all-purpose response—and more practical than earplugs. Still, if your mother-in-law just won't quit, don't be shy about respectfully letting her know that while you appreciate her input, you need to make your own decisions.

When a Baby *Doesn't* Draw Your Family Together

Having a child will enrich your life immeasurably—but don't expect it to heal all wounds. While a new baby may foster unexpected closeness or

BabyCenter Buzz

My Relatives Are Trying to Take Over!

"I'm expecting twins and my in-laws are generous to a fault, but very controlling. They went shopping and bought *all* the furniture for the babies' room without even asking us! These are my first, and I was excited to pick out furniture and decorate the nursery myself." —*Anonymous*

"My mother-in-law thinks she's entitled to name the baby!" —*Bridgette*

"My mother-in-law wants to be in the room when I deliver. I absolutely know I wouldn't feel comfortable with her there." —*April*

"We told everybody that we needed two weeks to settle in before anybody was welcome to stay at our home. I didn't need to add the stress of houseguests to my life so soon after the baby was born." —*Anonymous*

offer a joyful buffer between you and your relatives, it can also trigger feelings of loneliness, isolation, and loss. You may grieve anew for a dead parent, long for more attention from a living one, or crave greater contact with a distant sibling. Reach out, if you can. "I really want you to be part of this baby's life" might be the simplest way to express your feelings right now.

At the same time, be realistic about what others can—and can't—offer, and don't expect long-standing differences to suddenly disappear or a longed-for closeness to magically develop. Give it time, but be prepared to move on (or simply stop trying so hard) if it becomes too difficult or painful to keep the door open.

How Your Friendships Are About to Change

Many of your friendships will thrive now like never before. With friends who already have babies, you may feel like you're finally becoming a member of an exclusive "moms only" club, or you may delight in the outpouring of support when they throw you a baby shower or help out after the birth (even if their previously cute toddler suddenly seems like a menacing giant next to your newborn!).

On the downside, you may find yourself straining to stay close to child-

BabyCenter Buzz

How I Deal with 'Distant' Relatives

"I think the only answer is to talk to your family about how you feel and ask them to be more involved by requesting their help on specific things." —Kate

"My family can't be here for me, except for occasional phone calls. My new family is my husband, my baby, and me. The more I focus on that, the better I feel." —Janna

"I always felt that I was the one making all the effort and phone calls. Then one day, I just told my mother that I need attention and needed to feel included. Things have been great ever since I expressed what I wanted." —Amber

less friends—feeling overwhelmed with guilt if they long to be parents themselves, or simply being unavailable for the kinds of activities that you used to enjoy before (at this point, all-night dancing likely isn't at the top of your to-do list).

For better or worse, change is a given now—keep an open mind and an open heart, and try to roll with it.

Joining the "New Mom" Circuit

Once the baby arrives, other new mothers will become your life raft—floating you safely through the postpartum rapids of hormonal blues and new-baby fretting. So try to meet a few future comrades *now*—luckily, other hugely pregnant women are easy to spot!

Get phone numbers. If you're hitting it off with the women in your childbirth or prenatal exercise class, trade information so you can get in touch after your babies are born, or have a lunch date while you're still waiting.

Overlook superficial differences. This isn't the time to get too hung up on things like personal style or different life situations. You'll be amazed at how much you'll have in common with other new mothers. Nobody else understands as well as someone who's in the trenches of new parenthood right along with you—and these friendships often produce lifelong friends for your kids as well.

Cruise local mom hangouts. Spend a postpartum afternoon at the play-

Ask the Experts

Why Am I Drifting Apart from My (Childless) Best Friend?

Karen Kleiman, clinical social worker: Unfortunately, this isn't unusual. You're each focusing on different, although parallel, paths in your lives. You're preoccupied with your new family, as one would expect. But your friend may not be able to relate and may wonder if you still have room left for her in your life. You'd like her to join you in your new world, but she'd like you back in hers—hence the push and pull. Inevitably, you both feel misunderstood and perhaps a bit resentful of the other's inability to compromise. The more you allow yourselves to drift apart, the greater the chances the friendship will fizzle out. The key is to fight the inclination to pull away from each other and instead put energy back into the relationship.

First, sit down and assess whether you really want to save the friendship. Be honest with yourself because to work this out, you may need to compromise more than you're willing to right now. You may feel too tired or too resentful to do that. Think about it.

If you want to mend the rift, the best thing to do is talk to her about it. This may require taking the first step and saying, "I miss you." Since the two of you were close before, she's probably feeling the same loss you are. When you talk to her, be clear about what you miss—whether it's laughing together, talking on the phone, or going out to special places together. You'll be surprised how quickly your negative feelings transform into a gentler realization that you truly do miss and need your friend.

Next, decide on a plan of action. Figure out together what you can do to get back on track and make time for each other. For instance, plan on spending time alone, just the two of you, and other times with the baby after she arrives.

No matter what you do, your relationship will change. You're growing and need new and different things from each other. Most healthy, substantial friendships can endure the challenge of this major life transition—but it takes work. It also requires honesty, patience, compromise, flexibility, and, most important, an ongoing commitment to the relationship.

ground or the public library, and you'll likely meet dozens of mothers, some with new babies. Express your interest in getting together, or find out if there's a playgroup you might be able to join.

Consider joining a support group. In large cities, medium-size suburbs—and even the occasional small town—pregnancy and new-mom support groups are plentiful. These are usually moderated by a mental health professional, and most charge a small fee to participate. Even if the "group therapy" aspect doesn't appeal to you, these groups are usually more social than psychological, and many eventually evolve into informal mothers' groups (and then playgroups) once you get to know one another well enough to meet up on your own.

Start your own mothers' group. If you're just looking for a way to socialize with new moms and can't find any existing groups in your community, think about putting together one of your own. Start by asking the women in your childbirth or prenatal exercise classes, or put up a notice in your midwife's or doctor's office.

Getting Your Home Baby-Ready

Do you obsessively count and refold teeny-tiny onesies? Does 3 A.M. seem like a good time to hang a mobile in the nursery? Do you spend half your workday online, scoping out changing tables and diaper pails? Don't worry—you're not alone. Prepare sensibly and indulge your nesting passion, as long as it's fun. But try to hold off on that shopping spree until

BabyCenter Buzz

How My Friendships Changed

"Maintaining a friendship through pregnancy and a new baby is hard, but it's well worth it, especially if it's a lifelong friend. Sometimes all you can manage in those early months after having the baby is a brief phone call or e-mail—just enough to stay in touch. It does get easier as the baby gets older." —*Tamra*

"I had no idea why my friends flaked out on me until I examined our past and realized that they weren't very good friends to begin with! I've accepted it (it took time), moved on, and made friends with other new moms." —*Kayleen*

"I let my childless friends know that although I have a baby now, I still value their friendship and would like to get together. Sometimes I let the grandparents watch the baby for a few hours so that we can catch up a bit. Even a few hours together can strengthen a relationship." —*Angie*

"With friends who don't have kids, it's really important to remind yourself that their lives are still going on and that you need to ask about the things you know are important to them—work, relationship stuff, spiritual growth, even trying to get pregnant. If you just talk about your baby all the time, they'll start to resent you." —*Anonymous*

after the gifts and baby equipment loans have all rolled in. When the baby *does* come, all he really needs—besides diapers and a car seat!—is a warm place to sleep. And you.

Helping Your Older Child Prepare for the New Arrival

There's no way to predict how your child will respond when you bring home the new baby. Some kids feel like they've been demoted from their royal status to something more like a foot servant. For other children, the baby is a joyful reminder of their own growth and burgeoning place in the world. Some kids will be eager to help, while others may seem utterly oblivious to the intruder. Don't be surprised if your child has all of these feelings at different times. At this point, your best bet is to prepare your child with age-appropriate facts about the birth and the baby, and to reassure her (and yourself!) that there will always be plenty of love to go around.

Change is in the air, and your child may be feeling a little bewildered about what's going to happen soon. Giving her clear information on what to expect—both during the birth and when the baby comes home—may put to rest her fears about being out of the loop. Plus, it will remind her that she can always depend on you to include her and keep her needs in mind—something she'll surely draw on in the months to come.

Finish transitions now. Now is *not* the time to start any major changes—like moving your toddler from a crib to a bed or beginning potty training—even if you think it could make your postpartum life easier. Give it some time—there's enough change going on already—and expect some re-

---

Just the Facts

The Nesting Instinct

It's commonly believed that a sudden spurt of nesting means that labor's just around the corner. A poll of 33,000 women revealed that 71 percent of mothers-to-be "nested" before giving birth. If you're close to your due date and find yourself frantically cleaning out drawers and organizing cupboards, tidy and decorate while you feel up to it, but take the time to rest, too. Alphabetizing the canned foods can wait. If the baby really *is* on her way, you'll want to save some of your energy for the birth!

Just for Dad

Your New Role at Home

When that new pair of lungs cries out in the delivery room, expect your role to change. For many dads, the arrival of the second baby fosters an even more intimate relationship with their first child than they had before. While your partner recovers from birth and feeds your youngest, you'll likely become Daddy the Great Entertainer, keeping your older child too busy to notice Mom's preoccupation: Ta-da! Pizza for dinner (again)! Presto! A Lego model of the Golden Gate Bridge! If you're not already in charge of the bedtime routine, you may take over many of Mom's former jobs, like tooth brushing and story time, and, depending on your work schedule, you may become more involved in school drop-offs and playdates. If all of this is new to you, it can be a rude awakening.

So starting now, create some special time with your child—because you both need it and because it will ease the transition later. Sneak off for breakfast, just the two of you; finish that treehouse you started last summer; or (with her blessing) take over a routine that your partner usually handles. As the birth approaches, help your child make a card—or select a simple gift—for Mom and the new baby. And take time to relax—after all, you've done this before. Pity the poor guys who don't yet know about the 1 A.M. feeding. And the 3 A.M. one . . .

gression. It's not uncommon for young children to revert to baby talk or bed-wetting as a response to the new baby.

Visit the hospital or birth center together. Many hospitals now offer sibling programs especially designed for new sisters- and brothers-to-be and their parents. They usually take about two hours, during which your child will see a room like the one you'll be in, talk about her fears and concerns surrounding the new arrival, and visit the nursery to see what a real newborn looks like.

Line up child care for your hospital stay. Pick someone not only whom your child knows and likes but who's close enough that they won't mind a middle-of-the-night rendezvous. It's probably best to have them come to your house, rather than have your child go to a less familiar place. But many families find that an overnight works if you turn it into an occasion—making popcorn, using flashlights, allowing everyone to giggle a little later than their usual bedtime.

Explain what will happen while you're away. A few weeks before your due date, talk to your child about your upcoming absence. Discuss the arrangements as clearly and simply as you can. Though you may be in the

BabyCenter Buzz

Showers for Second (and Subsequent) Babies

"Becoming a first-time parent is a right of passage. Therefore, a baby shower should be for a first-time mother. Never to be repeated." —*Anonymous*

"Each child is special and deserves a shower. It doesn't have to be as elaborate as the first, but he still deserves a shower." —*C.*

"I'm expecting my third girl. I didn't want a shower with this one because I still have all the stuff from my older kids. But a friend insisted on giving me one and came up with the idea of having a 'Diaper Shower.' There was food and baby games, and for gifts people brought diapers of all sizes (wipes as well, if they wanted). I loved it because what more do you need than that, really?" —*Anonymous*

hospital only a day or two, he may still be upset by your absence (especially if this is your first night apart). Let him know that he can come to see you right after the baby's born.

Explain what will happen when you return home. Young children, especially, need to be reminded that the baby will be pretty bloblike at first. If he's been longing for a playmate, your child will be aghast (and probably annoyed) at the drooling, shrieking bundle that arrives instead. Reading books about newborns, looking at pictures of your own child as a new baby, and brushing up on the facts (babies poop, nurse, and cry a lot) will help create an accurate portrait of newborn life, as will clear explanations of any other significant changes: "When the baby comes, Daddy will take you to preschool, instead of Mommy."

Kids in the Birth Room

Whether to invite children to witness the arrival of their new brother or sister is a very personal decision. Some parents want to give their kids the chance to see the miracle of birth. Others are uncomfortable with the idea, and nervous about how their child may react. The experts, too, are divided. Some say that children under five are too young to attend; others disagree. There's no magic age: Some younger children might be comfortable, and some older children might not (and some hospitals may not allow it).

Ultimately, the choice for a child to be present at a birth depends not only on your child's comfort level but on yours as well. (If you have a hunch

BabyCenter Buzz

How I Made My Firstborn Feel Special

"We made big-sister T-shirts together and froze cupcakes for the girls to frost and take to school to celebrate with their friends after the birth." —*Anonymous*

"We assured our oldest daughter that she'll be the first one into the delivery room after the baby comes; then she'll get to go out and make the big announcement to all of the grandparents and friends who are awaiting the baby's information (sex, weight, length, name)." —*Wende*

"Let your kids help you pack all the stuff you're taking to the hospital. It made my older ones feel involved. I also took them to the store and let them pick out a little present for the baby, like a bottle, a small toy, or a blanket." —*Anonymous*

"I've secretly packed goody bags for my boys along with my hospital bag. Each contains a disposable flash camera, a coloring/activity book, crayons, a few different snacks, and a juice box. This should help them pass the time in the waiting room with their grandma and also allow them to take their very own pictures of their brother after he's born." —*Mary Beth*

that inviting your firstborn into the room will make you feel self-conscious, distracted, or emotionally constricted, then it's probably not a good idea.) If you do decide to explore the possibility with your child, present the idea without exerting any pressure. And let him know that he's allowed to change his mind at any time—up to and including the day you deliver.

Discuss the mechanics of labor. Read simple books about birth, and consider watching a video on childbirth together. Explain to your child that there will be blood and that you'll be making unfamiliar—and possibly alarming—sounds, but that all moms do that when they have babies. Birth centers and some hospitals offer one-session classes specifically designed to prepare siblings who are going to be present at births. You and your partner, your child, and the adult who will be *his* support person should all plan to attend together.

Assign one adult to care exclusively for your child during the birth. Choose someone with whom he has a positive relationship and feels comfortable talking. Keep in mind that childbirth is a powerful experience and that this adult will need to pay close attention to your child's cues. If he's uncomfortable and shows signs of wanting to leave the room (or even go

(continued on page 350)

Checklist

Nursery and Layette Essentials

What will you need for those first few weeks after you bring your baby home? We read what the experts had to say, and then we checked in with parents—and found that almost everyone has a different idea about what's essential. (And when you consider that people raised babies for thousands of years without plastic bottles or rubber crib sheets, it becomes clear that "need" is a fuzzy concept!) Still, your baby will require a few basics for wearing, feeding, getting around, and staying safe. Invest first and foremost in a reliable baby-care book (one that includes good information on breastfeeding if you plan to nurse); then consider the following:

CLOTHING

In general, you want soft, comfortable clothing with no irritating tags or seams—in other words, think comfort over cuteness (although most items will offer both!). You'll be changing your baby's clothes several times a day—newborns are messy and diapers do leak—so make sure outfits are uncomplicated and open easily. Babies outgrow newborn sizes quickly, so buy big—at least three months ahead. While we've included rough guidelines on quantity, how many of each item *you* need will depend on your own preferences, the climate, and how often you plan to do laundry.

___ One-piece outfits (4–7)
___ One-piece pajamas or nightgowns (4–7)
___ Cotton undershirts (6–10)
___ Sweater or jacket (1)
___ Fleecewear or snowsuit
___ Socks and booties (4–7)
___ Cap or bonnet (1–3)

DIAPERING

Prepare to be boggled by the number of diapers you'll change in those early weeks! Stock up now. Most parents these days opt for disposables; some choose a professional diaper service; and a few even wash their own at home. Decide which kind of diapers you want to use, and buy some.

___ Diapers
___ Changing table or pad
___ Diaper bag
___ Wipes

BATHING

___ Plastic bathtub
___ Towels and washcloths (4-6 of each)

OTHER TOILETRIES

Despite the store shelves buckling under baby creams, lotions, balms, and powders, you don't actually need much:

__ Diaper ointment (for rashes)
__ Baby nail clippers
__ Cotton balls and swabs
__ Gentle baby shampoo

MEDICINE CABINET SUPPLIES

__ Infant acetaminophen (consult with your baby's doctor about dosage)
__ A baby thermometer (rectal is still best for newborns)
__ Petroleum jelly (to lubricate the thermometer)
__ Nasal aspirator

GETTING AROUND

__ Car seat
__ Front pack or sling
__ Stroller

FEEDING

__ Bibs (4)
__ Cloth diapers for general mopping up (12)
__ Bottles and nipples
__ Breast pump

SLEEPING

__ Crib
__ Receiving blankets (4–6)
__ Waterproof pads (2–6)

FOR YOU

You'll need to stock up on a few things as well, especially if you plan to breastfeed.

__ Nursing bras (2–4)
__ Nursing pads for inside your bra (6 or more)
__ Nursing pillow to support your baby
__ Maxi-pads/panty liners for postpartum discharge

home), she must follow his lead. Make sure the person you choose isn't so invested in seeing the birth herself that she forgets to pay attention to your child's needs.

Help your child pack *his* bag. You can't predict how long your labor is going to last, so it's a good idea for your child to bring some books, cards, or other diversions in case your labor progresses slowly. Plan to bring some food for him, too. (He may not want to leave your room to go to the cafeteria, or it might be closed.)

Make the Birth Special for Your New Big Brother or Sister

Try the following ideas to help your child get excited about the upcoming arrival—but give her a rest from all the baby talk, too. Likewise, you might encourage well-meaning friends and relatives to lay off a little—kids get tired of being asked how it feels to have a brother or sister on the way.

Involve her. Invite your child to help you make simple decisions about the baby's room or to pick out furniture or supplies: "Should we put the rocking chair here or there?" "Do you think we should buy this bunny comforter or the one with the ducks?" Or ask if she'd like to do your prenatal exercise tape along with you.

Make a card for while you're gone. A simple message of "I love you," to be read to your child while you're away at the hospital, can go a long way toward reassuring her. Tuck a photo inside, for added comfort.

Reassure her after the birth, too. No doubt the highlight for your child will be meeting the baby—and seeing you again. To ease this first encounter, give her a small present "from the baby." Prop a picture of her by your bed, and make sure she sees it. Snap a new photo of her with the baby, and do whatever else you can to convey to her that she's still at the center of your life.

Your Job

Making it through the last few months, weeks, and days on the job can be either a welcome distraction or sheer torture, depending on how you're feeling and the kind of work you do. But like most things in pregnancy, it's probably a little of both! Here's how to leave work on a high note:

Sign off on last-minute benefits paperwork. Meet with someone from your human resources department to double-check all of your leave documentation. Decide whether you should add your baby to your health insurance policy or to your partner's, and alert both HR and your insurance provider about your decision. Some employers request a note from your doctor or midwife announcing your due date or the birth of your baby to "officially" start your maternity leave; find out if you need one.

Create a hand-off memo for your replacement(s). Make a list of everything you do over the course of a day, week, month, or project. Then explain each of these things in a clear way, in as much depth as you think your replacement (or replacements, if your tasks are getting divvied up among colleagues) will need. Give your supervisor a copy of the memo, too, so everyone's on the same page.

Meet with colleagues and supervisees who depend on you. They're sure to have questions about when you're coming back or about whether you'll be accessible for questions while you're out.

Arrange for a contact person to keep you in the loop while you're away. Ideally, this is a workplace friend, someone who can dish on what's really going on in your absence. Did a new contract come in? Is your replacement not up to snuff? Is your supervisor tearing her hair out because she's afraid you won't come back? These are the things you want to be up on so you can hit the ground running when you return.

Meet with your supervisor. Come prepared with your hand-off memo and a plan detailing how you see the work getting done while you're away. Don't get guilt-tripped into accepting some take-home work during your maternity leave unless you're absolutely sure you want to take it on. You need and deserve this time with your new family.

Tidy up your work space. Depending on how organized you are, this could take an hour or a month. Are things filed in ways that your coworkers will understand? Are there any personal items in your desk you don't want kicking around the office? And don't forget your computer: If there are things on there you'd rather someone else not see—say, your résumé and cover letter to a competitor, or digital photos from your friend's wild bachelorette party—be sure to delete them before your last day.

The Dilemma: Staying Home versus Returning to Work
Whether you continue to work, take extended time off, or quit "forever" is probably the most heated work-family issue you'll face. A topic of debate,

BabyCenter Buzz

Taking Time Off

"Stay home as long as you can! I'm a teacher and had my baby in May—then had all summer off with him. I *still* wasn't ready to leave him in late August when I had to return to school." —*Debbie*

"With my first child, I stayed home for three months. I went a little stir-crazy, but felt my baby was still too young to leave with someone else." —*Gayla*

"Depending on your financial situation, I suggest staying home for at least six months. I took off ten months and then went back part-time, which is wonderful. I still get a lot of quality time with my daughter and also some adult interaction to keep me sane." —*Conni*

"I took six weeks off with my first son and was ready to return to work by week seven. I enjoy working and don't feel it has hindered my parenting or my children in any way! I have two beautiful, energetic, healthy, well-adjusted sons. Don't be made to feel guilty about returning to work." —*Anonymous*

"Everyone's situation is different, of course. I was sure that I'd be back on the job within three months, but after having my baby, I decided I'd much rather stay home full-time. We had to make some changes to our spending habits, but it's been worth it!" —*Donna*

"I went back to work with my first. I think it was good for me to go back because I felt productive making money and accomplishing more. Now that I am about to have my second, I'm planning to stay home. Evenings and weekends are just too short to give my complete attention to more than one child." —*Marla*

controversy, and sometimes-harsh judgment from all sides, the decision is first and foremost a personal one, informed by a wide range of circumstances—most notably financial. And no matter what you decide, the grass often seems greener on the other side: Even the most die-hard worker bee has days when she wishes she were on indefinite maternity leave, and even the most enthusiastic stay-at-home mom sometimes looks longingly at her dressed-for-work neighbors pulling out of their driveways in the morning.

How to Make Up *Your* Mind

Regardless of what coworkers, relatives, or politicians might think, whether or not to go back to work is a personal decision. Some factors to consider before you decide:

Family finances. It may be that your salary forms the bulk of your family's income, or at least contributes a big enough chunk that you can't see doing without. On the other hand, with adequate savings and a reasonable cost-cutting plan, you may decide that taking an extended leave is not only doable but actually *more* affordable (when you factor in the costs of work: child care, transportation, clothing, dry cleaning, taxes, and lunches out).

Your childhood. Did your mother stay at home when you were little? Did your partner's? And does that make you inclined to run screaming to the commuter train (because she seemed unfulfilled)? On the other hand, maybe your mom worked and your memories of being a lonely latchkey kid are influencing your feelings now. Or maybe—whatever your mother's choice—she and you were happy with it, and you plan to follow in her footsteps now.

Your ability to be the only adult in the room for hours on end. Stay-at-home parents will tell you that their jobs are difficult mostly because they can go all day without interacting with another adult. For some, this isn't as much of a problem. They're great at networking at the playground, staying in touch with former colleagues via e-mail and phone, and most important, *getting out of the house.* New parents who are on the shy side may find this more difficult and could end up making a new best friend in *Oprah*, instead of the gregarious mom down the street.

Your willingness to let other people care for your child. Depending on when you're due back from maternity leave, finding quality care for an infant is no easy feat. Sometimes no caregiver feels right to you, no matter what their qualifications. If you're going to be tortured by the thought of leaving your child in someone else's care, you may need to take extra time off to sort through those feelings.

Whether you *like* your job. If the answer's no—and you have the financial resources to swing it—maybe this is the time to consider taking a break. You can look for a new position when your baby is older.

How easy will it be to go back to work after six months, a year, five years, ten? Depending on your job and the industry you're in, slipping back into your cubicle after an extended leave could either be a no-brainer or a serious hassle. If you're concerned that stepping off the ladder for even a year could jeopardize your ability to jump back on where you left off, speak frankly with people in your field. Are there extracurricular activities you could do if you quit—attend conferences, stay up on newsletters, con-

Just for Dad

All about Paternity Leave

Paternity leave is the time a new dad takes off work after the arrival of a new child. It's rarely paid, though a few progressive companies do offer paid paternity leave programs ranging from a few days to a few weeks. So most men have to take vacation time or sick days when their children are born, and a growing number of new dads are taking unpaid family leave to spend more time with their newborns. Here, a paternity leave primer:

- Ask your human resources department if you're eligible for paid or unpaid leave. Read up on your company's policy on paid leave; be aware that if your company doesn't have one, many employers are required by federal law to allow their employees (both men and women) 12 weeks of *unpaid* family leave after the birth of a child, under the Family and Medical Leave Act (FMLA). At the end of your leave, your employer must allow you to return to your job or a similar job with the same salary, benefits, working conditions, and seniority. (And if you're eligible for *paid* leave, you may be able to combine it with a few additional weeks of unpaid FMLA leave.)

- Federal guidelines require you to request leave 30 days before you plan to take it, but try to give your boss more advance notice if you can. You'll be in a stronger position to negotiate leave if you approach your supervisor with a specific plan and allow him plenty of time to help you implement it.

- It's illegal for an employer to discriminate against an employee who's taking leave. Still, many fathers fear fallout from taking time off—from snide remarks in the men's room to a high-profile project conveniently being given to somebody else. To find out how taking leave might play at your company, look into whether other men have done it—and how they were treated by their colleagues and supervisors. If others have gone before you, pick their brains about what worked for them and what didn't, which colleagues were most supportive and which weren't. If you're a trailblazer, try shoring up support among coworkers, especially other dads or dads-to-be. A national survey showed that most men agree that it's important for employers to give workers time off to meet family responsibilities, and support expansion of the FMLA—so others will be grateful for any steps you take in that direction. (If you do qualify for the FMLA and your employer refuses to allow you to take it, contact your regional office of the Wage and Hour Division of the Labor Department. A phone call from the Labor Department to your employer can resolve most problems. If not, the Labor Department will investigate your complaint and may sue your employer on your behalf.)

- If you work part-time or for a small company and you *don't* qualify for paternity leave under the FMLA, it can't hurt to ask your boss for a leave of absence anyway. Some companies may be willing to negotiate time off for a valued employee. Highlight the hard work you've done for them over the years, and stress how this time will end up *helping* your productivity, not hurting it—and the earlier you start making a case, the better your bargaining position. If you're affiliated with a labor union, ask your representative or manager whether you qualify for leave under union rules. Look into your state's laws on leave, too; sometimes these benefits are more generous than the FMLA.

tinue to network—that mitigate how big a deal it would be to take time off?

Your partner's take on the subject. Whatever the decision, clearly this is a major one for your relationship. Aside from the "Can we afford it?" question come all sorts of other issues: Does your partner feel anxious about being the only breadwinner? Do you think you'll be able to feel like a "real grown-up" when your partner walks in the door after a long day of work, and "all" you have to show for your day is a pile of half-folded laundry? (Because that will be a day of real achievement with a newborn!)

Whether there's room for compromise. Staying home with your baby versus returning to work doesn't have to be an all-or-nothing decision. Perhaps—depending on your employer and financial situation—you can strike a balance between having lots of time with your baby and keeping your career going, at least on some level. Maybe you can take an extended leave of absence—if your employer is very progressive or absolutely adores you—of 6 months or even a year. Maybe you can go back part-time for several months (or several years). Maybe you can resign your position but still take regular work from your former employer on a contract basis. Or maybe now's your chance to try out that consulting, catering, or other small-business scheme you've been dreaming about for years (note, though, that some child care will still be a necessity).

Preparing for Your Return

Though you may be daydreaming about that blissful time at home with your baby (just remember, we said *day*dreaming . . .), your first day back at work will come sooner than you realize—and probably sooner than you're ready for it. To help make your transition back as easy as it can be, start laying the groundwork now.

Just the Facts

Paid Paternity Leave

In 2004, California became the first state to offer paid family leave. Now Californian parents—regardless of gender—can take up to six weeks at partial pay to care for their new baby. Paid family-leave bills have been introduced in other states as well.

Just for Dads

Making the Most of Family Time If You Can't Take Leave

- Try working overtime before your baby comes, and exchange it for time off after the birth.

- Have your partner wake you up when the baby's finished nursing so you can be the one to lull her back to sleep. If your partner's pumping or the baby's on formula, take turns getting up for feedings.

- Take a good, hard look at extracurricular activities that steal your time with baby, and consider putting them off for now—this first year is going to be a very special one, and you don't want to miss out.

If you plan to breastfeed, find out how feasible it will be to pump. Have other new moms pumped breast milk in your workplace? If so, ask them how it went. Were supervisors and coworkers understanding? Was there any awkwardness, or is it an accepted practice?

Then figure out where you'll pump. If your company doesn't have a designated pumping space, ask your supervisor, the building manager, or the human resources staff for suggestions. Any private room—an unused office or conference room, or even a large, clean closet with a chair, a countertop, and an electrical outlet—will do. (Don't settle for a bathroom stall unless there's truly no other option.)

Explore your company's flexible-work policy. You may think you know all you need to about the various options your workplace offers, just from observing your coworkers. But you may be surprised. Reading the fine print on your human resources department Web page or doing a little digging with sympathetic managers may yield encouraging results. Especially if you're a valued employee, ideas like going part-time, job sharing, working from home, or switching to a three- or four-day workweek may be an option. Find a supervisor with whom you have a good rapport, and sketch out some options. If she knows that it means keeping you as a happy camper— and if she fears that otherwise you'll simply quit after your maternity leave runs out—she just might be willing to work with you to keep you on in whatever capacity you propose.

Decide on a start date and a schedule. Ask around, and experienced moms will tell you: Set your first day back at work for a Wednesday or a

Thursday. That way, you only have to get through a few days before the welcome reprieve of the weekend. And even if you're planning to return to work full-time, find out now if it may be possible to ease back in those first few weeks—working part-time at first and gradually upping your hours until you're back at your regular schedule, or working from home at first and then adding back days at the office as you get acclimated.

Start looking for child care *now*. A spot in a sought-after daycare center or family daycare home may mean getting on the waiting list while you're still pregnant. Alternatively, if you plan to hire an in-home provider, start networking with new and expectant mothers you know to get the scoop on how to go about finding and hiring a nanny when the time comes.

Your Finances

With the clock ticking quickly toward the start of your maternity leave (and the temporary or permanent loss of your paycheck)—and with all those baby necessities to buy now—it's high time to take a hard look at your finances. Whether it's figuring out if you can really afford to stay home, calculating how much you'll need to spend on nursery essentials, or budgeting for child care, think about how you'll cope with the extra expenses parenthood will bring.

Organizing Your Finances Before the Baby Arrives

While you may need to invest a few hours up front to get your financial system in place, once it's up and running, you'll save both time *and* money.

Pay bills in advance. Paying important bills—mortgage, telephone, and electric—before you give birth can help lighten your worrying load while you're in the throes of new parenthood. Use a bill-pay software program to schedule your payments in advance, and have them registered in your account. Many banks offer free online bill paying, and you can set up scheduled payments before your bills are due. If electronic solutions aren't for you, create your own tangible schedule (post it where you can see it) and pay bills as they arrive.

Create a bill-reminder list. Personal-finance software can alert you when your bills are due, and some credit card companies will even send out reminder e-mails. Online bill-payment systems usually have a bill-reminder feature, as well. Take advantage of these options so you don't have to rely on your sleep-deprived memory to make sure bills get taken care of.

Create a financial system. Office-supply stores offer a host of paper organizing systems created just for organizing financial records. If you're more tech-inclined, money-management software is a popular choice. Or you can create your own spreadsheet with expenses, due dates, account numbers, and phone numbers to help you keep on top of things.

Pay down debt. While you're still collecting a paycheck, use as much of it as you comfortably can to pay off credit card and other consumer debt. The last thing you need when you have a new baby—and a reduced income—are those unpaid balances and that ever-accruing interest.

A First-Month Fund: Start Saving *Now*

While you're still pulling down a paycheck, start socking away some extra dollars to give yourself a break after bringing your baby home. A sampling of what you might want to save for:

Occasional childcare or a baby nurse. If you don't have family nearby, hiring someone to watch your baby while you get some much-needed time alone or with your partner is essential. Prices can run anywhere from $5 an hour for your neighbor's teenager to $300 a day for a professional baby nurse.

Another way to get the help you'll need is to hire a postpartum-care doula, who can run errands, do light housekeeping, prepare meals, take care of older siblings, provide emotional support, and help with breastfeeding. The National Association of Postpartum Care and Services (800-453-6852; www.napcs.org) can help you find a doula in your area.

A cleaning service. Keeping the dust bunnies from accumulating under your couch won't be a priority while you're recovering from birth. But if a messy house drives you batty, you may want to hire a cleaning person or team to come in for a few hours.

Wash-and-fold laundry service. If you're already buried under a pile of laundry—even *without* a newborn around—consider using a laundry service, which will pick up dirty clothes and drop them off after they've been cleaned. Or you may be able to leave your clothes at a Laundromat and pick up your clean, folded laundry a few days later. Fees are usually determined by pound.

Meal delivery. Pizza delivery and Chinese takeout can get old quickly. Many metropolitan areas are home to restaurants and catering companies that specialize in delivering freshly prepared meals to your doorstep. Most companies offer side dishes and kids' meals and require a minimum order amount. Look online or in your local phone book for possibilities.

How to Lighten Your Credit Card Debt

Don't let guilt stop you from taking positive steps. The average family with credit cards carries a whopping $8,000 in debt. It's easy to fall into the I'm-way-over-my-head-so-what's-a-little-more thinking. But moving in the right direction now can help you reach other important financial goals.

Leave all but one card at home. Keep one card—the one with the best rates and terms—to keep better track of your spending. If you're the type who likes to bump up against your cards' spending limits, you'll also contain the damage to one card.

Use your debit card. Train yourself to use your debit card instead of your credit card when you're short on cash. You avoid running up balances, there's no monthly fee, and because the money comes right out of your checking account, you'll think twice before you buy something.

Know the score. Credit card interest rates can range from zero to 28 percent. If you're not sure why your interest rate is so important, here's an example: Let's say you have a balance of $1,000 and your interest rate is 22 percent. It would take you 12 years to pay off that balance if you made only the minimum payment of 3 percent. During that time, you'd pay $1,234.17 in interest. The same balance at 12 percent interest would take you 8 years to pay off, and you'd pay only $407.54 in interest. That's still not a great deal, but it represents a savings of more than 50 percent.

Don't miss those payment deadlines. Typical credit card late fees are in the $25-to-$30 range. If you remember to pay your bill on the due date or a day or two before, call the credit card company. Some will let you pay over the phone with a checking account number; others have Web sites where you can pay electronically (and instantaneously).

Lower the interest rate on your current card. Call your credit card company and tell them you want to cancel your card because a competitor has offered you a lower interest rate. They might offer to lower your rate on the spot, and if they don't, you've cancelled this credit card.

Get a lower-interest card. Unless you're already paying the lowest rate available, think about transferring your balance to a lower-rate card. Be careful about so-called introductory rates, though. They usually last only for four to six months, then can jump to 15 percent or higher.

Watch those annual fees. Cards with annual fees often have lower interest rates, but do the math to make sure they're worth it. If you carry a balance of $1,000 a month on a card with a 6.9 percent interest rate and a $50 annual fee, for instance, that's the equivalent of a no-fee card with a 12 percent interest rate.

Consolidate debt. If you're really in over your head, there are plenty of debt-consolidation companies eager to help you. Generally, they offer you one big loan—usually at a lower rate of interest and with a longer payment schedule than your credit cards. Make sure you read the fine print, though. These companies typically charge such high fees that even if the interest rate on the loan is lower, you may end up paying out more money than if you were to tackle your debts on your own. (Uncle Sam's consumer protection division—www.ftc.gov/bcp/menu-credit.htm—has helpful information on credit and debt issues.)

Calculating the Cost of Childcare

While it may seem too early to start thinking about who will care for your baby when you go back to work, it's not! Some daycare centers have long waiting lists and it can take months to find a caregiver you like and trust. Be prepared for a shock: Paying for a caregiver will take a big bite out of your monthly paycheck. Exactly how much you'll end up paying depends on where you live, what type of childcare you choose, how many hours a

Just the Facts

Paying a Childcare Provider "Under the Table"

Though you might be tempted to avoid the taxes (and tax-related paperwork) involved in officially hiring a nanny or home childcare provider, be warned: Skipping this crucial step is illegal, and the IRS is on the lookout for this kind of tax evasion. Also, if you don't pay the proper taxes and your caregiver later decides to file for social security and claims prior earnings, you'll be liable for unpaid taxes, interest, *and* penalties.

Finally, you won't be able to claim any childcare-related expenses when you file your income taxes or take advantage of your employer's dependent-care flexible spending account unless both you and your caregiver keep everything legit.

The Cost of Childcare

Type of Childcare	Average Cost	Advantages	Disadvantages
Daycare Center	$250 to $1,250 a month	More affordable than nanny care Reliable (won't call in sick) Ample supervision Staff members are often trained in early childhood education Licensed and regulated Child will have social interaction Some employers provide daycare on-site; drop-offs and pickups are super convenient and allow you to visit your baby on breaks Some are government-funded and have sliding-scale fees for middle- and low-income parents	Teachers care for more than one child; recommended ratios are typically 1:3 for babies Centers that care for infants can be hard to find Kids get sick more often Centers usually won't provide care for sick children Rigid pickup/drop-off times
Home Daycare	$700 a month for infants	Nurturing, homelike atmosphere Smaller groups of children Less expensive than most other childcare Kids socialize with other children Usually more flexible pickup and drop-off times	No backup if provider gets sick Most providers don't have formal early childhood education No caregiver supervision Less stringent licensing requirements Kids get sick more often Many won't take sick children
Nanny	$300 to $700 a week	More personalized attention In-home care is more convenient than out-of-home care More flexible than daycare and home daycare centers Children stay in familiar surroundings	Most expensive option No nanny supervision Playtime with other children must be arranged separately Extensive paperwork and taxes Can leave you in the lurch if your nanny quits or gets sick
Relative Care	Often free, but if you choose to pay, aim for at least minimum wage	More personalized care; ratio is usually 1:1 Caregiver has personal interest in your child You often share values with your caregiver Usually inexpensive	Employee-employer relationship is hard to establish Child-care philosophies may conflict Playtime with other children must be arranged separately No caregiver supervision May be exhausting for older relatives
Stay-at-Home Parent	No extra cost, but you'll be a one-income family and will likely have to make some lifestyle changes	No one truly replaces Mom or Dad You'll be there for your child's developmental milestones You're assured of loving, attentive care You don't have to explain your parenting philosophy You avoid the work-family tug-of-war	Isolation and loneliness, especially for dads Physical and emotional strain on caregiver Some loss of identity in giving up career Playtime with other children must be arranged Loss of income

week your baby will spend in childcare, and your income level (some centers have sliding scale fees for families who can't afford full price).

Third-Trimester Travel: Keep It Simple

Getting there *used* to be half the fun; now it may be no fun at all, especially when complaints such as back pain and swelling team up to make a car or plane ride more punishing than pleasurable. Even if you're an avid traveler having a normal pregnancy, your doctor or midwife will probably recommend that you put all trips on hold once you hit week 36, to minimize the chance that you'll be away from home when you go into labor.

Even before your final month, it's a good idea to check in with your caregiver before making travel plans. If you have medical or obstetric problems—such as an increased risk of preterm labor, poorly controlled diabetes or diabetes requiring insulin, placental problems, hypertension, twins (or anything else that makes your pregnancy high risk)—travel isn't a great idea because you'll probably need to take it easy and you and your baby will need to be monitored more closely now. Plus, if an emergency arises, you'll want to be near your regular practitioner and the hospital where she practices.

BY THE NUMBERS

Third-Trimester Travel

48% of moms-to-be don't squelch their wanderlust in late pregnancy

27% hit the road because of work or family commitments

17% just want to hunker down at home

8% stay put for financial, health, or personal reasons

Source: *A BabyCenter poll of more than 5,800 women*

Third-Trimester Travel Tips

As long as your practitioner gives the okay and you still feel up to it, go ahead and enjoy your last fling. Just be sure to listen to your body and take care not to overdo any activities. In addition to the precautions you've been taking throughout your pregnancy, pay particular attention now to the what-ifs:

Plan for an emergency. Figure out where the closest hospital or medical facility is at your destination. Think about where to go and whom to call if you sud-

Just the Facts

Airline Restrictions for Pregnant Passengers

Up until your last weeks of pregnancy, you needn't worry about commercial airline restrictions on pregnant passengers. But take your due date into consideration for the *return* trip. In an effort to prevent airborne births, many airlines won't board pregnant women who are due to deliver within seven days (or, for some, an entire month) of the flight.

Airlines won't quiz you on your pregnancy status when you book your trip, and they won't mention travel restrictions unless you ask, so ask about them when you reserve your seat. Play it safe by getting a letter from your caregiver verifying your due date and granting medical permission to travel (most airlines want it signed and dated a few days before your departure)—and keep it in your carry-on bag so you can access it quickly.

denly start having contractions or other complications in an unfamiliar place.

Travel with your partner or a pal. Cell phones are great, but they can't drive you to a hospital or offer a helping hand if a problem crops up. You don't want to go into labor on your own on a lonely stretch of highway.

Continue to pay attention to what you eat and drink. Give the fast-food joints a pass, and focus on eating several small, nutritious meals throughout the day—your digestive system will thank you at bedtime.

Dress for comfort. It's more important than ever to shelve your heels in favor of solid athletic or walking shoes. You don't want to risk a fall while hurrying to catch a plane or visiting sites around town. Pack loose, comfortable clothing, and dress in layers to prepare for changes in temperature.

Have a realistic itinerary. Forget about signing up for a planned tour—you don't want to become prisoner to someone else's idea of a good time, and you simply won't have the energy to pack in a full day of sightseeing. Make sure your travel plans include downtime for naps and snacks.

Go for a walk or swim when you arrive. You can walk or swim right up to your due date. A 15-minute walk around the block or dip in the hotel pool may be all it takes to feel refreshed after a long journey. And if you've changed time zones, spending some time outside during daylight hours will help combat jet lag.

BabyCenter Buzz

I Vacationed Close to (or Even at) Home

"My husband and I took one last trip before our daughter was born—without leaving town. We reserved the honeymoon suite at a local hotel. After dinner at the fanciest restaurant in town, we went swimming and then had some sparkling cider and strawberries sent up to our room. What a wonderful splurge!" —N.J.

"Having our parents watch our 2-year-old over the weekend was vacation enough for us! We slept in, went out to eat, and went to a movie. Very relaxing—without the hassle of planning a trip." —June

"We played tourist for the day. We live just outside of Washington, DC, and had never been to some of its most famous sites!" —Gretchen

"I had a spa day at my house and invited a few friends over for an afternoon of manicures, pedicures, and facials." —Susan

Don't Leave Home Without . . .

Your medical records and vital health information. Carry your health insurance card and a copy of your medical history, which should include your due date, risk factors, blood type, a list of any medications you're taking, and any that you're allergic to. Keep it with you at all times during your trip.

Your medications. Pack a sufficient supply of any prescribed medications, prenatal vitamins, and even over-the-counter remedies you may need during your trip, especially if you're going someplace where those medications aren't readily available.

Emergency contact numbers. Before you leave, prepare a complete list of names and phone numbers to contact in case of emergency, and keep the list in your purse or carry-on.

Extra pillows or your favorite maternity pillow. Sitting for long stretches in the car or sleeping in your in-laws' lumpy guest bed can put a damper on an otherwise fun trip. A comfy pillow will take some of the pressure off your aching back and hips.

Ask the Experts

What Should I Do If I Have Contractions When I'm Away from Home?

Ann Linden, certified nurse-midwife: If you're having contractions at regular intervals, if you've had more than four in an hour, or if you have any other signs of preterm labor, head to a hospital so you can be examined and monitored right away. If you aren't sure about the frequency of your contractions, do the following: Empty your bladder, drink a couple of glasses of water or juice, then lie down on your left side and count your contractions for an hour. If you haven't yet hit week 37 and they continue at a regular pace or happen more than four times in 60 minutes, go to the hospital immediately.

If you're at term (week 37 and beyond) and have just started having contractions, give your caregiver a call. Depending on your particular situation—including how far away you are, how frequently you're contracting, whether or not you've given birth before, and whether you have any complications—she may advise you to get into the car and head for home, or she may suggest going to a local hospital. (In either case, someone else should be at the wheel!)

A supply of bottled water and snacks. Dehydration can bring on contractions, so you'll want to make sure you're getting plenty of fluids while on the road. Bring some fruit, a few granola bars, or a bag of trail mix to munch on to keep your energy up, too.

PART IV

LABOR AND BIRTH

Your pregnancy—these nine long months of mind-boggling physical and emotional metamorphosis—will soon be reaching its finale: the day your squalling newborn is finally placed into your waiting arms. Make no mistake, though. As miraculous as that moment will be, it won't happen magically. There's a lot of hard work involved in bringing a baby into the world—laying the groundwork for a positive, healthy birth and getting through the sheer marathon of labor and delivery itself (no matter how much you read about the process and how many friends regale you with their own birth stories, childbirth is like nothing you can possibly imagine—in both back-breaking ways and beautiful ones). What's more, no matter how much you plan for the "perfect" birth, things can and sometimes do go awry. Knowing what's in store—and how your caregiver will manage any problems that crop up—will go a long way toward easing your mind and helping you feel ready for your baby's birth day.

Labor and Birth Checklist

Here are a few things to consider as you prepare for your baby's arrival:

▶ Find out what you can about the childbirth education classes offered in your area and then sign up for the one you want. Good classes fill up fast.

▶ Talk over your options for labor pain management and other interventions with your caregiver. She can answer your questions and help you create a birth plan to guide your big day.

▶ Research the pros and cons of circumcision and cord blood banking, and interview and choose a caregiver for your baby.

▶ Arrange for a support network to help you during the birth and the first few weeks at home. Ask friends and family to do specific things, such as bring you a hot meal during those early weeks at home, care for your other children, or run errands.

▶ Pack your bag early. You may feel a little less stressed if you're ready to go at a moment's notice.

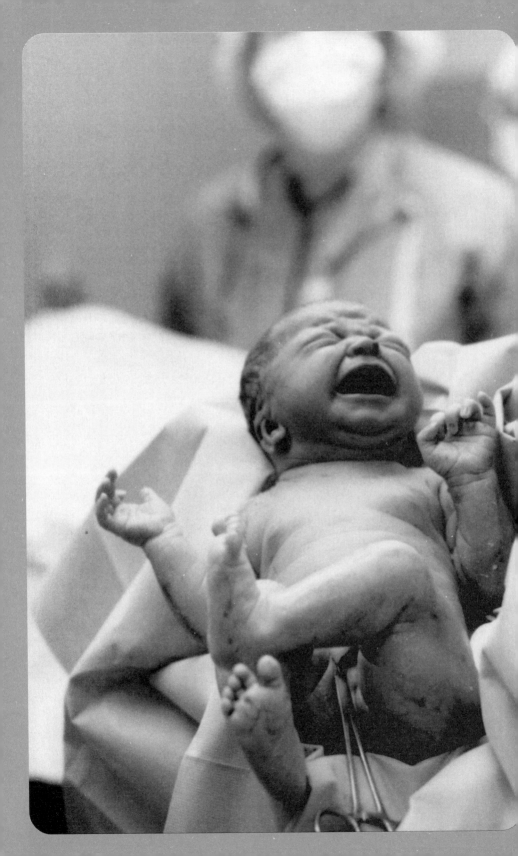

GETTING READY FOR LABOR DAY

This biding-our-time-until-the-birth period can seem unbearably long—even as you keep busy with last-minute preparations. Some things to do and think about as you count down to the big day:

Where to Have Your Baby: Hospital, Birth Center, or Home

Your choice of *who* will deliver your baby will likely determine *where* you'll deliver. Almost all obstetricians and family physicians operate out of hospitals (though a small percentage may deliver in birth centers); certified nurse-midwives work in hospitals and birth centers, and may attend home births; and direct-entry midwives tend to do home births exclusively.

Having a Hospital Birth

It wasn't always so, of course—but a hospital is where the vast majority of women deliver their babies these days. Giving birth in a hospital means you'll have plenty of "just in case" help at hand: trained medical staff, epidurals, c-section capability, and in many cases access to newborn intensive care. (Note, though, that not all hospitals have 24/7 in-house anesthesia cover-

BY THE NUMBERS

Where Women Deliver

More than 99%	deliver in a hospital.
0.2%	have their baby at a freestanding birth center.
0.57%	give birth at home.

Source: *National Center for Health Statistics*

QUICK TIPS

Getting to Know Your Hospital

Fill out paperwork in advance. You don't want to have to sign releases and permissions forms when you're in labor. Ask if you can preregister in the weeks before your delivery to get this red tape out of the way. Also, find out if you'll need to notify your insurance company when you're admitted to the hospital.

Request a private postpartum room if you can afford it. Sharing a room with a stranger can be noisy and nerve-racking. Ask the hospital what the chances are that you'll get a private room if you request one. As a rule, you'll be required to pay the difference between the cost of a private and a shared room.

Plan your route—and an alternate route. Getting lost on the way to the hospital may become a funny anecdote to tell later in your baby's life, but it won't seem funny at all while you're panting through contractions. (Also find out where you should park and how to access the mother-baby unit after hours.)

Understand routine rules and details. Find out where to check in if you go into labor in the middle of the night. Ask about visiting hours for siblings, relatives, and friends. Don't be shy about calling with follow-up questions. You won't be in any mood to figure this stuff out when you're in labor.

age, so you may have to wait for an anesthesiologist to come in if you want an epidural or need an emergency c-section. If you're high risk or if you've had a previous c-section and want to try for a vaginal birth (VBAC) this time, make sure your provider practices at a hospital with a round-the-clock anesthesiologist.) And if you're having a complicated pregnancy, a hospital may be your only option—birth centers won't accept women with certain conditions, and midwives won't advise a home birth, either.

Even if you live in an area with more than one hospital, you'll give birth wherever your midwife or doctor has admitting privileges. If you have a choice between hospitals, take a tour of their maternity wards before making your decision. (Even if you *don't* have a choice, take advantage of this opportunity to get familiar with the place you'll be delivering. The more comfortable you are, the less intimidating the experience will be on delivery day.)

Having Your Baby at a Birth Center

Are you a healthy woman at low risk for pregnancy and birth complications who wants a more natural, family-centered experience without having routine medical interventions (such as IVs and continuous elec-

Just the Facts

What to Ask About the Hospital

Before you settle on a particular facility, ask:

- How many laboring women does each nurse typically take care of?
- What's the hospital's policy on doulas?
- Is there an anesthesiologist on-site around the clock?
- Will I labor and deliver in the same room?
- How many support people are allowed in my room?
- Are siblings allowed to attend the birth?
- Is vaginal birth after cesarean (VBAC) allowed?
- What are the hospital's policies regarding continuous electronic fetal monitoring and routine IVs?
- Is there a newborn intensive care unit?
- Can my baby stay in my room with me? Part-time or round-the-clock?
- Are private postpartum rooms available?
- Are lactation consultants available? How often are they on-site?
- Are there specific visiting hours?
- Is early discharge allowed if I feel up to it?

tronic fetal monitoring)? If so, a birth center may be right for you. Birth centers offer a low-tech, high-touch, personalized, and comfortable place to have babies. If you choose an accredited birth center, you'll be cared for by licensed professionals—usually a midwife and a nurse, with a backup hospital nearby and a physician on call in case of an emergency. Birth centers aren't "mini-hospitals"—your labor will never be induced or "helped along" here, and c-sections are never done at a birth center—but they are equipped with IVs, oxygen, medication, and infant resuscitation equipment, so if need be, emergency care can be started while you or baby are awaiting transport to the hospital.

Typically, a birth center is an independent facility, though a growing number are affiliated with (and often housed inside) hospitals themselves. At a freestanding birth center, you'll get prenatal care there

BabyCenter Buzz

Why I Opted for a Hospital Birth

"I thought about having a home birth (there's no birthing center around here), but given that I live near a hospital with a great midwifery practice, I decided to go the 'normal' route. My mother is relieved!" —*Emily*

"I know for sure that I want an epidural. Why go anywhere else?" —*Anonymous*

"I'm going to try for a vaginal birth after cesarean, and my local birth center won't admit VBAC moms. I'm hoping for the best." —*Nora*

"I tend to worry, so having my baby where there's up-to-date medical equipment and plenty of expertise goes a long way toward easing my mind. I know that if something goes wrong, a hospital is the best place to be." —*Dawn*

throughout your pregnancy and, if there are no complications, give birth there when the time comes. Birth centers also offer childbirth education and breastfeeding classes, and you'll have your postpartum visits there as well. (In-hospital birth centers operate a little differently—they're usually available to any midwife or doctor who has admitting privileges at the hospital, but your prenatal visits will likely be at your caregiver's office.)

BabyCenter Buzz

Why I Chose a Birth Center

"It was really important to me to work with midwives and have natural childbirth in a friendly environment." —*Laurie*

"When I toured my local birth center, I couldn't believe how comfortable and warm it felt—so different from the way I felt when visiting the hospital. I was sold instantly." —*Dori*

"I wanted to be part of the team, not told what to do. For the first time (after two previous children), I felt that *I* gave birth. I could tell others what I needed and not vice versa! I felt medically safe at all times and very emotionally satisfied." —*Anonymous*

Just the Facts

The Benefits of a Birth Center

Birth centers provide:

A comfortable environment. A typical private room has carpeting, plants, pictures, a rocking chair, and a bed large enough for your partner to share with you. Birth centers usually have kitchens where you can store or prepare food, too, and some also have large whirlpool tubs.

Your pick of invitees. While some hospitals limit how many people you can have present at the birth, you get to decide who's with you at a birth center. And if you'd like your children present, they'll be warmly welcomed.

Freedom of movement and more. You can move around freely, choose the position you'd like to be in for labor and birth, and eat and drink anything you choose during labor.

Lots of encouragement to have a drug-free birth. Analgesic drugs, such as Demerol, are often available if you want them, but epidurals—which require an anesthesiologist—are not.

A sense of control and involvement. Birth centers never routinely use interventions such as IV hydration. And instead of continuous electronic fetal monitoring, a midwife or nurse will monitor your baby's heartbeat intermittently with a handheld Doppler (like the one your caregiver uses during prenatal visits). Birth centers do have IVs, oxygen, medication, and infant resuscitation equipment.

Breastfeeding help and encouragement. Birth centers make it a priority to provide breastfeeding education and support during the prenatal period, in the first hours after birth, and later in the postpartum period as well.

Lower costs. Because women who deliver in birth centers usually stay for less time and use fewer interventions, the average cost is about a third less than a hospital birth.

Hospital backup. All accredited birth centers have a backup arrangement with doctors and a nearby hospital. One in eight women who starts labor in a birth center ends up needing to transfer to a hospital. In most cases, they transfer for nonemergency reasons, such as when labor isn't progressing and Pitocin is required. (Still, moving in midlabor is discouraging and uncomfortable. Also, while some birth center midwives have admitting privileges at hospitals, many don't—so it's possible that a physician you've never met will deliver your baby.)

Speedier checkout. You'll be allowed to go home within 12 to 24 hours of delivery, with the idea that sticking around really isn't necessary—or good—for you or your baby. The birth center staff may call you to see how things are going, and you're always welcome to call them with questions. Some offer the option of a home visit a day or two after you give birth, as well.

Having a Home Birth

If you're healthy, have a normal obstetric and medical history and haven't had a previous c-section, home birth may be an option for you. But giving birth at home definitely isn't for everyone—and the American College of Obstetricians and Gynecologists officially opposes home births. If you have a chronic health or pregnancy-related problem such as high blood pressure, diabetes, a twin pregnancy, or any other complications, you'll have to stick to a hospital. And even if you are a good candidate for home birth, you must be committed to going it 100 percent natural and understand the medical risks involved. Also know that most health insurance policies do *not* cover the cost of home births.

Just the Facts

What to Ask About the Birth Center

Before you settle on a birth center, get the following questions answered—many recommended by the National Association of Childbearing Centers (NACC):

• Is the birth center accredited by the Commission for the Accreditation of Birth Centers? What's the staff's qualifications and experience, and are they all licensed healthcare providers?

• What happens if I develop a problem during pregnancy?

• How does the Center help women manage labor pain? What medications are available, and how often do women use them?

• What are the arrangements for care if complications arise? How often are women transferred to a hospital during labor or postpartum? What percentage of these are emergency transfers? How long does it take to get to the backup hospital?

• If I need to be transferred during labor, will the midwife come with me? Does she have admitting privileges at the hospital? If not, will she stay with me for support?

• Who's the backup physician, and can I meet her during my pregnancy?

• What kind of problems has the Center encountered? How often have babies had to be transferred to the hospital?

• What kind of postpartum care do babies and mothers receive? What's the minimum—and maximum—allowable postpartum stay?

• Will my health insurance cover your services? (You should also speak to your insurance company and find out what's covered if you start at the birth center and end up giving birth at the hospital.)

BabyCenter Buzz

Why I Chose a Home Birth

"My baby's home birth was the single most beautiful experience of my life. My daughter came into the world surrounded by those who love her." —*Anonymous*

"My husband and I not only felt comfortable being in our own home, but we also had a say in how our birth went. It was refreshing to be treated as an educated individual rather than a mindless number."   —*Melinda*

"Even though I had to transfer to the hospital for an emergency c-section (the baby turned at the last minute, and stuck her feet down my birth canal), I still value my home birth experience. I felt so comfortable and at ease during my labor. It was easy, fast, and less painful than my first two deliveries in the hospital."   —*Anonymous*

"My third child was my best birthing experience ever. My oldest children got to be there, and they still talk about the experience. I was ready to push before I even knew it."   —*Amanda*

Other factors to consider:

• You'll be in familiar and comfortable surroundings.

• You'll have more control over your birth experience and won't have any routine medical interventions.

• You can have any number of family members or friends in attendance.

• You won't have to endure interruptions from hospital staff and other patients.

• You may need the expertise of hospital staff and certain equipment at your disposal if something goes wrong. For this reason, it's wise to deliver at home only if you're within 20 minutes of the nearest hospital—and if your transportation there is fail-safe. And be sure your midwife is licensed and experienced, carries equipment and supplies to start emergency treatment if needed, and has an arrangement with a backup physician and hospital in case you need to be transferred.

• The lack of medical and support staff at your disposal after the birth means that you'll probably want some extra help in the days following delivery. Consider having a relative or friend come to stay for a few days, or hire a postpartum doula.

Checklist

What to Pack for the Hospital or Birth Center

A list of items you shouldn't leave home without:

FOR LABOR

____ Birth plan

____ Insurance card and any hospital paperwork if you've preregistered

____ Bathrobe

____ Slippers with nonskid bottoms

____ Socks (a few pairs)

____ Eyeglasses, if you need them (even if you usually wear contacts)

____ Hair band, if you need one

____ Hairbrush

____ Lip balm

____ Nonperishable snacks and drinks

____ Massage oils or lotions

____ Extra pillow (in a patterned or colored pillowcase so it doesn't get mixed up with hospital laundry)

____ Relaxation materials: books, magazines, games, music (and a small music player)

____ Pictures of someone or something you love

____ Lucky charm of some sort—jewelry, or a special stone from your favorite beach, for instance

Do You Need a Doula?

Faced with the uncertainty of birth, many women find enormous reassurance in seeking out a private labor coach, or doula, to assist them during labor and delivery. In fact, some research has found that women attended by labor support professionals have shorter labors, fewer complications, and healthier newborns. The theory is that mothers who have

FOR YOUR COACH

____ Camera or camcorder, film, tape, memory cards or sticks, and extra batteries (if your hospital allows births to be photographed or filmed)

____ Toiletries

____ Change of clothes

____ Snacks and reading material

____ Wallet with money for parking and change for vending machines

POSTPARTUM

____ Nursing bras

____ Breast pads

____ Maternity underwear

____ Nursing nightgown or pajamas

____ Toiletries

____ Address book and prepaid phone card or cell phone (though some hospitals won't allow you to use cell phones in certain areas)

____ Roomy going-home outfit and comfortable shoes

FOR YOUR BABY

____ Infant car seat

____ Outfit for the trip home

____ Receiving blanket (a heavy one if weather is cold)

____ Socks or booties

____ Cap

____ Bunting or snowsuit (for cold weather)

one-on-one professional support in labor produce lower levels of stress hormones than women left alone or attended by inexperienced coaches.

Because labor-and-delivery nurses often must split their time among several laboring patients—not to mention coming and going according to their shifts—hiring a doula may be the only guaranteed way to assure that someone who knows what they're doing will be with you throughout the labor-and-delivery process. Most doulas are certified labor support special-

BY THE NUMBERS

Using a Doula

48% of mothers-to-be say
they plan to have a
doula for labor support
and to help postpartum

Source: *A BabyCenter poll of
more than 38,000 women*

ists and have coached dozens of women through birth. Their fees—which are typically several hundred dollars (though a few pioneering hospitals are starting to provide doulas to all laboring patients)—include the delivery as well as preparatory and follow-up visits. (Unfortunately, a doula's services are seldom covered by health insurance.)

Creating a Birth Plan

While there's no way you can control every aspect of labor and delivery, writing a birth plan gives you an opportunity to think about and discuss with your partner and your caregiver how—ideally—you'd like your baby's birth to be handled. Plus, having a printed document will help refresh your caregiver's memory when the time comes, and bring new members of your medical team—such as your practice's on-call practitioner and your labor and delivery nurse—up to speed about your preferences when you're in active labor (and probably not in the mood for drawn-out

BabyCenter Buzz

Why I Loved Having a Doula

"When it came to the nitty-gritty parts of labor, I'm so glad that we had a doula. All the book smarts in the world can fly out the window when you're tired and emotional. Our doula suggested comfort strategies and offered encouragement. She also gave my husband the chance to take a break without leaving me alone." —*Beth*

"My husband wasn't in favor of having a doula 'replace' him, but after we hired her, he was so glad we did. She took the beating from me so my husband didn't have to!" —*Jenny*

"My doula stayed with me all through labor and for about two hours after the birth. Then she came back that evening to help with the whole nursing thing!" —*Leah*

conversation). Keep in mind, though, that you'll need to stay flexible in case something comes up that requires your birth team to depart from your plan.

Because so much depends on your doctor or midwife, where you decide to give birth, and even where you live (an urban, suburban, or rural area), you'll need to do some research to find out what's possible before you begin creating your birth plan. Once you've filled this worksheet out, take it with you to your next prenatal checkup. After going over it with your doctor or midwife, revise it if you need to, and then give a copy to her, have one put in your file at the hospital or birth center, and put one in the packed bag you'll take with you when you go into labor.

Other Big Decisions to Make Now

Circumcision

If you're having a boy, you'll need to decide whether to have him circumcised. The procedure—which is often done in the hospital a day or two after delivery—involves removing his foreskin, the covering of the head of his penis. Some parents choose circumcision because it's an important cultural or religious ritual, while others opt for it because they believe it has health advantages. Some medical evidence suggests that circumcision lowers the risk of sexually transmitted in-

---

QUICK TIPS

Packing Some Labor Props

It's nice to come prepared in case you want a little extra something to help yourself cope with the pain of labor. Comfort items to consider:

Tennis ball. Rolled around firmly on your lower back, this provides a soothing, deep massage that may feel especially good if you have back labor.

Hot-water bottle. This can feel heavenly pressed against your lower back during contractions.

Ice packs or a frozen water bottle. Applied to your lower back, these offer pain relief and a cooling distraction. You may also want an ice pack or cold washcloth to drape over your forehead.

A rice-filled sock. Instead of a heating pad, try filling a clean sock with raw rice, knotting it closed, and then heating it in the microwave for two to three minutes. Applied to your lower back, this can offer warmth and gentle pressure.

Birthing ball. This is a large, inflatable exercise ball that provides a flexible place to sit, or can serve as a useful prop to kneel against or drape yourself over during contractions. (It's also great to sit on when you're bouncing a fussy newborn!)

Birthing chair or stool. A low stool with a padded, U-shaped seat that supports you in a squatting position can help ease back pain.

fections, urinary tract infections, and penile cancer (though this type of cancer is very rare in any case, circumcised or not), but the issue is by no means clear-cut. And, like any surgical procedure, circumcision isn't without risk, albeit a very small one. (The American Academy of Pediatrics says that the choice is best left up to parents. But the organization does recommend that if you circumcise your son, he should be given pain relief during the procedure.) Before making your decision, discuss the issue with your partner, your pediatrician, your family and friends, and, if you're religious, the leader of your congregation.

Cord Blood Banking or Donation

Cord blood banking is a procedure in which the blood left in your baby's umbilical cord and placenta after birth is collected, frozen, and stored for future medical use.

Cord blood is prized because it's a rich source of hematopoietic stem cells—the building blocks of our blood and immune systems. These stem

BabyCenter Buzz

What I Wish I'd Known *Before* I Went into Labor!"

"I wish I'd known that there were better childbirth classes *not* affiliated with my hospital." —*Anonymous*

"I wish someone would've told me to have a bag packed about two months ahead of time. I went into labor early and my husband had to run home to get some stuff for me. He brought me *thong* underwear!" —*Devan*

"I wish I'd spent more time researching pain-relief medications. I want an epidural, but I know now that I do *not* want anything like Demerol because of the effect it had on me during my first daughter's birth." —*Anonymous*

"I wish I'd known to bring more food to eat after delivery. I was starving!" —*Anonymous*

cells have the ability to differentiate and mature into many different kinds of blood cells, so they can be used to treat a host of diseases. Cord blood has been used successfully as part of the treatment for cancers like leukemia and lymphoma, certain immune deficiency problems, inherited blood disorders like sickle-cell anemia and thalassemia, and other conditions. (*Note:* Chances are your baby cannot be treated with his own cord blood.) Promising new research indicates that cord blood may eventually be used to treat conditions as varied as diabetes, spinal cord injuries, heart failure, stroke, and neurological disorders—though this research is still in its infancy. Estimates vary widely about the chance that one of your children will develop a disease that could be treated with cord blood stem cells—ranging from one in 1,000 to one in 200,000, depending on whom you ask.

> ## QUICK TIP
>
> ### Getting in Touch When the Big Day Arrives
>
> Make sure that everyone on your birth team—your caregiver, partner, and doula, as well as any friends or loved ones joining you in the delivery room—knows how to get in touch with each other when your labor starts. Write out a list of numbers (including cell phone, pager, work, and other numbers), or program them right into your cell phone. Also decide on a point person to contact your extended family and circle of friends and let them know when your baby is here—and provide that person with all the necessary phone numbers and/or e-mail addresses she'll need to spread the news.

The process of collecting cord blood is painless and safe. After you've delivered your baby and the umbilical cord has been clamped and cut, your doctor or midwife will insert a needle into the umbilical vein (on the part of the cord that's still attached to your placenta—the needle doesn't go anywhere near your baby). Typically, the entire process takes less than ten minutes. Once the blood is sealed in a bag, it's shipped to a cord blood bank, where it's processed and frozen for long-term storage.

To store cord blood, you have two options: public cord blood banks, where you donate the blood for the good of the public—though these banks are still few and far between—and private cord blood banks, where you pay a hefty fee (initial processing fees in 2004 ranged from $800 to $1,800, with a subsequent yearly storage fee of about $100) to store the blood for your family's personal use. (Note: If you have a child with a disease like sickle-cell anemia or leukemia who could benefit from a sibling's cord blood, but you can't afford the fee, talk to your caregiver and your

(continued on page 385)

WORKSHEET: PREPARING A BIRTH PLAN

Name: _____

Partner's name: _____

Today's date: _____

Doctor or midwife's name: _____

Name of birth facility: _____

ATTENDANTS AND AMENITIES

I'd like the following people present during labor and/or birth:

Partner: _____

Friend(s): _____

Relative(s): _____

Doula: _____

Child(ren): _____

I'd like to bring music: yes/no

I'd like the lights dimmed: yes/no

I'd like to wear my own clothes during labor and delivery: yes/no

We'd like to take pictures and/or film during labor and delivery: yes/no

LABOR

I'd like to wear contact lenses during labor and birth, as long as I don't need a c-section: yes/no

I'd like the option of returning home if I'm not in active labor: yes/no

I'd prefer that my partner be allowed to stay with me at all times: yes/no

I prefer than only my practitioner, labor-and-delivery nurse, and personal guests be present (that is, no residents, medical students, or other hospital personnel): yes/no

I'd like to eat during labor: yes/no

I'd like to stay hydrated by drinking clear fluids instead of having an IV: yes/no

I'd like to be free to walk and move around during labor: yes/no

As long as my baby is doing fine, I'd prefer to have intermittent monitoring instead of continuous electronic fetal monitoring: yes/no

As long as my baby and I are doing fine, I'd like my labor to be allowed to progress free of stringent time limits: yes/no

PAIN RELIEF

I'd like to try the following pain-management techniques:

Acupressure ___   Hypnosis ___

Bath/shower ___   Massage ___

Breathing techniques/distraction ___   Medication ___

Hot/cold therapy ___

I'm interested in pain medication only if I request it—I do *not* want pain medication *offered* to me: yes/no

If I decide I want medicinal pain relief, I'd prefer:

Regional analgesia (an epidural and/or spinal block) ___

Systemic medication ___

If they're available, I'd like to try:

A birthing stool ___

A squatting bar ___

A birthing ball ___

A birthing pool/tub ___

A birthing chair ___

Other _____

A beanbag chair ___

I'd like to bring the following birthing equipment with me:

Birthing stool ___

Birthing pool/tub ___

Beanbag chair ___

Other _____

When it's time to push, I'd like to:

Do so instinctively ___

Be coached on when to push and for how long ___

I'd like to try the following positions for pushing (and birth):

Semireclining ___

Hands and knees ___

Side-lying position ___

Whatever feels right at the time ___

Squatting ___

As long as my baby and I are doing fine, I'd like the pushing stage to be allowed to progress free of stringent time limits: yes/no

VAGINAL BIRTH

I'd like to view the birth using a mirror: yes/no

I'd like to touch my baby's head as it crowns: yes/no

I'd like the room to be as quiet as possible while I give birth: yes/no

I'd rather risk a tear than have an episiotomy: yes/no

My partner would like to help "catch" our baby: yes/no

I'd like my baby placed on my abdomen or chest as soon as she's born: yes/no

I'd like to hold my baby immediately after birth—putting off any nonurgent tests and other procedures: yes/no

I'd like to breastfeed as soon as possible: yes/no

I'd like to wait until the umbilical cord stops pulsating before it's clamped and cut: yes/no

My partner would like to cut the umbilical cord: yes/no

I'd prefer not to get routine Pitocin after I deliver the placenta: yes/no

(continued)

WORKSHEET: PREPARING A BIRTH PLAN (CONT.)

C-SECTION

I'd like my partner present at all times during the operation: yes/no

I'd like to remain conscious if possible: yes/no

I'd like the screen lowered a bit so I can see my baby coming out: yes/no

As soon as my baby is dried (and as long as she's in good health), I'd like her given to my partner so he can hold her close to me in the operating room: yes/no

I'd like to breastfeed my baby in the recovery room: yes/no

POSTPARTUM

I'd like to spend as much time as possible with my baby before she's taken to the nursery for newborn evaluations and other procedures: yes/no

I'd like all newborn procedures to take place in my presence: yes/no

If I can't be with my baby for newborn procedures, my partner would like to stay with the baby at all times: yes/no

I'd like to stay in a private room: yes/no

I'd like a cot provided for my partner: yes/no

I plan to:
Breastfeed exclusively ____   Formula-feed exclusively ____
Combine breast- and formula-feeding ____

The following can be offered to my baby:
Formula ____   Sugar water ____   Pacifier ____
I would prefer that nothing be offered to my baby at any point ____

I'd like my baby fed:
On demand ____   On a schedule ____

I'd like:
24-hour rooming in with my baby ____
My baby to room in with me only when I'm awake ____
My baby brought to me for feedings only ____
To make my decision later, depending on how I'm feeling ____

If my baby's a boy:
I want him to be circumcised at the hospital ____
I want some type of analgesic for my baby during circumcision ____
I'll have him circumcised later ____
I don't want him circumcised ____

I'd like my other child(ren) brought in to see me and meet the new baby as soon as possible after the birth: yes/no

I'm interested in checking out of the hospital early: yes/no

child's doctors. There may be programs available to help you with the cost of cord blood storage.)

Choosing a Doctor for Your Baby

Choosing the right pediatrician or family doctor is more important than you might think: The average new parent and baby visit the doctor's office *11 times* in the first year alone! Choose well, and the doctor you pick might treat your child all the way from first cold to precollege physical. Most parents start the search during pregnancy and arrive at their final choice during the third trimester. Making a decision well in advance of labor and delivery allows for an informed—not hasty—choice.

Once you've drawn up your short list, make an appointment to interview prospective candidates. Most doctors have only about ten to 15 minutes to spare for a meeting. If the interview takes longer, some may charge a consultation fee.

WHAT TO ASK PROSPECTIVE PEDIATRICIANS/FAMILY PHYSICIANS

Name: _____

Location: _____

BASICS

How long have you been in practice?

What do you like best about your job?

Do you have any sub-specialties?

Are you a solo or group practice?

If you're solo, who covers for you if you're not available?

If you're in a group practice, how often will other practitioners see my baby?

What are your hours?

Are any evening or weekend hours available?

How are appointments handled for contagious kids? Do they share the same waiting room as healthy children?

How can I reach you in an emergency?

What hospitals are you affiliated with?

How do you feel about parents calling with routine/nonemergency questions?

Do you have an advice nurse or special calling hours for such questions?

How comfortable are you discussing a child's behavior—tantrums, discipline issues, social development, and so on?

BABY CARE

Where do you stand on:

Breastfeeding?

Formula-feeding?

Circumcision?

Sleep training methods?

Cosleeping?

Use of antibiotics?

The use of alternative medicine?

QUESTIONS TO ASK YOURSELF:

Did you feel comfortable with the doctor?

Is the office conveniently located?

How long were you kept waiting?

Did the waiting room and the exam rooms have toys and books to occupy young patients?

Did the office seem clean?

How helpful were the nurses and support staff?

CHAPTER 17

GIVING BIRTH: NORMAL LABOR AND DELIVERY

This is it! Whether you're waiting by the door with a packed bag or caught completely off guard, the beginning of labor is an astonishing thing. Your entire pregnancy and all of your preparations have led to this moment, and your baby will be in your arms before you know it! But as you embark on this final, thrilling phase of your pregnancy, bear in mind that there's no one "normal" labor or birth and that your experience may differ significantly from the "typical" scenario outlined here. And even if labor and birth feel like an endpoint, they're actually the furthest thing from it: the beginning of your new life as a mother—and the beginning of a lifelong journey you'll take with your child.

Is Labor Close at Hand?

On TV shows, it's always so simple: A hugely pregnant woman wakes with a start, grasps her belly, and shakes her sleeping mate awake with the announcement "Honey, it's time." In real life, though, the beginning of labor can be a bit harder to suss out. For one thing, labor is a complex process that can take weeks to fully kick in. For another, the hallmark signs of impending labor can sometimes be hard to distinguish from the many normal symptoms of late pregnancy. Some clues that your body is gearing up for delivery day:

Your baby "drops." If this is your first pregnancy, you may feel what's known as "lightening" a few weeks before labor starts. You might detect a heaviness in your pelvis as this happens and notice less pressure just below your rib cage, making it easier to catch your breath.

You note an uptick in Braxton Hicks contractions. An increase in the frequency and intensity of Braxton Hicks can signal prelabor, during which your cervix ripens and the stage is set for true labor. Or you may notice a crampy, menstrual-like feeling during this time. Sometimes as true labor draws near, Braxton Hicks contractions can become relatively painful and strike as often as every ten to 20 minutes, making you wonder if "this is it." (*Hint:* If they don't get longer, stronger, and closer together, probably what you're feeling is "false labor.")

Your cervix starts to ripen. In the days and weeks before delivery, Braxton Hicks do some of their preliminary work of softening, thinning, and perhaps opening your cervix a bit. (If you've given birth before, your cervix is more likely to dilate a centimeter or two before labor starts—but keep in mind that even being 40 weeks pregnant with your first baby and one centimeter dilated is no guarantee that labor's imminent.) During your last few prenatal visits, your practitioner may do vaginal exams to note any cervical changes that could be happening.

You notice "bloody show." If you pass your mucus plug—the thickened mucus that's sealed your cervical canal during the past nine months (it may be tinged with blood)—labor is probably just around the corner. You might lose your plug all at once, or notice increased vaginal discharge over the course of several days. (Note, though, that having sex or a vaginal exam can also disturb your mucus plug and cause you to see some show even when labor isn't about to start.)

Labor begins. Although it's not always possible to pinpoint exactly when "true" labor begins, you can be pretty sure labor has started when the sporadic Braxton Hicks you've been noticing for weeks gradually become longer, stronger, and closer together. They may be as far

QUICK TIPS

False versus True Labor

The signs of false labor include:

- Irregular (unpredictable and nonrhythmic) contractions that don't seem to increase in frequency or intensity. True labor contractions, on the other hand, hit at regular intervals, which shorten over time while the intensity of the contractions increases.

- Pain centered on your lower belly and groin—rather than pain in your back and abdomen.

- Contractions that subside when you start or stop an activity or change position.

BabyCenter Buzz

My Water Broke at the . . .

"My water broke while I was in the emergency room with my brother-in-law, who was having an appendicitis attack. The funny thing about it is that yes, I was at the hospital—but I was at the *wrong* hospital!" —*Beth*

"I was at my final childbirth education class. Now the teacher has a great story to tell her other classes!" —*Gisele*

"My water broke in the middle of the night while I was sleeping—before I'd had any noticeable contractions. I rode to the hospital sitting on towels!" —*Holly*

"My water broke during the pushing phase of labor. I was really starting to wonder if my baby would be delivered in the bag of waters!" —*Anonymous*

apart as every ten to 20 minutes in the beginning, but they won't stop or ease up no matter what you do, and in time the interval between contractions will lessen. In some cases, though, the onset of strong, regular contractions comes with little or no warning—it's different for every woman and with every pregnancy.

Your water breaks. When the fluid-filled amniotic sac surrounding your baby ruptures, you might feel a large gush or a small trickle. In either case, though, it should prompt a call to your doctor or midwife. Most women start having regular contractions sometime *before* their water breaks—but in some cases the water breaks first. When this happens, labor usually soon follows. If you don't start having contractions on your own within a certain amount of time, (depending on the particulars of your situation and your caregiver's normal MO), you'll need to be induced because—without the amniotic sac's built-in protection against germs—your baby will be at increased risk for infection.

When to Call Your Doctor or Midwife

Toward the end of your pregnancy, your practitioner should give you a clear set of guidelines about when it's time to let her know that you're having contractions. These instructions will depend on your individual sit-

Call Your Caregiver If . . .

- Your water breaks or if you suspect that you're leaking amniotic fluid. The color and consistency may be important. Let your caregiver know if your fluid is yellowish or greenish, thick or thin.
- You notice a decrease in your baby's activity.
- You have vaginal bleeding (unless it's just bloody show—mucus with a spot or streak of blood), fever, severe headaches, vision changes, or abdominal pain.
- The signs aren't clear but you think the time may have come. Don't be embarrassed; doctors and midwives are used to getting calls from women who aren't sure if they're in labor and who need guidance—it's part of their job.

uation—whether you've had pregnancy complications or are otherwise considered high risk, whether this is your first baby, and practical matters like how far you live from the hospital or birth center—and your caregiver's personal preference (some prefer an early heads-up). If you have an uncomplicated pregnancy, she'll likely have you wait to head in until your contractions have been coming every five minutes for an hour. (Or course, if anything else is going on—your baby isn't moving enough, you're bleeding, or you think your water has broken—you'll need to call right away.) As a rule, if you're high risk, she'll want to hear from you earlier in labor.

When You Arrive at the Hospital or Birth Center

Protocol differs from facility to facility. Upon your arrival at the hospital or birth center, you'll likely face:

Paperwork. If you haven't preregistered, your partner can take care of any forms that need immediate attention while you're being checked in.

Urine test and a change of clothes. A nurse or your provider will have

BabyCenter Buzz

How I Knew I Was Really in Labor

"I was eight days overdue, five centimeters dilated, and I still didn't know I was in labor until my sister (who'd given birth before) told me I was. I thought I had gas!" —*Anonymous*

"I knew I was in labor when I couldn't sleep because of the contractions." —*Anonymous*

"My back really hurt, the contractions continued and became closer together, and I couldn't walk or talk through them. Then I knew it was time to head to the hospital." —*Kelli*

you pee into a cup so she can test your urine for protein, sugar, and ketones and then will give you a gown to change into. (If you'd prefer, most hospitals—and all birth centers—will allow you to wear your own clothes.)

A check of your vital signs and more. Your caregiver will take your pulse, blood pressure, respiration, and temperature, and ask about your due date, whether your baby's been moving, when your contractions started, how far apart they are, whether your water's broken or if you have any vaginal bleeding, and whether you've recently had anything to eat or drink. She'll also want to know about any previous pregnancies and births, whether you have any health problems or allergies, whether you're currently taking any medication, and whether you've had any pregnancy complications.

A check of your contractions and your baby's heart rate. If you're at a hospital, you'll be attached to an electronic fetal monitor—at least initially, and possibly for your entire labor. But if you're at a birth center, your caregiver will periodically listen to your baby's heartbeat with a handheld Doppler like the one used during your prenatal visits. She'll also periodically put her hands on your belly to feel your contractions.

A vaginal exam. Your provider will want to check your cervix for dilation and effacement and feel how low your baby is. (If your caregiver isn't certain that it's a *head* she's feeling, she'll do an ultrasound to confirm your baby's position.)

At this point, if it looks like you're not in labor or are still in early labor—and everything is okay with you and your baby—you'll probably be

Just the Facts

Fetal Monitoring

Your practitioner or a nurse will check your baby's heart rate during labor to keep close tabs on how he's doing and see how he's tolerating your contractions. This can be done with an electronic fetal monitor—either periodically or continuously—or intermittently with a handheld Doppler.

In hospitals, electronic fetal monitoring is a routine practice, but—as with most aspects of labor and delivery—policies vary. Some providers (and some hospitals) require that you be attached to a monitor throughout active labor and birth; others will hook you up for an initial 15- to 30-minute check and then, as long as everything is progressing smoothly, have only intermittent checks thereafter. (If you're at a birth center, you'll be monitored intermittently with a handheld Doppler.) If you get an epidural or need Pitocin, you'll be monitored continuously for the rest of your labor.

Electronic fetal monitoring itself is painless—though being tethered to a monitor can limit your movement and for some women make it more difficult to cope with contractions. Two electronic devices (one for your baby's heartbeat and another for your contractions) are held in place by a wide stretch band placed around your belly. They'll pick up and transmit information to a machine by your bedside. You'll hear the galloping of your baby's heartbeat (for many women, this is the soundtrack they'll associate most poignantly with labor), and the monitor will record both your baby's heart rate and your contractions. In certain circumstances, your caregiver may choose to do internal monitoring—by attaching a tiny electrode to your baby's scalp—to get a more accurate reading.

A baby's heart rate normally drops slightly during a contraction and then rises again afterward. Certain types of decreases in your baby's heart rate, on the other hand, may signal a possible problem. A "nonreassuring" heart rate pattern may precipitate a change in the course of the delivery: anything from a vacuum-assisted vaginal birth to an unplanned or even emergency c-section.

sent home until your labor is further along. (In some cases, you may be asked to stay for an hour or two so you can be reexamined to see if there's been any change since the initial evaluation.)

If it turns out that it's time for you to be admitted, the nurse or your midwife or doctor may:

Ask if you have a birth plan. If you're not asked, bring it up! Even if you don't have a written plan, you should share your needs and preferences with those in attendance, including the labor nurse and the doctor or midwife. It's also a good time to let the staff know if you hope to labor without

BabyCenter Buzz

My Caregiver Wasn't on Call When I Went into Labor

"My usual midwife wasn't on call when I went into labor. But the midwife covering for her shared the same philosophy, so I got the kind of care I'd hoped for anyway. Plus, she stayed with me all through my labor, so by the time my baby was born, we'd really bonded." —*Ann*

"When you go into labor, the most important people to you will be your coach and your nurse. Doctors rarely stay in the room throughout." —*Jacyln*

"I hired a doula—I highly recommend getting one—because I was concerned about ending up with a doctor I didn't know. She was there the whole time; my OB only came in for the last 10 minutes." —*Riono*

"I cried when I went into labor because the person I liked least from my practice was on call. Little did I know I wouldn't be delivering my baby for another 30 hours, by which point our favorite doctor had arrived!" —*Megan*

medication or if you have your heart set on an epidural—or if you're not set on one route or the other.

Possibly recommend an enema. Though an enema is no longer routine, some nurses or providers may still offer one in early labor. This will cleanse your bowels and help prevent bowel movements during the pushing stage. But there's no *medical* reason to have an enema and they can be uncomfortable, so feel free to refuse. (Rest assured: Labor-and-delivery nurses are well prepared to deal with this common side effect of giving birth, and won't bat an eye if it happens.)

Draw some blood. She'll send a sample to the lab so your blood can be typed (in case you need a transfusion) and tested for various infections and other problems.

Possibly start an IV. At many hospitals, IVs are a matter of course. And you'll definitely need an IV:

- to get antibiotics if you test positive for Group B strep
- for hydration if you can't keep fluids down
- if you want a spinal or an epidural
- if you need Pitocin
- if you have any health problems or pregnancy complications

But if your pregnancy has been normal thus far and no labor compli-cations are expected, you can—with your practitioner's approval—ask to hold off on the IV. That way, you'll be freer to move around as the urge strikes you, without having to contend with tubing and an IV pole. You can also ask for a saline or hep lock—which allows for IV access if needed later but leaves you free to move around.

Your Pain-Management Options

Whether you ultimately have an unmedicated birth or go for the drugs, labor pain and its management looms large for any expecting mother—especially if this is your first time. Whatever your hopes or expectations, prepare to be taken by surprise: Labor is hard to imagine and even harder to predict. And not only is every labor different, but everyone experiences—and copes with—pain differently. Even though labor is unpredictable, it's important to spend some time thinking about your choices beforehand so you approach the experience with a plan that makes the most sense for *you*. There is no "right" way to have a baby.

If you want an unmedicated birth, you'll need to actively prepare for it—by developing a birth plan and making sure you'll be giving birth with a supportive caregiver in the right environment, ensuring that you have good labor coaching, and educating yourself about childbirth and coping tech-niques. On the other hand, if you know you're interested in numbing pain instead of working through it, you'll want to give birth in a hospital where epidurals are available around the clock.

You can't predict the future, so no matter which camp you find your-self in, learn as much as you can ahead of time about both natural and med-icinal pain management. Tension and fear tend to heighten the perception of pain, and anything you can do to lessen the anxiety you feel will help with the challenges ahead. (It may even help the *progress* of your labor, since high levels of stress hormones can affect your uterus's ability to contract.)

Even if you signed up for an epidural the day you learned you were pregnant, you'll still benefit from having some natural approaches in your bag of tricks, whether to use at home in early labor (or during bouts of false labor), in the hospital during your wait for the anesthesiologist, or in the un-likely event that your epidural doesn't provide total pain coverage.

And even if you'd hoped for an unmedicated birth, your plans may change if you have a much longer or more painful labor than you imagined or if you need medical interventions that interfere with your ability to manage pain naturally. Even if you have firm beliefs now about how you'd like to deal with labor pain when the time comes, a willingness to roll with the reality of your own labor and birth as it unfolds may ultimately be your greatest strength (and also help you avoid disappointment later if you don't have the "ideal" birth you'd imagined).

A look at your pain-management choices:

Natural Approaches to Controlling Pain

If you want to remain in control of your body to the greatest extent possible, be an active participant throughout labor, and have minimal interventions in the birth process, a natural, unmedicated approach will suit you best. If you choose to go this route, you accept the potential for pain and discomfort as part and parcel of the birth experience—an experience that includes working with complete awareness through each stage of labor. But with the right preparation and support, pain isn't all you'll take away from the experience; you'll likely feel empowered and deeply satisfied by it.

As long as your pregnancy (and labor) are problem-free, you can have a natural experience at a childbirth center, at home, or at a hospital. But if you're planning a hospital birth, you'll need to explicitly discuss your wishes and goals with your caregiver and find out what interventions are routine and how you might get around them. (Women with complications may need a variety of interventions, which tend to make it harder—though certainly not impossible—to cope without pain medication.)

Pros

• Most of these techniques are noninvasive, so there's little potential for harm or side effects for you or your baby.

• Many women have a real sense of empowerment during labor and accomplishment afterward—and many report that they'd opt for an unmedicated birth again the next time. For some women, being in charge helps lessen their perception of pain.

• There's no loss of sensation or alertness. You'll be awake and active during labor and birth, enabling you to move around more freely and to find positions that help you stay comfortable during labor and

BabyCenter Buzz

Giving Birth without Drugs

"When a contraction started, I'd imagine a huge, moonlit wave rising up, up, up—and then crashing down. Then my imaginary sea would be calm again until the next contraction started. I also made a strange groaning sound that helped a lot. I labored this way, drug-free, for 20 hours!" —*Anonymous*

"I didn't have drugs and I'm proud of it. It hurt like heck, but I felt every bit of my daughter being born, and I would never, ever exchange that for anything in the world." —*Anonymous*

"I had natural births with my daughter and son. Toward the end, the contractions really hurt—but I just kept thinking of all of the women who'd labored before me, and that gave me more energy to push." —*Anonymous*

"Believe me, you're no wimp if you opt for the epidural. But if you think you can stand it, consider going natural. You won't be sorry!" —*Anonymous*

"Have an open mind and see what happens. I'm having my first child, and will attempt a natural birth—but won't be disappointed if I wind up opting for an epidural." —*Catherine*

"I loved how I was able to be in control and let my body dictate positions and comfort techniques. But even more, I found giving birth without drugs to be a bonding experience—my husband and I worked through the most difficult task of our lives together. The feelings were overwhelming, but after giving all I had and more for this precious little child to be placed in my arms, I couldn't imagine it any other way." —*Aubrie*

that aid the delivery process when it's time to push your baby out.

• Your partner may feel more involved as you work together to manage your pain.

• You're not required to be hooked up to an IV or monitoring machines, so you'll be free to move around—walk if you'd like, take a shower or a bath, and use the toilet instead of a bedpan.

• You're less likely than women who get epidurals to need Pitocin, a vacuum extraction or forceps delivery, or bladder catheterization.

• You can practice breathing exercises, visualization, and self-hypnosis ahead of time—and use them again later. Many new mothers find themselves drawing on their relaxation techniques in the early days of breastfeeding, while coping with postpartum discomfort, or when caring for their newborn feels especially stressful.

Cons

• Unlike an epidural, these techniques don't eliminate pain—so if you're not willing to feel and work *with* the pain, you'll be happier with an epidural.

• Natural approaches may not offer adequate pain management if you end up with a complicated labor that requires a lot of interventions or if you're exhausted from a prolonged labor and really need to sleep.

Breathing Exercises and Visualization

Most childbirth classes cover breathing and visualization techniques. You and your partner may be given specific breathing patterns to practice, and your instructor may coach you on using visualization (of a place that soothes you— or of the safe, easy birth of your baby) to help you work through the pain. You may also learn techniques like progressive or controlled relaxation—where you learn how to focus on and then release tension by zeroing in on a particular muscle, tightening it up, and then letting it go until it's as loose as possible. These techniques draw on relaxation and partnership as a way to manage your contractions, and they may work especially well if your labor progresses as it should. If you've ever studied yoga, a martial art, or meditation, you may already have the practice you need to breathe through your birth. You may find, too, that bringing something special to look at (a favorite photograph, for instance) and having soothing music also help you relax.

One-to-One Labor Support

Having someone at your side who's committed to giving you emotional reassurance as well as helping you be as comfortable as possible can dramatically reduce your anxiety and stress level and help you get through the rigors of labor without drugs. Some research shows that women who have continuous support are less likely to need systemic pain medication or an epidural during labor and are more likely to have a normal vaginal birth than those who don't have such support.

Positioning and Movement

When you're unmedicated and not tethered to a monitor, you can try a variety of positions during labor, including standing or leaning on your partner, sitting, and kneeling (either upright or on all fours).

You may find movement comforting, too, and want to try walking or rocking in a chair or on a birth ball. Moving around can make you feel more in control, thus lessening your anxiety and discomfort. (Some high-tech hos-

BabyCenter Buzz

Giving Birth Using Hypnosis

"I had an epidural with my first, but used hypnosis with my second and had virtually no pain. What I did feel was less painful than menstrual cramps." —*Anonymous*

"Hypnobirthing taught me to be confident in my body and my baby's ability to birth in a gentle, calm way." —*Mel*

"The less fear you have, the less you'll tense up—and the less you tense up, the easier your birth will be. It totally worked for me—I got to the hospital at 8 centimeters and was never in major pain. It was an awesome experience." —*Anonymous*

"I was very happy with the feeling of control that hypnobirthing gave me. Even though I ended up being induced with Pitocin—which resulted in a hard labor—I was able to keep myself together with meditation and the self-confidence I learned. Hypnobirth doesn't take away the pain; instead, it gives you the coping techniques you need to ride it out with purpose and dignity." —*Lisa*

pitals have wireless monitoring systems, so even if you have complications that require continuous monitoring, you may still be able to move about freely.)

During the pushing stage, an upright position may help your baby descend, and squatting or kneeling may help to open your pelvic outlet. That said, the differences aren't that great—so feel free to try a variety of positions and settle on the ones that make you most comfortable.

Hypnosis

Some studies suggest that hypnosis decreases the sensation of pain during labor. To use self-hypnosis, you'll need training and practice ahead of time so you can learn how to focus and relax your muscles during labor.

Massage, Touch, and Hot and Cold Therapy

Massage promotes relaxation, soothes tense muscles, and may decrease your perception of labor pain. You can get a massage from your partner—human touch by a loved one can be very reassuring if you're feeling anxious—or another support person. You may be comforted by light stroking (called effleurage), or you may prefer a stronger touch. If you're having back labor, you'll likely want firm massage or steady counterpressure applied to your lower back. At times during your labor, though, you may find that massage is annoying and will need to communicate that to your support team.

BabyCenter Buzz

Laboring in Water

"I had a very quick labor and only got to stay in the tub for about ten minutes, but even two years later, I remember that as the most blissful, pain-free time in my labor." —*Jen*

"I had difficult back labor, and the only time I could relax was in the tub, with warm water pouring over my back from the faucet." —*Anonymous*

"The water provided amazing pain relief, and I found the freedom of movement very comforting. I could change position easily because the tub I delivered in was large and round—not a regular bathtub." —*Anonymous*

"My last baby was a water birth. It was totally unplanned (my hospital only lets you *labor* in the water). But I suddenly had to push my baby out, and my midwife caught her underwater. I wasn't going to hold her in so they could drain the tub!" —*Christy*

Many women also swear by warm compresses or a hot-water bottle used on an aching lower belly or back—or anywhere else they're feeling discomfort—to help them relax and reduce pain. Some find that cold packs are more soothing, and others find that alternating hot and cold is helpful. It's worth giving both a try—just be sure to protect your skin from direct contact with heat or cold.

Hydrotherapy

Hydrotherapy—using water to help ease the discomforts of labor—may mean soaking in a bath during early labor or letting soothing shower water run over your belly and back in active labor. Most birth centers and some hospitals provide extra-large or Jacuzzi-style tubs for laboring women—and some of those that don't may let you bring your own.

Like other drug-free options, hydrotherapy allows you to remain alert and in control, and the soothing and pressure-relieving effects of the water promote muscle relaxation and may decrease pain and anxiety and lessen the need for medication. One study suggests that continuous soaking in early labor may slow labor a bit, so some caregivers recommend limiting the length of your baths early on or waiting until labor is well-established to take a long soak. (That said, a warm bath is a great way to deal with false labor pains.) Make sure, too, that the tub water is at body temperature (98.6°F)

Just the Facts

Water Births

While hydrotherapy during labor is almost universally accepted, actually giving *birth* underwater is controversial. Proponents contend that babies won't try to breathe in the few seconds they're underwater after they emerge from the birth canal, and cite the fact that many women have safely given birth underwater. But opponents point out that babies who are short of oxygen after birth may gasp while still immersed and inhale water into their lungs. Fresh water isn't the same as amniotic fluid, and there are cases—albeit very rare—of babies dying from drowning during water births. There's also a concern about an increased risk of infection from bacteria that may be in the tub.

or less, because anything higher can raise your temperature—and your baby's temperature and heart rate as well.

Not all women are good candidates for water therapy during labor, though—it's clearly not an option if you have complications that necessitate continuous electronic monitoring, for instance. And most caregivers advise against immersion if your water's already broken, due to the risk of infection from bacteria lurking in the tub, water jets, or hosing. (A shower, though, is fine.)

Drugs for Labor Pain

Natural childbirth certainly isn't for everyone, of course. In fact, the majority of women in the United States opt for some kind of pain medication—most commonly an epidural—to help them cope with labor. You may decide well before delivery day that you want pain medication, may ask for relief when you find that labor isn't at all what you imagined, or may end up opting for medication if nature throws you a curveball and you end up with a long or complicated labor. Your choices for pain relief include:

Systemic Medication

Systemic painkillers such as narcotics dull your pain but don't completely eliminate it. (You may also be given a tranquilizer—alone or in combination with a narcotic—to reduce anxiety or nausea, or for sedation.) Systemic drugs are either given through an IV line into your bloodstream or are injected into a muscle, and they affect your entire body rather than just your lower abdomen

Just the Facts

Acupuncture

Acupuncture, which has been used for centuries in traditional Chinese medicine, involves inserting and manipulating fine needles into specific points on your body. There's evidence that acupuncture is useful in relieving things such as dental pain and lower-back pain, but there are fewer studies about its effectiveness in labor. Though most experts agree that more research is needed, the evidence does suggest that acupuncture may work for some women—promoting relaxation, alleviating some pain, and reducing the need for medication.

No one really knows *how* acupuncture works to decrease pain, but two common theories are that the technique either blocks certain pain impulses to your brain or stimulates the release of natural pain relievers called endorphins. The acupuncture points commonly used in labor include spots on your hands, feet, and ears. The downside of this technique is that it requires a skilled practitioner, and few doctors or midwives are trained acupuncturists. If you're interested in trying this method and you're having your baby at a birth center or at home, you may be able to arrange for a certified acupuncturist to be on hand.

and pelvis. They may make you feel sleepy, but unlike the general anesthesia that's often given for surgery, they won't completely knock you out.

PROS

• Systemic pain relief may help if you can cope with some pain but need to take the edge off.

• It's easier and less invasive to insert an IV or give an injection than it is to put in an epidural or a spinal block, and it doesn't require an anesthesiologist.

• Women using systemic medication are less likely to end up needing Pitocin or having their babies delivered with forceps or a vacuum than those who opt for an epidural.

CONS

• In the doses commonly used for labor, systemic medication is much less effective than an epidural or a spinal block for pain relief. (The dose must be relatively small because these drugs cross the placenta and can affect your baby.)

• Systemic medication can cause a variety of unpleasant side effects, such as drowsiness, dizziness, and disorientation. Because of this, you'll have to stay in bed. Some of these drugs can also cause nausea and itchiness.

BabyCenter Buzz

Giving Birth with Systemic Medication

"After 11 hours of labor, I couldn't endure my back pain any longer. My doctor gave me Demerol. I should have asked for it much, much sooner. I'm now pregnant with my second child and will definitely request something before the pain becomes unbearable." —Pat

"I had two pain shots in my IV, which helped me sleep a little (I was in labor for 19 hours!)." —Jen

"My contractions were so intense that I couldn't relax even between them, so I asked for a narcotic. Right after the nurse put in the IV and the drugs kicked in, I told her I had to push." —Callie

"I was in a lot of pain, dying for an epidural—but the anesthesiologist was busy with another patient. I was given a mild narcotic to help me cope while I waited. It was just enough to help me handle the big contractions that were starting to come on very quickly." —Lorraine

"I had a dose of Nubain and later had trouble remembering the details of my delivery. The whole thing is still fuzzy." —Cheri

• Narcotics can sometimes slow labor, especially if given too soon.

• In large doses, narcotics can interfere with your breathing. (This happens only rarely, in part because it's unusual to get high doses during labor. If it does happen, you'll need medication to reverse the effects of the narcotic.)

• Systemic pain medication can affect your baby's heart rate in such a way that your practitioner or labor nurse may have trouble interpreting the results of fetal heart rate monitoring.

• Narcotics sometimes make it harder for your baby to start breathing on his own after birth, particularly if you're given a large dose within a few hours of delivery. For this reason, your practitioner will be stingy with narcotics late in your labor. Sometimes, though, labor will progress much more quickly than expected. If this happens, your baby may need medication to counteract the effects of the narcotic. (If your baby is premature or otherwise at risk, your practitioner may recommend an epidural instead of systemic pain relief.)

• Systemic narcotics can interfere with your baby's alertness at birth and may make your early attempts to breastfeed more difficult.

Epidural

An epidural block (often just called an "epidural") delivers continuous pain relief to the lower part of your body while allowing you to remain fully conscious. Medication is delivered through a very thin, flexible tube (called a catheter) that's inserted into the epidural space just outside the membrane that surrounds your spine. You lie curled on your side or sit on the edge of the bed while an anesthesiologist or nurse anesthetist cleans your back, injects the area with numbing medicine, and carefully guides a needle into your lower back. She then passes a catheter through it, withdraws the needle, and tapes the catheter in place so she can administer medication through it as needed. You can lie down at this point without disturbing the catheter.

BabyCenter Buzz

Giving Birth with an Epidural

"I had a wonderful experience because of my epidural. I was pain-free for six of the seven hours of my labor. My husband and I had some relaxing quality time together. I pushed for about 45 minutes and delivered a healthy boy. I was able to go to the bathroom and shower within two hours of my son's birth. I'm still amazed at how much I enjoyed the labor and delivery because of my epidural." —*Anonymous*

"I wish someone would've told me that delivery can go well. I had myself all worked up for a long, drawn-out, painful birth experience. My labor and delivery went off without a hitch and, thanks to the epidural, was relatively pain-free. If I'd known it was possible to actually *enjoy* giving birth, I would've done it years ago!" —*Anonymous*

"I'm going into labor listening to my body, and if it says 'epidural,' then that's what I'm getting." —*Anonymous*

"I can't imagine why you'd choose any other option. I was given just enough medication to ease the pain, but I could definitely tell when I was having a contraction and when it was time to push." —*Anonymous*

"My anesthesiologist went too far with the needle and punctured the sac that protects my spinal cord. She didn't mention that I might have a terrible headache for the next few days as a result. I had to go back to the hospital four days later so they could take blood out of my arm and inject it into my spine to clot over the puncture. That hurt more than the epidural placement, but within an hour, the headache was gone. This is supposed to be a rare problem, but the doctor who fixed it said he sees it all the time." —*Kate*

You'll first be given a small "test dose" of medicine to be sure the epidural was placed correctly, followed by a full dose if there are no problems. Your baby's heart rate will be monitored continuously, and you'll have your blood pressure taken every five minutes or so for a while after the epidural is in to make sure it isn't having any negative effects. The medication you'll receive through the epidural will likely be a combination of a local anesthetic and a narcotic. Local anesthetics block sensations of pain, touch, movement, and temperature, and narcotics blunt pain without affecting your ability to move your legs. Used together, they provide good pain relief with less loss of sensation in your legs and at a lower total dose than you'd need with just one or the other.

PROS

• An epidural provides a route for very effective pain relief that can be used throughout your labor.

• The anesthesiologist or nurse anesthetist can control the effects by adjusting the type, amount, and strength of the medication. This is important because as your labor progresses and your baby moves further down into your birth canal, you may find that the dose you've been getting no longer covers the pain or that you're suddenly having pain in a different area.

• Because the effect of the medication is localized, you'll be awake and alert during labor and birth. And because you're pain-free, you can rest if you want (or even sleep!) as your cervix dilates, which means you may have more energy when it comes time to push.

• Unlike systemic narcotics, only a tiny amount of medication reaches your baby.

• Once the epidural's in place, it can be used to provide anesthesia if you need a c-section or if you're having your tubes tied after delivery.

CONS

• You have to stay in an awkward position for ten to 15 minutes while the epidural is put in, and then wait another five to 20 minutes before the medication takes full effect.

• Depending on the type and amount of medication you're getting, you may lose some sensation in your legs, so you won't be able to stand. Sometimes, particularly in early labor, so little anesthetic is needed to make you comfortable that you have normal strength and sensation in your legs and can move around without difficulty. (This is called a "walking epidural.")

Still, many practitioners and hospitals won't allow you to get out of bed once you've had an epidural, whether you think you can walk or not.

• An epidural requires that you have an IV, frequent blood pressure monitoring, and continuous electronic fetal monitoring.

• An epidural may slow your labor, in which case you may need Pitocin to get it back on track.

• The loss of sensation in your lower body lessens the bearing-down reflex and may make it harder for you to push your baby out, so it often lengthens the pushing stage of labor. You may want to have the epidural dose decreased while you're pushing so you can participate more actively in your baby's delivery. It can take time for the pain medication to wear off enough that you can feel what you're doing, and there's no evidence that decreasing the epidural dose actually shortens this stage of labor.

• Having an epidural increases your chance of having a vacuum extraction or forceps delivery, which in turn increases your risk for serious tears (page 441).

• In some cases, an epidural provides spotty pain relief. This can happen because of variations in anatomy from one woman to the next or if the medication doesn't manage to bathe all of your spinal nerves as it spreads through your epidural space. The catheter can also "drift" slightly, so the pain relief might get spotty after starting out fine. (If you notice that you're starting to have pain in certain places, ask for the anesthesiologist or nurse anesthetist to be paged so your dose can be adjusted or your catheter reinserted.)

• The drugs used in your epidural may temporarily lower your blood pressure, decreasing blood flow to your baby, which in turn slows his heart rate. (This is treated with fluids and sometimes medication.)

• Narcotics delivered through an epidural can cause itchiness, particularly in your face. They can also bring on nausea—though this is less likely with an epidural than with systemic medication, and some women feel nauseated and throw up during labor even *without* pain medication.

• Anesthetics delivered through an epidural can make it more difficult to tell when you need to pee. Also, if you can't pee into a bedpan (which for many people is harder than letting go on a toilet), you may need to be catheterized.

• No one knows exactly why, but an epidural raises your risk of running a fever in labor. It doesn't boost your or your baby's odds of getting an *infection*—but because it's unclear at first whether the fever is from the

epidural or from an infection, you and your baby may wind up getting un-
necessary antibiotics.

• In one in 100 women, an epidural causes a bad headache that may
last for days. (You can reduce the risk of headache by lying as still as possible while the needle is being placed.)

• In very rare cases, an epidural can affect your breathing, and in extremely rare cases it can cause nerve injury or infection.

Spinal Block

A spinal block (or "spinal") quickly delivers pain relief to your lower body
for a limited period of time. An anesthesiologist or nurse anesthetist inserts
a needle into your lower back, guides it through the membrane surrounding
your spine, and injects an anesthetic with or without a narcotic into your
spinal fluid. This effectively eliminates pain from your waist down. A spinal
differs from an epidural in two ways: It's delivered directly into the spinal
fluid (and not into the space surrounding your spine), and it's a onetime injection rather than a continuous feed through a catheter. As a result, relief is
rapid and complete, but lasts only a few hours.

Your practitioner may order a spinal block if you decide you want pain
relief late in labor or if you're progressing so rapidly that delivery is likely to
be sooner rather than later and you can't wait for an epidural. It's also an
option if you need to have a c-section or if you're having your tubes tied after
delivery and you don't already have an epidural in place.

PROS
• Complete pain relief kicks in after only a few minutes.
• In contrast to systemic narcotics, only a tiny amount of medication
reaches your baby.

CONS
• You have to stay in an awkward position for five to ten minutes
during the procedure.
• You'll need an IV and continuous electronic fetal monitoring, and
you won't be able to get out of bed.
• The decrease in sensation may make it harder for you to push your
baby out, which can lengthen the pushing stage and increase your odds of
needing a vacuum extraction or forceps delivery (which, in turn, increases
your risk of serious tears).

• The drugs may temporarily lower your blood pressure, decreasing blood flow to your baby, which in turn slows his heart rate. (This is treated with fluids and sometimes medication.)

• If a narcotic is used, it can cause itchiness, particularly in your face. It can also bring on nausea—though this is less likely with a spinal than with systemic medication, and some women feel nauseated and throw up during labor even *without* pain medication.

• In rare cases, a spinal can cause an uncomfortable tingling sensation in your legs or buttocks that lasts a couple of days.

• In one in 100 women, a spinal causes a bad headache that may last for several days.

• In very rare cases, a spinal can affect your breathing, and in extremely rare cases, it can cause nerve injury or infection.

Combined Spinal-Epidural

Some anesthesiologists offer what's called a combined spinal-epidural, in which an epidural needle is inserted into your lower back and a narrower spinal needle is inserted through the epidural needle (so you're only stuck once). After medication is given through the spinal needle, it's removed, and a catheter is passed through the epidural needle before that needle is withdrawn. This technique offers the rapid pain relief of a spinal combined with the continuous relief of an epidural.

The Three Stages of Labor

Labor and birth are divided into three stages. The first stage actually has two *phases*, beginning with the onset of contractions and the gradual effacement and dilation of your cervix (early or "latent" labor). That's followed by active labor, when your cervix begins to dilate more rapidly and contractions are longer, stronger, and closer together (this is when it's usually time to call your doctor or midwife). The active phase ends when your cervix is fully dilated to ten centimeters, and the last part of this phase is called transition. The second *stage* of labor (pushing) begins once you're fully dilated and ends with the birth of your baby. The third and final stage begins right after the birth and involves the separation and delivery of the placenta.

Take It Easy

Don't become a slave to your stopwatch just yet—it's stressful and exhausting to record every contraction over the many long hours of labor, and it isn't necessary. Instead, you may want to time them periodically to get a sense of what's going on. In most cases, your contractions will let you know (in no uncertain terms) when it's time to take them more seriously! Meanwhile, stay rested because you may have a long day (or night) ahead of you, drink plenty of fluids to stay well-hydrated, and don't forget to go to the bathroom often (even if you don't feel the urge)—a full bladder may make it more difficult for your uterus to contract efficiently; plus, an empty bladder leaves more room for your baby to descend.

First Stage: Early Labor

Once your contractions are coming at regular intervals and your cervix begins to progressively dilate and efface, you're officially in labor. That said, unless your labor starts with a bang—from essentially having no contractions to having fairly regular contractions—it's sometimes tricky to determine *exactly* when true labor starts because these early labor contractions can be hard to distinguish from the Braxton Hicks contractions that contribute to false labor.

For this reason—and because every labor is so different—it's not easy to say how long this phase typically lasts or even (after the fact) how long it lasted for a particular woman. The length of early labor depends in large part on how ripe your cervix is at the beginning of labor and how frequent and strong your contractions are. With a first baby, if your cervix isn't effaced or dilated to begin with, this phase may take about eight hours—or even longer—though it can be significantly shorter, too. But if your cervix is already very ripe or if this isn't your first baby, it's likely to go much more quickly.

During the course of early labor, your contractions will gradually become longer, stronger, and closer together. While the experience of labor can vary widely, a typical one might start out with contractions coming every ten minutes and lasting 30 seconds each, and eventually increasing to every five minutes and lasting 40 to 60 seconds each as you reach the end of early labor. Some women have much more frequent contractions during this phase, though the contractions will still tend to be mild and last less than a minute.

Sometimes early labor contractions can be quite painful, though they may be dilating your cervix much more slowly than you'd like! If your labor is typical, though, your contractions now won't require the same attention that they will later in labor. You'll probably find that you can still talk through them and putter around the house. You may even feel like taking a short walk. If you feel inclined to relax instead, take a warm bath, watch a video, or doze between your contractions if you can.

You may also notice increasingly mucousy vaginal discharge, which may be tinged with blood—the so-called "bloody show." This is perfectly normal, but if you see more than a tinge of blood, call your caregiver. (Also call if your water breaks, even if you're not having contractions yet.) Early labor ends when your cervix is three to four centimeters dilated and your progress starts to accelerate.

First Stage: Active Labor

Active labor is when things *really* get rolling. Your contractions become more frequent, longer, and stronger, your cervix begins dilating faster— going from 3 to 4 centimeters to 10 centimeters—and toward the end of active labor, your baby begins to descend, too. As a general rule, once you've had regular, painful contractions (each lasting about 60 seconds)

Just the Facts

Back Labor

Having intense lower-back pain during contractions is relatively common, and you may have heard that it means your baby is facing up toward your pubic bone with the back of his head resting on the bony part of your spine—a position known as "sunny-side up," or posterior.

While it's true that women with posterior babies are likely to have intense back labor, you can have back pain during contractions even if your baby isn't posterior. Only about 15 percent of babies are posterior at the beginning of labor, yet far more than 15 percent of laboring women complain of intense back pain. This pain is usually attributed to the pressure your baby's head is putting on your lower back, though there may be other factors at work as well, including pain that's "referred" from your uterus.

That said, women whose babies remain posterior have longer labors, tend to need Pitocin more often, and have a significantly higher rater of c-sections. The good news is that almost 90 percent of babies who are posterior at the start of labor rotate and deliver in the more typical, facedown (anterior) position. Only about 5 percent of babies are posterior at birth—and many of them were facedown at the beginning of labor and later rotated to the sunny-side up position.

every five minutes for an hour, it's time to call your midwife or doctor and head to the hospital or birth center. (Some providers prefer a call sooner; when to call is something to discuss with your caregiver ahead of time.) In most cases, the frequency of contractions eventually increases to every two-and-a-half to three minutes. Still, some women may never have contractions more often than every five minutes.

Though labors vary widely, on *average* (and without Pitocin or an epidural) it takes about six hours for a woman having her first baby to go from four centimeters to full dilation. (Pitocin generally speeds up the active phase, while epidurals tend to make it last longer.) If you've already had a vaginal birth, active labor is likely to go more quickly. In contrast to early labor, you'll no longer be able to talk through your contractions. Breathing exercises, relaxation techniques, and a good labor coach can be a huge help now. Massage and lots of gentle encouragement are lifesavers, too.

When you get to the hospital or birth center, you should be able to move freely around the room as long as you don't have any medical or obstetric complications. You may find that it feels good to walk, but you'll probably want to stop and lean against someone (or something) during each contraction. If you're tired, sitting in a rocking chair or lying in bed on your side works as well. This might be a good time to take a warm shower or bath (if you have access to a tub) or to ask your partner for a massage. If you've already decided you want pain medication or you're having a hard time coping with contractions and nothing else seems to help, now's the time to talk to your provider about getting an epidural or systemic medication.

BabyCenter Buzz

How I Coped with Back Labor

"During a 38-hour back labor with my first child, my husband used a rolling pin, believe it or not, on my lower back for counterpressure, which helped immensely. Another lifesaver was having my doula stand behind me and firmly press my hips together during contractions to help relieve some of the pressure of the baby's skull on my tailbone!" —*Anonymous*

"I never thought I'd find myself laboring on all fours, but that's what it took to make the pain manageable. I didn't even care what I looked like." —*Anonymous*

The Second Stage: Pushing

By the end of transition, your baby has usually descended somewhat into your pelvis. This is when you might begin to feel rectal pressure, as if you have to move your bowels. Some women begin to bear down spontaneously and may even start making deep grunting sounds at this point. There's often a lot of bloody show. You may also feel nauseated or even vomit now.

If you've had an epidural, you'll feel varying amounts of presure, depending on the type and amount of medication you're getting. If you'd like to be a more active participant in the pushing stage, ask to have your epidural dose lowered at the end of transition.

POSITIONS FOR PUSHING

Though the classic image of birth has a sweaty, panting mother-to-be propped up in a hospital bed, there are actually a variety of positions you may want to try for the pushing stage. (Of course, if you've had an epidural or a spinal, remaining in bed may be your only option. You shouldn't lie flat on your back, though—the head of the bed can be raised so you're semisitting, or you can lie on your left side and your partner can help support your upper leg when you push):

• Squatting, upright kneeling, sitting, or even standing is more comfortable than lying down for some women, and it puts gravity to work assisting your weary muscles. What's more, squatting helps open your pelvic outlet as much as possible, giving your baby more room to maneuver his way through your pelvis and out into the world.

- Pushing on all fours is another comfortable, effective option—especially if you have back labor. Getting on all fours helps to relieve the pressure of your baby's head against your lower back.
- Lying on your side works well and allows you to rest between contractions—helpful if it's been a long or difficult labor and your energy is waning.

Once your cervix is fully dilated, the work of the second stage of labor begins: the final descent and ultimate birth of your baby. At the beginning of the second stage, your contractions may be easier to handle than they were during transition and may be a little further apart, giving you the chance for a much-needed (and well-deserved!) rest in between them. As your uterus contracts, it exerts pressure on your baby, moving him down the birth canal.

Some women—those whose babies are very low in their pelvis—feel an involuntary urge to push early in the second stage (and sometimes even before), while those whose babies are still relatively high won't have this sensation right away. If everything's going well, you might want to take it slowly and let your uterus do the work by itself until you spontaneously feel the urge to push—waiting a while may make you less exhausted and frus-

Just the Facts

Transition

The last part of the active phase—when your cervix dilates from 8 to a full 10 centimeters—is called the transitional period because it marks the "transition" to the second stage of labor. This is the most intense part of labor, with contractions coming hard and fast and with symptoms that can include shaking and shivering. Contractions are usually very strong during transition, coming about every 2½ to 3 minutes and lasting a minute or more.

If you're laboring without an epidural, now's the time when you may begin to lose faith in your ability to cope, so you'll need lots of extra encouragement and support from those around you. The good news is that if you've made it this far without medication, you can usually be coached through transition—one contraction at a time—with constant reminders that you're doing a great job and that the end is near.

BabyCenter Buzz

What Transition Is *Really* Like

"My contractions felt like a series of waves, each one bigger and more intense than the last. The pain was overwhelming, but I was surprised to find that the breathing and meditation techniques I learned in childbirth class helped me ride each contraction out." —*Anonymous*

"To me, transition wasn't so much painful as incredibly *intense*. The contractions didn't feel like a sharp, stabbing pain—but rather a whole-body experience. My brain would sort of shut off, and my entire being would revolve around the tightening and then release of the contraction. It was primal, for sure—but for me it wasn't 'pain' in the classic sense." —*Anonymous*

"I knew I was in active labor when I had a hard time focusing during contractions. When a bad one would hit, I'd squirm around because it felt like if I found the exact right position, it wouldn't hurt so bad. (There *is* no exact right position, though!) Later, during transition, I couldn't squirm, couldn't count, couldn't concentrate—all I could do was grip the bed, writhe in pain, and moan that I was ready to be done. I could feel intense pressure in my pelvis, almost down in my anus, and I was seriously reconsidering my no-epidural decision. Luckily, shortly thereafter the nurses told me it was time to push!" —*Emily*

"I've discovered one thing that's helped ease my anxiety about labor pain: reading other women's birth stories. Every one relays different experiences. This helped me realize that when the time comes, you can take it one step at a time, coping with whatever's going on at the moment in whatever way you can to get through." —*Anonymous*

---

trated in the end. That said, in many hospitals it's still routine practice to coach you to push with each contraction in an effort to speed up the baby's descent.

Your baby's descent can be rapid or (especially if this is your first) gradual. The entire second stage can last anywhere from a few minutes to several hours. Without an epidural, the average duration is close to an hour for a first-timer and 20 minutes if you've had a previous vaginal delivery. (If you have an epidural, the second stage generally lasts longer.) With each contraction, the force of your uterus—combined with the force of your abdominal muscles if you're actively pushing—exerts pressure on your baby to continue to move down through the birth canal. When a contraction is over and your uterus is relaxed, your baby's head will re-

Just for Dad

Ten Tips to Help Her Through

As hard as it may be to watch your mate in pain, most fathers find the birth of their child one of life's most powerful and satisfying moments. To help you be the kind of labor coach your partner dreams of:

Know what to expect. Labor is *not* the time to be flipping through this book, so bone up on your reading beforehand. And go to a childbirth class with an open mind—you'll get solid, basic information, as well as a sense of how other dads-to-be are planning to get through the big event.

Be ready to wait. Unlike what you see in the movies, most women labor for hours before they even *go* to the hospital. Indeed, many couples find it more comfortable to spend the early stages of labor at home. Besides, many hospitals won't let you check in until your contractions are regular and close together. So watch TV, cuddle on the bed, or find another relaxing way to pass the hours; this isn't the time for finishing up last-minute projects or doing household chores.

Be flexible. Well before your baby's due date, take time to discuss with your partner her expectations and options; later, you can take the initiative with her wishes in mind. But be prepared to change course—part of a labor coach's job is to discern what works and drop what doesn't.

Don't take things personally. Your partner may seem to be in her own world during labor and she may become outwardly irritable at times. Giving birth is a long, hard job, and some women cope by reaching deep inside themselves. She may love having you massage her early in labor, for instance, and then during transition find being touched intolerable and let you know that in no uncertain terms! It's important not to misconstrue her behavior as a rejection of *you*.

Bring a few things for yourself. Your partner is the center of attention, but you may be spending the night at the hospital, too, so don't forget to pack some things for yourself. Essentials: A clean shirt, comfortable shoes, and a sustaining snack (one with no strong odors, please!). Bring a bathing suit, too, in case you decide to join your partner in the tub or shower.

Ask questions. Doctors and nurses don't always explain everything they're doing or whether it's mandatory. Don't be shy about seeking out information— especially if your mate's not up to asking questions herself.

Be her advocate. Only you and your partner know what you both want, but she may not be in the best condition to make hard decisions. Be ready to step in if the situation calls for it. You may need to request that the doctor cut short a nap, that an anesthesiologist be paged, or that a mirror be brought in. And if your partner plans to breastfeed, help make sure that she has a chance to do so soon after your baby's born, and that someone's there to help her out if she's having trouble.

Know your capabilities. There's a lot going on in the birthing room. Know what you're willing to do during the process and what you want to leave to the professionals. Maybe you're comfortable cutting the umbilical cord, but not "catching" your baby. If that's the case, say so.

Just *be* there. This is one of those events when showing up is the most important thing of all. Even if you want—or have—to leave most of the hands-on stuff to the pros, your presence matters. And no matter how you really feel, project a sense of confidence and calm reassurance: "You're doing great! Everything's going fine." There'll be time for you to unravel later.

cede slightly—a "two steps forward, one step backward" progression.

After a time, your perineum—the tissue between your vagina and rectum—will begin to bulge with each push, and before long, your baby's scalp will become visible. You can ask for a mirror to get that first glimpse of your baby, or you may simply want to reach down and touch the top of his head. It may sound scary right now, but it's a very exciting moment.

Now the urge to push becomes even more compelling. With each contraction, more and more of your baby's head becomes visible. The pressure of his head on your perineum feels very intense, and you may notice a strong burning or stinging sensation as your tissue begins to stretch. At some point, your practitioner may ask you to push more gently (or not to push at all) so your baby's head has a chance to gradually stretch out your vagina and perineum—a slow, controlled birth is essential to prevent tearing. By now, the urge to push can become so overwhelming that to help counter it, you'll be coached to blow or pant during contractions.

Your baby's head continues to advance with each push until it "crowns"—the time when the widest part of his head is finally visible. The excitement in the room will be palpable as your baby's face begins to appear: his forehead, nose, mouth, and, finally, his chin.

After his head emerges, your doctor or midwife will suction his mouth and nose and feel around his neck for the umbilical cord. (No need to worry—

Just the Facts

Perineal Tears

As your baby's head pushes out into the world, it might tear the perineum—the area between your vagina and your anus. Tears range in severity, but many women have only slight tearing and relatively speedy healing.

The most superficial tears are called first-degree lacerations, which involve skin but no muscle. These tears are often so small that few or no stitches are required, and they generally heal quickly and cause little or no discomfort. Some women end up with deeper, skin-and-muscle tears that require stitches and may cause some postpartum discomfort—these are called second-degree lacerations. Occasionally, women have more extensive tearing that may extend all the way through their rectum (page 441).

BabyCenter Buzz

I Pushed That Baby Out!

"The urge to push was overwhelming and uncontrollable. After hours of contractions, it was such a relief to be able to *do* something each time they hit." —*Beth*

"The epidural made it hard to feel my contractions, and I had zero urge to push. In the end, I pushed for 4 hours before my baby was finally born." —*Anonymous*

"When the baby was crowning, my midwife kept saying, 'Here's her head—she's crowning. This is the ring of fire.' And it really was like a fire down there! I was terrified that I was just going to rip in half. But then it was over, and I only had a little tear—and a great, big baby!" —*Megan*

"For me, pushing was the hardest part. I thought that once you got to that point, it all happened pretty fast. But it was, hands-down, the most challenging part of my labor." —*Anonymous*

"I'd always assumed that the pushing would be the most painful part (I mean, I'd seen a baby's head, and I *knew* how big my vagina was!), but then it turned out to be the labor that blew me away and the pushing that seemed easier by comparison. At least I was finally *doing* something." —*Cat*

if the cord is around his neck, it's either slipped over his head or, if need be, clamped and cut.) His head then turns to the side as his shoulders rotate inside your pelvis to get into position for their exit. With the next contraction, you'll be coached to push as his shoulders emerge, one at a time, followed by his body.

Once he hits the atmosphere, your baby needs to be kept warm and will be dried off with a towel. Your doctor or midwife may quickly suction your baby's mouth and nasal passages again if he seems to have a lot of mucus. If there are no complications, he'll be lifted onto your bare belly so you can touch, kiss, and simply marvel at him. The skin-to-skin contact will keep your baby nice and toasty, and he'll be covered with a warm blanket-and perhaps given his first hat—to prevent any heat loss. Your practitioner will clamp the umbilical cord in two places and then cut between the two clamps. (Or your partner can do the honors!)

You may feel a wide range of emotions now: euphoria, awe, pride, disbelief, excitement (to name but a few), and, of course, intense relief that it's all over. Exhausted as you may be, you'll also likely feel a burst of energy, and any thoughts of sleep will vanish for the time being.

The Third Stage: Delivering the Placenta

> ### BY THE NUMBERS
>
> **Lacerations During Birth**
>
> Women who experience injury to the perineum during birth, either from tearing or having an episiotomy: **85%**
>
> Source: *The American Urogynecologic Society*

Within minutes after giving birth, your uterus begins to contract again. The first few contractions usually separate the placenta from your uterine wall. When your practitioner sees signs of separation, she may ask you to gently push to help expel the placenta. (This is usually one short push that's not at all difficult or painful.) This usually happens within 5 to 10 minutes of your baby's birth, though it may take as long as 30 minutes.

After you deliver the placenta, your uterus should contract and get very firm. You'll be able to feel the top of it in your belly, around the level of your navel. Your practitioner, and later your nurse, will periodically check to see that it remains firm, and massage your uterus if it isn't. A well-contracted uterus helps prevent continued bleeding from the place where the placenta was attached.

If you're planning to breastfeed, you can do so right away if you and your baby are both willing. It's a good idea for the baby (and often deeply satisfying for you) to get an early start. Not only that, but nursing your baby triggers your body to release oxytocin (the same hormone that causes contractions) and helps your uterus contract so it can lessen bleeding. If you aren't nursing or are bleeding excessively, you may need medication to help your uterus contract.

Your contractions at this point are relatively mild. By now your focus has shifted to your baby, and you may be oblivious to everything else going on around you. If this is your first baby, you may feel only a few contractions after you've delivered the placenta. (If you've had a baby before, you may continue to feel occasional contractions for the next day or two.) These so-called afterbirth pains can feel like strong menstrual cramps. If they bother you, ask for pain medication. You may also find that you get

Just the Facts

Episiotomy

An episiotomy is a cut that your practitioner may make in your perineum right before delivery to enlarge your vaginal opening. Obstetricians used to cut episiotomies routinely to speed delivery and prevent tearing, particularly during first births. That's because experts believed that the "clean" incision of an episiotomy would heal more easily than a spontaneous tear. But a great many studies over the past 20 years have disproved this theory, and most experts now agree that this procedure shouldn't be done routinely.

In fact, research has shown that women with spontaneous tears generally recover in the same or less time and often with less pain and fewer complications than those with episiotomies. What's more, women who get episiotomies are more likely to end up with serious tears (known as third- or fourth-degree lacerations) than those who deliver without being cut. These lacerations result in more pain after the birth, require a significantly longer recovery period, and are more likely than smaller tears to affect the strength of your pelvic-floor muscles. And a serious tear may cause problems with fecal incontinence. Even so, there are a few situations in which an episiotomy is still necessary for your or your baby's well-being:

- If your baby's heart rate shows that he isn't tolerating the last minutes of labor well and needs to be born as quickly as possible.

- If your baby is very large and your practitioner needs a little extra room to manipulate him so he can come out.

- If your practitioner needs more space to use forceps to help deliver your baby.

- If your perineal tissue is starting to bleed or not stretching well as your baby's head begins to crown. The idea here is that being cut in *one* place may allow you to avoid tearing in more than one place. That said, a few shallow tears may still be preferable to an episiotomy, so your practitioner will have to make the call.

If your doctor or midwife decides to do an episiotomy, she'll give you an injection of a local anesthetic and use surgical scissors to make a small cut. (Sometimes, if your perineum is already numb and thinned out from the pressure of your baby's head, she may be able to do the episiotomy without any pain medication.) Afterward, you'll get another shot of local anesthesia to be sure you're completely numb before your practitioner stitches you up.

a case of the chills or feel very shaky. This is perfectly normal and won't last long.

Your caregiver will examine the placenta to make sure it's all there. Then she'll check you thoroughly to see if you have any tears that need to be stitched. If you tore or had an episiotomy, you'll get an injection of a local anesthetic before being sutured. You may want to hold your newborn while

Ask the Experts

How Can I Avoid an Episiotomy?

Suzanne Powell, childbirth educator: Starting around week 34, you could try massaging your perineum. Daily massage may increase the area's stretching ability, leading to less need for an episiotomy and fewer natural tears.

Have your partner use this technique with clean hands and trimmed nails—or try it yourself. (If you're going solo, have a large mirror handy so you can see what you're doing and to help familiarize yourself with your perineal area.)

- Sit in a semireclined position in a warm, comfortable area, and spread your legs apart. Lubricate your fingers, thumbs, and perineal area with vitamin E oil (from punctured vitamin E capsules), pure vegetable oil, or personal lubricant. (Don't use baby oil, mineral oil, or petroleum jelly.)

- Place your thumbs 1 to 1½ inches (or to just past your first knuckle) inside your vagina. Press down toward your rectum and out to the sides of your vagina at the same time. Gently and firmly continue stretching until you feel a slight burning or tingling sensation.

- Hold this stretch for about two minutes—until the tingling starts to subside.

- Now slowly and gently massage the lower part of your vagina back and forth, hooking your thumbs onto the sides of your vagina and gently pulling the tissue forward, as your baby's head will do during delivery. Keep this up for three to four minutes.

- Finally, massage the tissue between the thumb and forefinger back and forth for about a minute.

- Be gentle because a vigorous touch could cause bruising or swelling. During the massage, avoid pressure on your urethra (urinary opening) because this can lead to irritation or infection.

Of course, perineal massage isn't for everyone, and it may not help in every case. The most important thing you can do is to choose a midwife or doctor who's experienced and comfortable delivering babies without performing episiotomies. In general, midwives tend to do episiotomies less often than physicians. But regardless of the type of practitioner you choose, discuss your wishes and expectations with her before the birth.

you're getting stitches—it can be a great distraction. Or, if you feel too shaky, ask your partner to sit by your side and hold your new arrival while you look at him.

If you had an epidural, the anesthesiologist or nurse anesthetist will come by and remove the catheter from your back. (This takes just a second and doesn't hurt.) Unless your baby needs special care, insist on some quiet time together. The routine eyedrops, vitamin K shot, and footprints can wait

BabyCenter Buzz

I Had an Episiotomy

"I had an episiotomy when my daughter was born. She's 13 months old, and I still find that certain positions during sex hurt. I'm beginning to wonder if it'll ever go away!" —*Anonymous*

"It has been six weeks since my episiotomy. I feel fine, except for a little itching at the scar. I figure that's just part of the healing." —*Liana*

"I had just a few stitches for my small cut. My doctor gave me a pain reliever, cold packs for the area, and a water bottle to wash off with. I only had pain for the first two days when I was going to the bathroom—it really stung." —*Anonymous*

"I had an episiotomy four weeks ago. It didn't hurt when they made the incision, but the pain afterward was the worst. I'm still recovering. My advice: Stay off your feet, drink lots of fluids, and relax!" —*Welma*

a while—you and your partner will want to share this special time with each other as you get acquainted with your new baby and revel in the miracle of his birth.

What Happens to Your Baby Immediately after Birth

In the moments after you give birth, your medical team will:

Assign your baby an Apgar score. Your practitioner or labor nurse will be observing your baby closely from the moment he's born. At one and then at five minutes after birth, she'll do an Apgar assessment— a scoring system that's been widely used for more than 50 years—to evaluate your baby's heart rate, breathing, muscle tone, reflex response, and color. It's a way of quantifying his initial condition—but it does not predict his long-term health. If your baby's doing well, your nurse or caregiver will do these simple assessments while your baby is resting on your belly.

In the first hour after birth, a nurse will also:

Footprint your baby. And—if you're in a hospital—she'll put an ID

Just the Facts

Adding Up the Apgar

As your practitioner checks each of the following factors, she assigns it a score between zero and 2. Afterward, the scores are totaled (10 is highest).

HEART RATE
0: No heart rate
1: Fewer than 100 beats a minute
2: More than 100 beats a minute

RESPIRATION
0: Not breathing
1: Weak cry or slow, irregular breathing
2: Good, strong cry

MUSCLE TONE
0: Limp
1: Some bending of arms and legs
2: Active motion

REFLEX RESPONSE
0: No response to airways being suctioned
1: Grimace during suctioning
2: Grimace and cough or sneeze during suctioning

COLOR
0: The baby's whole body is completely blue or pale
1: Good color in body with blue hands or feet
2: Completely pink (for dark-skinned babies, pink on palms, soles, lips, and mouth)

The one-minute Apgar score conveys information about your baby's condition after his first minute of life and helps your practitioner assess how he's adapting outside the womb and whether extra observation or treatment is needed. (If your baby is distressed at birth, though, resuscitation efforts will begin even before he's a minute old.)

Newborns who score between 7 and 10 are in good to excellent condition and usually need only routine postdelivery care. (Don't be disappointed if your baby doesn't get a 10; a "perfect" score is unusual at this point because a baby's extremities are almost never completely pink after only one minute out of the birth canal.) Babies who score just under 7 may need oxygen, and those with lower scores might need further interventions as well. Still, a low score at this time has no bearing on your baby's long-term health or development.

The 5-minute Apgar score helps your doctor or midwife determine how your baby has responded to any resuscitative efforts and whether he'll continue to need monitoring. A score of 7 to 10 is considered normal. If the score is less than 7 at this point, your baby will still need to be watched closely and an Apgar may be done again every five minutes for up to 20 minutes to monitor his changing condition. Again, a lower-than-normal score, on its own, doesn't necessarily signal long-term problems.

BabyCenter Buzz

Meeting My Baby for the First Time

"No one told me how great it would be to watch my baby being born with a mirror! A doctor brought one in for me. I was able to see that little face come out and look at it for the first time. Those are memories that a lot of women just don't have—and that I will never forget."   —*Anonymous*

"I lost a lot of blood during the delivery, so I was too out of it right after my son was born to hold him. My husband did the holding for me, and once my condition had stabilized, he placed the baby in my arms. Our first meeting may have been a bit delayed, but it was no less sweet."   —*Laurel*

"I sang to my baby girl immediately after her birth as I had done all along during my wife's pregnancy. She looked intently at me and seemed to recognize my voice. I was totally and immediately smitten. She's so beautiful!"   —*Steve*

"I had a long, hard labor—and when my baby was first born, I didn't feel much of anything other than exhaustion. It definitely wasn't love at first sight, or that 'instant' bond you hear about so often. It took a few days for me to totally fall in love, but when I did, I fell hard. Don't feel guilty if it's not all rainbows and butterflies the instant your baby is born. Bonding takes time."   —*Anonymous*

band on his wrist or ankle (and matching ones on you and possibly your partner, too).

Weigh and measure your baby. She'll make a note of how much he weighs (and may also measure his length and head circumference).

Administer eyedrops. Your baby needs antibiotic ointment or eyedrops within an hour after birth to protect against any exposure to bacteria in your birth canal.

GIVING BIRTH: SPECIAL SITUATIONS AND COMPLICATIONS

Mother Nature alone can't always guarantee an easy birth. Your practitioner may decide—either before or after you go into labor—that the best way to deliver your baby involves one or more medical interventions. That can mean anything from using drugs to keep your labor from stalling to having a scheduled c-section if a vaginal birth is deemed too risky. While it can be disappointing to find out that you need interventions that you neither expected nor desired, in the end what really matters is keeping you and your baby safe—a goal your doctor or midwife has uppermost in her mind.

Assisted Vaginal Delivery

Some babies need a little extra help coming into the world. If you're completely worn-out, if your baby's coming out face-up and the pushing stage of labor is prolonged, or if your baby's nearly out but his monitor readings aren't reassuring, your caregiver may use forceps or a vacuum device to help deliver him. Though they sound a bit frightening, these interventions are considered safe as long as your baby's head is low enough in your birth canal—and they may be preferable to a c-section.

The vast majority of forceps- and vacuum-assisted deliveries leave nothing more than a slight bruise or swelling on your baby's head that disappears within a couple of days. Unless you've already had an epidural, you may get a pudendal block before the procedure—local anesthetic is injected through your vaginal wall and bathes the area around your pudendal nerve to numb your entire genital area. You'll probably also get an episiotomy so there's room to insert the instrument. If you're concerned about these procedures, ask your practitioner to explain the risks and benefits in your particular case.

Forceps

Like a pair of spoon-shaped surgical tongs, forceps help your practitioner grasp your baby's head and gently pull her out of the birth canal. Forceps may be used when you're too exhausted to push any more, when you're having trouble pushing because of an epidural, or to speed your baby's delivery if needed. In addition to an obstetrician, it's routine for a pediatrician to be on hand for any delivery that requires instruments. (Midwives don't do forceps deliveries, so if a midwife's been attending you in labor and forceps are needed, her backup physician will step in.) If your baby still won't budge, you'll need to have a c-section.

After the sort of prolonged delivery that often requires forceps, you may find it difficult to go to the bathroom or experience urine leaks because of temporary changes in your pelvic and perineal nerves and muscles. Also, if you're feeling pain from your episiotomy and then resist moving your bowels, you'll become constipated.

Occasionally, forceps also can cause lacerations in your cervix and vagina, which may need stitches and which can take a few weeks to fully heal. If an episiotomy tears more during a forceps delivery, you may end up with a laceration that extends through your anal sphincter.

Finally, your baby may be slightly bruised from the forceps, but the bruises generally clear up in a few days. Sometimes, a scalp blister forms after the delivery. Such blisters look unsightly, but they heal in a few weeks. The risk of more serious problems for your baby is very low.

> ## BY THE NUMBERS
>
> **Assisted Vaginal Delivery**
>
> Vaginal deliveries in which a vacuum or forceps is used: **nearly 1 in 7**
>
> Sources: *American College of Obstetricians and Gynecologists, National Center for Health Statistics*

Vacuum Extraction

Your practitioner may opt for vacuum extraction instead of forceps if she needs to

BabyCenter Buzz

I Had an Assisted Vaginal Delivery

"Forceps saved my daughter's life. When she dropped, the umbilical cord was wrapped around her neck. Her heart rate dropped quickly. My doctor said, 'We need to get this baby out!' I pushed while she used the forceps. Three pushes and the baby was out. She was fine, other than small cuts on her forehead and near her eye." —Anonymous

"After a few hours of pushing, I was told it wasn't working. The doctor did a vacuum extraction with an episiotomy. My baby was literally sucked out of me! We're all fine now." —Anonymous

deliver your baby quickly. Like forceps, the vacuum allows the doctor to help your baby move down the birth canal faster than she would on her own.

If you need a vacuum extraction, your practitioner will attach a flexible, rounded cup to your baby's head in the birth canal and then either use a small hose to hook up the cup to a suction pump or operate a small handheld pump. The vacuum pulls while you push. The most common side effect for babies is a bruise on the top of their head that usually goes away in a few days. More serious complications are relatively rare.

And as with any delivery—particularly one that might follow a prolonged pushing stage or with a big baby—you may find it difficult to go to the bathroom or have some urine leaks because of temporary changes in your pelvic and perineal nerves. You may also have vaginal or perineal lacerations, which will eventually heal.

Breech Birth

Some babies never move into the textbook, head-down position. Instead, they stay feet- or bottom-down or even lie sideways (called the transverse position) as labor begins. Your practitioner will usually recommend trying to manually turn your baby via an external cephalic version (ECV) before you get to this point. But if the ECV

BY THE NUMBERS

Breech Births

Babies who are in a breech or transverse position at term: **about 4%**

Breech babies who are delivered via c-section: **86%**

Sources: *National Center for Health Statistics; American Academy of Family Physicians*

BabyCenter Buzz

Delivering My Breech Baby

"I had a c-section, and it was just fine. My water broke, and in I went. Recovery wasn't particularly bad for me—uncomfortable, but manageable." —*Anonymous*

"During my last pregnancy, we didn't find out that my baby was breech until after my water had broken. I choose to deliver her vaginally, and I was a good candidate for it, since I've already had several babies. I'm glad that I had a vaginal birth, and I'm grateful to my doctor for letting me deliver this way. Still, every woman needs to do what she thinks is best for her situation. So much depends on the doctor's skill and experience—if he or she isn't practiced in breech delivery, I wouldn't attempt it." —*Anonymous*

doesn't work, or if your baby decides to flip upright again, you'll need a c-section because it's less risky than a vaginal birth. (The exceptions: If birth is imminent when you arrive at the hospital or if you're having twins and your first baby is head-down but your second baby isn't, your practitioner may opt for a vaginal delivery.)

Cesarean Section

A c-section is a surgical procedure that involves making an incision in your abdomen and uterus through which your baby is delivered. Depending on your particular circumstances, a c-section may be scheduled in advance, unplanned, or done in an emergency. A look at this increasingly common mode of delivery:

A Step-by-Step Guide to Having a C-Section

If you need a c-section, the following steps will be taken (this is true even if you're having an emergency c-section—each step will just be done more quickly):

• Your doctor or midwife will explain why she believes a c-section is necessary as well as the risks and benefits of the surgery. (If your usual practitioner is a midwife, an obstetrician will perform the surgery and will explain the procedure to you as well.)

• You'll be asked to sign a consent form.

Just for Dad

When Your Partner Has a C-Section

If you've been diligently helping your partner practice her huffing and puffing, you may find yourself dismayed to be heading for the OR in scrubs—especially if she's having an emergency c-section. You'll need to keep your wits about you to reassure your partner, who may be exhausted and terrified. She'll be wheeled in ahead of you, and you'll be given scrubs, a cap, and booties to put on before you join her. Most likely, you'll be offered a seat by your partner's head, where you'll be able to hold her hand and talk to her.

A c-section is major surgery, so be prepared for a lot of cutting and a great deal of blood. If you're squeamish, don't peek over the surgical curtain to watch the proceedings; you won't be much good as a support person if you faint.

Afterward, your partner will need to spend three nights in the hospital to recover, so you may need to rethink previous childcare and work arrangements. And when she returns home, expect your mate to need a lot of extra TLC: She'll be sore and exhausted for a number of weeks. Recovering from surgery *and* caring for a new baby is not something she can do alone.

• An anesthesiologist will come by to review with you various pain-management options. It's rare these days to be given general anesthesia, which would knock you out completely, except in the most extreme emergency situations. More likely, you'll be given an epidural or spinal block, which numbs the lower half of your body but leaves you awake and alert for the birth of your baby. (If you already had an epidural for labor, it'll be used for your c-section, too. Before the surgery, you'll get extra medication through the catheter to ensure that you're completely numb.)

• You'll have a catheter placed to drain your urine during the procedure, and an IV will be started if you don't have one already.

• The top section of your pubic hair will be shaved.

• You'll be moved into an operating room.

BY THE NUMBERS

The Rising Rate of C-Sections

Women who delivered via c-section in 2003:	**28%**
Women who delivered via c-section in 1990:	**23%**
Women who delivered via c-section in 1980:	**17%**
Women who delivered via c-section in 1970:	**6%**

Source: *Centers for Disease Control and Prevention*

Just the Facts

Who'll Have a Scheduled C-Section

Your doctor will likely pencil you in for surgery if:

- You've had previous invasive uterine surgery.
- You've had previous c-sections (see vaginal birth after cesarean, below, for exceptions)—especially if you had a "classical" (vertical) uterine incision.
- You're carrying triplets or more.
- Your baby is very large, especially if you're diabetic.
- Your baby is breech.
- You have placenta previa.

• Pain relief will be administered and a screen raised above your waist so you won't see the incision being made. If you'd like to witness the moment of birth, ask a nurse to lower the screen slightly so you can see the baby but not much else. Your partner, freshly attired in operating room garb, may take a seat by your head.

• Your belly will be swabbed with an antiseptic.

• Once the anesthesia takes effect, the doctor will most likely make a

BabyCenter Buzz

I'm Disappointed That I Had a C-Section

"I had an emergency c-section. We're both safe and healthy, but I feel really cheated out of the whole delivery experience." —Nicole

"I had my first baby via an unplanned c-section because of fetal distress, and it took me a good six weeks to feel like myself again. I felt so guilty for not enjoying being a mother and not just being happy that I had a healthy baby." —Mally

"After more than three hours of pushing, the doctor intervened. At first, I felt as though I'd failed in some way. But this little miraculous boy has taught me that being a parent is all about losing that control. You can prepare all you like, but things will happen as they're meant to. You've got to be ready emotionally for the fact that you can't possibly prepare for all the challenges you'll face as a parent. Sometimes, you're going to have to wing it." —Anonymous

Just the Facts

Unplanned C-Sections

You may need to have a c-section if problems arise during labor. These can include:

Your labor stalls. If your cervix stops dilating or your baby stops moving down the birth canal—and your provider's attempts to stimulate contractions to get things moving again haven't worked—your baby will be delivered surgically.

Your baby's heart rate gives your caregiver cause for concern. If your practitioner decides that your baby can't withstand continued labor and a vaginal delivery, you'll be moved into the OR. Likewise, if the umbilical cord slips through your cervix (called a prolapsed cord), your baby will need to be delivered immediately because a prolapsed cord can cut off his oxygen supply.

Your placenta starts to separate from your uterine wall. If you have a significant placental abruption, your baby won't get enough oxygen unless he's delivered right away.

You have an active genital herpes infection. If you have a genital herpes outbreak when you go into labor, delivering your baby via c-section will protect him from contracting the infection himself.

---

small, horizontal incision in your skin above your pubic bone (called a bikini cut). She'll then make a second cut in the lower section of your uterus (this is called a low-transverse incision). In an extreme emergency, the doctor may opt for an up-and-down incision, which extends from your pubic bone to your navel and may allow your baby to be delivered more quickly—but such instances are rare.

• The doctor will reach in and pull your baby out. You'll get a chance to see him briefly before he's handed off to a pediatrician or nurse.

• While the staff is examining your baby, the doctor will deliver your placenta and stitch you up.

• When your baby's exam is complete, the pediatrician or nurse may hand him to your partner, who can hold him near you while you're being stitched up. This part of the surgery can take about 30 minutes because each layer of muscle and skin needs to be closed.

• After the surgery is complete, you'll be wheeled into a recovery room, where you can finally hold your baby. If you plan to breastfeed, give it a try now. You may find nursing more comfortable if both you and your newborn lie on your sides facing each other.

Vaginal Birth After Cesarean (VBAC)

Having a past c-section doesn't necessarily mean that you can't try for a vaginal birth this time around. With the proper preparation, many women go on to have a vaginal birth after c-section. As a rule, your chance of having a successful VBAC is higher if the reason a c-section was done with your last baby isn't an issue this time around—if your baby was delivered surgically because he was breech, for instance. If you've had a previous c-section but have also given birth vaginally before, your chance of a successful VBAC increases dramatically. Overall, an estimated 60 to 80 percent of women who attempt VBACs succeed.

If you try for a VBAC, you'll need continuous electronic fetal monitoring to make sure your baby's faring well. You'll also need an IV and will have to refrain from eating anything during labor in case you wind up needing an emergency c-section.

BY THE NUMBERS

VBACs on the Wane

The number of women having VBACs has declined markedly in recent years due to controversy about its safety, specifically the potential for uterine rupture (a rare injury, but one that can be catastrophic for mother and baby). Ultimately, you and your practitioner will need to determine if the benefits of a VBAC outweigh the risks.

Women with a previous c-section who delivered vaginally in 2003:   **11%**

Women with a previous c-section who delivered vaginally in 1996:   **28%**

Source: *National Center for Health Statistics*

The Benefits of VBAC

• A VBAC allows you to avoid major abdominal surgery and the risks associated with it, including possible blood transfusion, infection, and a longer hospital stay.

• Many women who have VBACs feel a tremendous sense of pride and accomplishment. If you were disappointed by a previous c-section, you may feel relief and joy about delivering this baby vaginally.

The Risks of VBAC

• For women with one prior low-transverse c-section, there's a small (usually less than 1 percent) but serious risk of uterine rupture, which can result in severe blood loss for you and oxygen deprivation for your baby.

Just the Facts

Who's a Candidate for VBAC

You and your practitioner may consider VBAC if:

- You've had one prior low-transverse cesarean delivery.
- Your pelvis seems large enough to allow your baby to safely pass through.
- You have no other uterine scars or previous ruptures.
- There's a physician on-site who's able to monitor your labor and perform an emergency c-section if necessary.
- There are an anesthesiologist, other medical personnel, and equipment available around the clock to handle an emergency situation for you or your baby.
- You have a caregiver who supports the idea. She also has to have admitting privileges at a hospital where appropriate coverage is available 24/7 and whose policies allow VBAC (an increasing number of hospitals don't). Needless to say, attempting a VBAC at a birth center or at home isn't safe.

- A planned c-section is safer and easier to recover from than an unplanned one. If you attempt a VBAC, you could endure hours of labor only to have an unplanned c-section anyway.

When VBAC *Isn't* an Option

You'll automatically be scheduled for another c-section if:

- You've had a prior c-section involving a vertical or T-shaped uterine incision (note that the type of scar you have on your belly may not match the one on your uterus) or other uterine surgery, such as a myomectomy to remove fibroids.
- You've never given birth vaginally and have had two prior c-sections (even if they're both low-transverse incisions).
- You have a small pelvis.
- You have a medical condition or obstetric problem that makes a vaginal delivery risky.
- You're giving birth in a situation where an emergency c-section isn't

BabyCenter Buzz

Delivering My Baby after a Previous C-Section

"We had our son last night by VBAC. Just me doing what my body told me. Just my hubby doing what I asked of him. He's beautiful. He cried, wiggled, nursed, and slept. And I feel so great about it, every bit of it." —*Anonymous*

"If you want a VBAC, believe in yourself and at least try. I wasn't really sure about it, but now I feel fulfilled and very happy." —*Annie*

"I was one of the unlucky 1 percent who have a uterine rupture after a previous c-section. I was rushed into emergency surgery, where my doctors discovered that I was bleeding internally. I lost so much blood that I needed a transfusion. Thank God they had doctors on hand to do the surgery." —*Rosie*

"One real benefit of VBAC over a c-section is that when you already have a child at home, recovery is much easier." —*Anonymous*

possible—there's no immediate access to a surgeon, anesthesia, sufficient staff, or a proper facility.

Delivering Twins or Multiples

If giving birth is unpredictable when it involves only *one* baby, it's even more so for twins, triplets, and higher-order multiples. If you're carrying triplets or more, you won't have to make any birth decisions: Your babies will most certainly arrive via c-section. But if you're carrying twins, you may be able to deliver vaginally (about 50 percent of twins arrive this way). The key is often how your babies are positioned. While most singletons are headfirst, twins can be positioned in many combinations—both headfirst (the most common scenario), one headfirst and one breech, both breech, or any combination in between. Problems with the umbilical cord or the placenta's position and postpartum bleeding are other potential complications.

With so many variables, you'll give birth in a delivery room that doubles as an operating room instead of a regular birthing room, and you'll be surrounded by high-tech equipment and a large team of medical personnel. Most twin births are attended by one or two obstetricians, a midwife (if you're using one), an anesthesiologist (in case you need to deliver

BabyCenter Buzz

Giving Birth to My Twins

"At 9:36 a.m., Alexander Ian was born. I got about six minutes of respite from pain and pushing until the doctor broke my second bag of water. I couldn't believe I had to push again. Joshua David was born at 9:49 A.M. The boys had to be in an incubator overnight to keep their body temps up, but they were in my room with me and were able to come home with me two days after their birth." —*Nichole*

"My twins were born via c-section. They were both head-down, but the doctor wasn't comfortable with a vaginal delivery." —*Jodi*

"I had my twins vaginally—actually, it was a VBAC! Baby A was head-down, and Baby B was transverse but slipped head-down after his brother delivered. It was my easiest delivery yet!" —*Lori*

by c-section), at least two nurses, and two pediatricians (one for each baby)—plus your partner or birthing coach, of course.

Emergency Home Birth

It's highly unlikely that you'll find yourself unexpectedly giving birth at home or in the backseat of a taxi—but it *can* happen. In less than 1 percent of births, a woman who's had no labor symptoms or only intermittent contractions suddenly feels an overwhelming urge to push, signaling her baby's imminent arrival.

If this is your second child and you first labor was fast and furious, be prepared to make a mad dash for the hospital or birth center, because subsequent labors can go even faster. But if it feels like you're not going to make it and you find yourself at home (or elsewhere!) with contractions coming fast and strong, the following step-by-step guide can help make your baby's delivery a safer one:

- Call 911 and ask the dispatcher to send an emergency medical squad.
- If your partner isn't right there with you, call a neighbor or nearby friend.

BabyCenter Buzz

I Never Made It to the Hospital . . .

"I was 12 days overdue with my second child when mild contractions finally kicked in. My midwife said to call her when they were coming every five minutes for an hour. Thinking we had a long day ahead of us, my husband and I turned in for the night. Occasional contractions would wake me up, but they were sporadic and still fairly mild, and I was able to doze between them. Finally, I woke up and had an overwhelming urge to push. Our daughter was born less than five minutes later, and my husband literally 'caught' her! Luckily, both the baby and I were perfectly fine." —Anonymous

"I somehow mustered the presence of mind to deliver my own baby at home. My water broke, and I had only five reeling contractions before I felt my body pushing. I screamed to the empty house as I felt my baby crown. I crawled to the bathroom and delivered her, pulling her to my chest for warmth as her first cry met my husband as he walked in. I knew not to cut the cord, and knew to cover us both with a towel and nurse her until the paramedics came. She's a perfect baby who decided that her birth would be a 'mommy and me' experience!" —Laura

"It didn't seem that I could possibly be ready to give birth—and my physician agreed, but also told me to go to the hospital if I felt it was necessary. Within an hour of that, my daughter was born in the backseat of my car, with the assistance and love of my husband. My advice is to be prepared for all contingencies." —Anonymous

---

• Call your doctor or midwife. She'll stay on the phone to guide you until help arrives.

• Unlock your door so the medical crew and your partner, neighbor, or friend can come in (you may not be in a position to get to the door later!).

• Grab a towel, sheet, or blanket so you can dry your baby immediately after birth. (If help doesn't arrive in time and you forget this step, you can use your clothes instead.)

• If you feel an overwhelming urge to push, try to delay it by panting, using breathing techniques, or lying on your side. Be sure to lie down or sit propped up; if you give birth standing up, your baby could fall and suffer a serious injury. And don't forget to take off your pants and underwear.

• If your baby arrives before the medical team does, do your best to guide her out as gently as possible.

• If the umbilical cord is around your baby's neck, either ease it over her head slowly or loosen it enough to form a loop so that the rest of her body can slip through. When she's fully out, don't pull the cord. Wait until you deliver the placenta, which you will shortly. *Don't try to tie off or cut the cord.* Leave it attached to your baby until help arrives.

• Dry your baby immediately. Then rest her on your tummy, skin-to-skin, and warm her with your body heat. Cover yourself and your baby with a dry blanket.

• Ease out any mucus or amniotic fluid from her nostrils by gently running your fingers down the side of her nose.

• If your baby doesn't cry spontaneously at birth, try to stimulate her by rubbing her back or flicking her heels.

• While you're waiting for medical help, try letting your baby nurse if she wants to—but only if you can keep the umbilical cord slack, not taut (sometimes, if the placenta is still inside you, the cord won't be long enough to allow you to bring your baby to your breast). Besides offering your baby comfort and security—and giving you a chance to see her close up—her sucking will tell your body to release oxytocin, the hormone that stimulates the delivery of the placenta and that helps your uterus contract back down to size. If you can't breastfeed your baby right away, rub your nipples to release the hormone.

• After you deliver the placenta, vigorously massage your belly right below your navel. This will help your uterus contract and cut down on bleeding.

Labor Augmentation or Induction

Not every woman has a textbook labor. Your practitioner may need to take steps to start or bolster contractions if you're well past your due date, if your baby isn't doing well in the womb, or if your labor isn't progressing the way it should.

Labor Augmentation

If you're already in labor but your contractions aren't coming frequently or forcefully enough to dilate your cervix or help move your baby down the birth canal, your practitioner may decide to start you on Pitocin—a synthetic form of the hormone oxytocin, which spurs uterine contractions. The medicine is given through an IV and adjusted as needed. (If you're at a birth center and your caregiver decides that you need Pitocin, you'll be transferred to the hospital.)

First, your doctor or midwife will carefully watch how your contractions are affecting you and your baby. If everything looks good, she'll start you off with a small dose of Pitocin, then gradually increase it until your uterus responds. How much you'll need depends on the quality of your contractions so far, how sensitive your uterus is to the drug, how much your cervix is dilated, and how far along you are in your pregnancy.

The goal is to give you just enough medication to bring on contractions that dilate your cervix quickly and help your baby descend—but not so much that your uterus becomes hyperstimulated, which could put stress on your baby. As a rule, your practitioner is shooting for three to five contractions every ten minutes. (Having more than five contractions in ten minutes or single contractions that last longer than two minutes means that your uterus is overstimulated.) While your labor is being augmented, your practitioner will use continuous electronic fetal monitoring to keep tabs on your contractions and your baby's well-being.

Labor Induction

If your labor hasn't started on its own, your practitioner can use certain techniques to "induce" contractions. Reasons she may do this include:

• Your water breaks and your labor doesn't start on its own within a certain amount of time. (Exactly how long that is depends on your practitioner and your particular situation.)

Just the Facts

Breaking Your Bag of Waters

Your practitioner can also get your labor in gear by breaking your bag of waters. She'll insert a small plastic hooked instrument through your vagina and cervix to rupture your amniotic sac, which should cause no more discomfort than a regular vaginal exam. Experts continue to debate the risks and benefits of the procedure: On one hand, it may mean a shorter labor and less need for Pitocin. But on the other hand, keeping your amniotic sac intact until it breaks on its own offers greater protection against infection and umbilical cord compression. Your practitioner will consider whether this procedure is a good choice for you based on, among other things, how much your cervix is dilated, how low the baby is in your pelvis, whether you need internal fetal monitoring, and your overall risk of infection.

Ask the Experts

How Can I Be Most Comfortable during a Scheduled Induction?

Suzanne Powell, childbirth educator: You'll be more comfortable if the induction is started slowly. This can be done by using a gel to help soften your cervix so that it will dilate more easily. And even with other induction techniques, like rupturing the amniotic sac or starting Pitocin, you can still use comfort measures like relaxation, massage, and positioning. If you want to, you can labor without pain medication, but you shouldn't feel bad if you opt for medication at some point.

• You're still pregnant one to two weeks past your due date. Most practitioners won't let you wait longer than this to give birth because it puts you and your baby at increased risk for problems.

• It's no longer safe for your baby to remain in your womb. This may be the case if tests show that your placenta isn't functioning properly, you have too little amniotic fluid, or your baby isn't thriving or growing as he should.

• You develop preeclampsia, a serious condition that can only be "cured" by delivery.

• You have a chronic or acute illness—such as high blood pressure, diabetes, or kidney disease—that threatens your health or your baby's.

• You've previously had a full-term stillbirth.

Just the Facts

The Risks of Inducing Labor

While it's generally safe, induction *does* carry risks—most notably the possibility that your uterus could become hyperstimulated (bringing on contractions that are too frequent, too long, or too strong—which in turn can affect your baby) or that you'll need a c-section if your labor doesn't progress as hoped. And in rare cases, prostaglandins or Pitocin can also cause placental abruption or uterine rupture (though ruptures are exceedingly uncommon). To check both the frequency and length of your contractions as well as your baby's heart rate, you'll need to have continuous electronic fetal monitoring during an induced labor.

Just the Facts

Techniques for Inducing Labor

The methods used to induce labor depend on your cervix's condition. If your cervix hasn't yet started to soften, thin out, or open up, it's "unripe" and not yet ready for labor. In this case, your practitioner will use either hormones or "mechanical" methods to ripen your cervix before the induction. Sometimes, these procedures end up jump-starting your labor as well. Some of the techniques used to ripen your cervix and induce labor are:

Stripping or sweeping the membranes. During a pelvic exam, your practitioner inserts her finger through your cervix and manually separates your bag of waters from the lower part of your uterus. This causes the release of natural prostaglandins, which can help ripen your cervix and possibly get contractions going. In most cases, this procedure is done during an office visit, and then you're sent home to wait for labor to start, usually within the next few days. Many women find the procedure uncomfortable or even painful.

Using prostaglandin medications. Your practitioner may try to ripen your cervix by inserting into your vagina medication that contains prostaglandins. This procedure can also stimulate contractions and get your labor going.

Using a Foley catheter. Your doctor or midwife will insert a catheter with a very small balloon at the end of it into your cervix. When the balloon is inflated with water, it puts pressure on your cervix, stimulating the release of prostaglandins, which cause it to open and soften. When your cervix begins to dilate, the balloon falls out and the catheter is removed.

Using Pitocin. Your practitioner may give you this drug through an IV pump to start your contractions. She can adjust the amount you need according to how your labor progresses.

Postpartum Hemorrhage

All women lose some blood after giving birth. And because your blood volume increases by almost 50 percent during the course of your pregnancy, your body is well-prepared to compensate for this blood loss. Unfortunately, though, some women bleed too much after birth and require special treatment. A postpartum hemorrhage (PPH) can happen right away or, rarely, not until several weeks after delivery.

Normal bleeding after childbirth is primarily from open blood vessels in your uterus where the placenta was attached. Usually, after the placenta is delivered, your uterus contracts, closing off those blood vessels. Your practitioner may massage your uterus and give you Pitocin as well to help it con-

BabyCenter Buzz

My Labor Was Induced

"My amniotic fluid level became dangerously low, so my doctor sent me straight to the hospital. They hooked me up to an IV and broke my water. I began to have strong contractions very quickly. I had an epidural, so the pain was really minimal. The whole process only took a few hours." —*Tonya*

"I have mixed feelings about my induction. It was kind of a disaster: a long, hard labor; fetal distress after the Pitocin; and an emergency c-section. But then again, we have a healthy baby now! And I'm not sure he was *ever* going to leave the premises voluntarily." —*Anonymous*

"With my first child, my water broke on its own and I went into labor. With my second, my fluid was low and I was induced. Honestly, there was no difference between these two labor experiences." —*Michele*

tract. Breastfeeding, which prompts your body to release natural oxytocin, can also aid in the process.

There are several things, though, that can increase your bleeding or make it hard to control. The most common is that your uterus is just too pooped to contract well, a condition known as "uterine atony." Special medication and uterine massage may be all that's needed to remedy the problem.

You're at increased risk for uterine atony if your uterus was overdistended during pregnancy, whether from having a big baby, twins or more, or too much amniotic fluid. You're also at higher risk if you've given birth many times before, have a very long labor or a very quick one, have been induced or augmented with Pitocin, have a uterine infection, or have preeclampsia and are getting magnesium sulfate (a medication that's used to prevent seizures but that can cause uterine relaxation).

Rarely, fragments of the placenta stay in your uterus and cause bleeding, so you'll need a dilation and curettage (D & C) to remove them. You may also suffer heavy bleeding if your uterus, cervix, or vagina tears during labor or if you've had a large episiotomy—in which case you'll need

BY THE NUMBERS

Hemorrhaging after Birth

Percent of pregnancies
complicated by PPH: **5%**

Source: *Williams Obstetrics,*
21st Edition

stitches to help staunch the flow. Sometimes uterine fibroids contribute to bleeding because they prevent your uterus from contracting the way it should.

You're also at increased risk for PPH if you have a systemic blood-clotting disorder, whether it's inherited or pregnancy-related (which might happen if you have severe preeclampsia or a placental abruption). A placenta that's implanted too deeply in your uterus can also be a culprit. Finally, a ruptured or inverted uterus can cause profuse bleeding, but these complications are rare.

Preterm Birth

If you deliver your baby before week 37, it's called a preterm birth and your newborn is considered premature. About a quarter of all preterm births are intentional—meaning that your medical team decides to induce labor early (or perform a c-section) because you have a serious medical condition, such as preeclampsia, or because your baby's stopped growing. The rest of these early deliveries are known as spontaneous preterm births. You may end up having a spontaneous preterm birth if you go into labor prematurely, if your water breaks early, or if you have a condition called cervical insufficiency, in which your cervix dilates too soon without contractions.

Preterm birth can be risky for your baby. A very premature baby needs to be in a hospital with a neonatal intensive care unit (NICU) so he can be cared for by doctors and nurses who specialize in high-risk newborn care. If your local hospital isn't equipped to handle your baby's needs, you may be transported to a different hospital for delivery. (If need be, your baby can be transported after birth, but if there's time, it's usually best to make the trip while he's still in your womb.)

If you go into labor before week 34 or if you need to deliver early for medical reasons, your caregiver will try to delay your labor for a few days so your baby can get corticosteroids to speed his lung development and help prevent complications. And no matter how far along you are, if you're positive for Group B strep or if your strep status isn't known, you'll get antibiotics to prevent infection in your baby.

During labor, you'll have continuous electronic monitoring to detect any problems with your baby's heart rate. If he doesn't seem to be tolerating labor well, you'll need a c-section. Whether you give birth vaginally or have a c-section, a pediatrician will be there for the birth so she can examine and care for your

BabyCenter Buzz

Delivering My Premature Baby

"My son was born at 24 weeks. After four months and six days in the NICU, he came home and is doing remarkably well." —*Trish*

"I gave birth to our daughter at 26 weeks. The birth was so surreal. I kept thinking: 'This can't be happening. It's way too early.' But nothing could stop her. She was in the NICU for four months, and everyone kept telling us these miracle stories ('Our neighbor had a baby at 25 weeks, but now she's healthy as an ox'). Our little early-bird special is seven months old now, and she's doing great! I never would've believed it." —*Anonymous*

"My baby was born at 34 weeks, and in his doctor's words, 'He's doing as well as full-term babies.' He was born with fully developed lungs, but for now he's in NICU until he's able to feed from a bottle and gain some weight." —*Anonymous*

baby as soon as he's born. It's impossible to predict exactly what kind of treatment a premature baby will need, how long he'll have to stay in the hospital, and whether he'll suffer from any long-term problems. The more developed your baby is at birth, though, the more likely he is to survive and the less likely he is to have health problems. Babies who are born between weeks 34 and 37 (anything after this is considered full-term) generally do very well.

If you're planning to breastfeed but your baby's in the NICU, be sure to let your caregiver and pediatrician know. If your baby's not yet ready to feed, you'll want to start using a breast pump to help your milk come in and to keep your supply up. The hospital can give you special containers for collecting and freezing your milk so you can give it to your baby later. When he's ready to start breastfeeding, you'll be able to feed him in the nursery. Most NICUs have rocking chairs for nursing moms, and the nurses there will help you and your baby get started.

Serious Perineal Tearing

It's common to have some minor tearing during childbirth, but about 4 percent of women who deliver vaginally end up with a serious tear in their perineum (the area between the vagina and the anus) when their baby's head

BabyCenter Buzz

I Had a Serious Tear

"I was completely unaware that I had had any tearing until my doctor started sewing me up in the delivery room. Even then, I didn't really understand what a third-degree tear meant. It took me a very long time—almost six months—to feel completely normal again and to even *think* about having sex. No one tells you that this might happen!" —*Anonymous*

emerges. These tears are called third- or fourth-degree lacerations. A third-degree laceration is a tear in your vaginal tissue, perineal skin, and perineal muscles that extends into your anal sphincter. A fourth-degree tear is a deeper cut that goes through your anal sphincter all the way to your rectum. These tears can happen to anyone, but they're more likely in the following situations:

- You have a forceps delivery
- You have an episiotomy (Although episiotomies are supposed to prevent tears, some women tear beyond the surgical cut and end up with even more serious lacerations than they would have if they'd torn naturally.)
- You deliver a very big baby
- Your baby is born face-up
- You have a shorter-than-average distance between your vaginal opening and your anus

If you have a serious tear, you'll need a fair number of stitches to sew up all the layers of tissue and muscle, so you'll be numbed beforehand with a local anesthetic or a pudendal block. Afterward, you'll need to apply ice packs to the area for the next 12 hours or so. Don't be shy about asking for pain medication if you're very uncomfortable (and chances are, you will be).

After a severe tear, urinating or having a bowel movement can be painful—and you may become constipated as a result. Later, you may have some involuntary flatulence or, more rarely, fecal incontinence. Make sure your practitioner gives you a stool softener so you can start taking it right away (you'll also want to take it for the first few weeks that you're home), and don't fight the urge to move your bowels. Avoid putting anything, including an enema, into your rectum. The pain will lessen over time, but your discomfort may last for three months or more.

Uterine Inversion

Normally within about 30 minutes of your baby's birth, your placenta detaches from the wall of your uterus and is "delivered" through your vagina. But sometimes the placenta doesn't completely separate on its own and your practitioner may try to help it along. In very rare cases (about one in 2,100 to 6,400), the uterus literally turns inside out and is pulled out of the vagina along with the placenta. This is called a uterine inversion.

Usually, your practitioner is able to detach the placenta from your uterus and essentially push your womb back into its proper place right away. In rare instances, though, she may need to perform abdominal surgery to return the uterus to its original position. Once your uterus has been repositioned, you'll be given a continuous IV infusion of oxytocin to firm it up, to control bleeding, and to help it stay where it belongs. You'll likely also get a blood transfusion, and perhaps antibiotics to prevent infection.

Uterine Rupture

When you attempt to give birth vaginally after a previous c-section, there's a small risk (less than 1 percent) that the old incision will give way and your uterus will rupture. You're also at risk for uterine rupture if you've had fibroids removed or had a surgical procedure to correct a misshapen uterus.

A spontaneous uterine rupture—that is, a rupture in a woman who's never had uterine surgery—is extremely rare (1 in 15,000 births). Those at risk include women with five or more children, an overly distended uterus, or a placenta that's implanted too deeply. Persistent, forceful contractions can also contribute to rupture, as can a difficult forceps delivery. Sometimes a rupture isn't discovered until after your baby's born and your bleeding doesn't taper off as it should.

If your uterus ruptures during labor, your baby will be delivered by emergency c-section, and your uterus will be repaired. (If the damage is extensive, though, you may need a hysterectomy.) You'll likely lose a lot of blood, so you may need a transfusion. You'll probably also get IV antibiotics to prevent infection.

Though uterine rupture can be terrifying, women who've had them can and do go on to have more children—though, for obvious reasons, they deliver any future babies via scheduled c-section.

PART V

RECOVERING FROM CHILDBIRTH: THE FIRST 6 WEEKS

Congratulations! Your precious baby is finally here. You're probably head over heels in love with the new little person in your life—and possibly feeling overwhelmed by the physical, emotional, and lifestyle changes you've undergone. Be kind to yourself as you adjust to your new role. Your body needs rest to recover from the rigors of childbirth and you need time to bond with your baby.

If you've had an uncomplicated vaginal birth, you'll probably be able to head home 24 hours after your baby arrives (or sooner if you're at a birthing center), although many new moms opt to stay at the hospital for about two days. If you had a c-section, you'll most likely have to stick around the hospital for three or four days.

Before you go home, you may need to take care of some final health matters. For instance, if you're Rh-negative and your baby is Rh-positive, you'll need an injection of Rh immune globulin within 72 hours of delivery. And, if you're not immune to rubella, now's a good time to get vaccinated. The rubella vaccine isn't safe during pregnancy and you can rest easy that you won't be conceiving again in the next month!

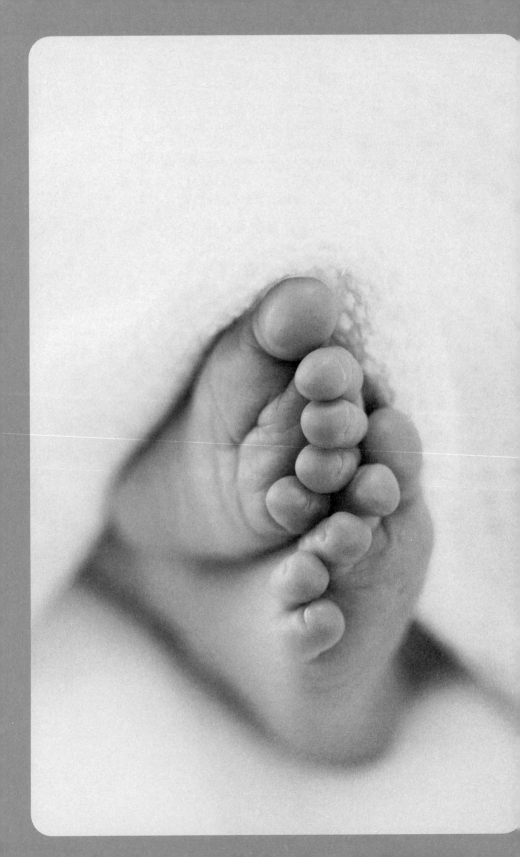

YOUR BODY
AFTER THE BABY

How Your Body Changes after Delivery

Giving birth is the first step in your physical recovery from pregnancy, but it's far from the last. It will take weeks (the official postpartum period lasts six weeks), and possibly even months, for you to feel like your "old self" again. Physically, that is. Emotionally, you're forever changed by the remarkable new life cradled in your arms.

The physical changes that begin immediately after birth are so dramatic and linked to pregnancy that many people refer to this time as the "fourth" trimester. A look at what's happening to your body in the first hours and weeks after childbirth:

Immediate Weight Loss

While you probably won't return to your prepregnancy weight for some time, you will lose a significant amount of weight immediately after delivery. Subtract one 7- to 9-pound baby, another pound or two of placenta, and at least a pound of blood and amniotic fluid, and that leaves most women 12 pounds lighter.

The weight keeps coming off, too. Throughout pregnancy, your body's cells were hard at work retaining water, and now all that extra fluid—along with the fluid from your increased blood volume—will be looking for a way out. You'll produce more urine than usual in the days after birth—an astounding 3 quarts a day—and you may notice yourself perspiring a lot (even while you sleep). By the end of the first week, you'll lose about 4 pounds of water weight. (The amount will depend on how much water you retained during pregnancy.)

Your Shrinking Uterus

At the time of delivery, your uterus is like a 2½-pound melon, 25 times its prepregnancy size. Within minutes after your baby is born, contractions cause it to begin to shrink, clenching itself like a fist, its crisscrossed fibers tightening in the same way they do during labor. This process can cause cramps known as afterpains.

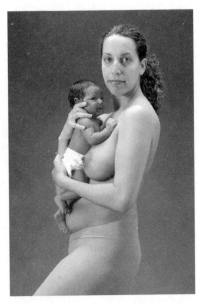

Your uterus retreats quickly. For the next couple of days after birth, you can feel the top of your uterus at—or a couple of finger widths below—the level of your belly button. Within a week your uterus is half the weight it was at delivery, and by week 2, it's down to a mere 11 ounces and located entirely within your pelvis. By weeks 4 to 6, it's back to its normal prepregnancy weight

Even if your labor and delivery was fast and easy, it'll take some time for your body to regain its strength and shape. Focus on your baby, but pamper yourself, too. Take it easy and give it time.

of 2 ounces. This process is called involution of the uterus.

After your baby is born, cells that form the lining of the uterus begin to slough off. It results in a discharge called lochia that lasts for weeks. At first, this discharge is mixed with blood so it appears bright red and menstrual-like; then it gradually gets lighter in color, finally fading to white or yellow before it stops.

A New Hormone Mix Comes into Play

After childbirth, there's a dramatic decline in progesterone and estrogen levels that will affect you physically and emotionally. One change you may notice: losing your hair. Many women shed handfuls beginning around one to four months after delivery. If you're breastfeeding, your baby's suckling will trigger the release of the hormones prolactin and oxytocin. Prolactin stimulates milk production, and oxytocin causes the milk-producing cells and ducts in your breast to contract and push milk to your nipple. If those first breastfeeding sessions cause some abdominal cramping, it's because oxytocin also triggers uterine contractions. These

Just the Facts

Your Bladder Just after Birth

It's not uncommon to feel as if you don't have to pee much in the first day after you give birth, especially if you had an epidural or a forceps or vacuum-assisted vaginal delivery. This is caused by a temporary decrease in bladder sensitivity. With all the extra fluid your kidneys are processing, your bladder will be filling up rapidly, so it's essential you urinate frequently even if you don't have the urge or haven't had much to drink. Overdistention of your bladder can cause urinary problems and will also make it harder for your uterus to contract, leading to more afterpains and bleeding. If you're unable to pee within a few hours after you give birth, your caregiver will put a catheter in your bladder to release the urine. (If you deliver by c-section, you'll have a urinary catheter for the surgery and the following 12 hours or so.) Let the nurse know if you're having difficulty urinating or are producing only a small amount of urine each time you pee. If your bladder gets too full, it can actually prevent you from going.

hormonal dips and surges may also contribute to the emotional swings you may be feeling now.

Postpartum Symptoms and Complaints

Afterpains

WHAT THEY ARE: Painful abdominal cramps caused by uterine contractions. Breastfeeding can bring on cramps or make them worse because your baby's nursing triggers the release of the hormone oxytocin, which causes contractions. Afterpains usually grow worse with each successive pregnancy.

HOW LONG THEY'LL LAST: The cramping will be most intense during the first day or two after you give birth and should taper off within two to three days. (If you're a first-time mom, you may barely feel them.)

HOW TO COPE:

• Try to pee as often as you can (even if you don't feel the urge to go). A full bladder displaces the uterus so it can't contract as well as it should.

• Some women find it helpful to lie on their stomach with a pillow under their lower belly. Gentle massage of this area can also help.

- Ibuprofen generally works well for afterpains and is safe for breast-feeding moms. If it doesn't give you enough relief, let your caregiver know.

- If the cramping hasn't started to ease up after a few days or the pain becomes unbearable, call your caregiver. It could be a sign of infection or another problem that requires medical attention.

Back Pain

WHAT IT IS: Postpartum back pain is caused by a number of factors, including weakened abdominal muscles, relaxation of pelvic ligaments, altered posture while you were pregnant, a long and difficult labor that taxes muscles you don't normally use, holding your baby in awkward positions

Just the Facts

When Can I . . .

Have sex? Generally, a few weeks after delivery, if you didn't have an episiotomy or any lacerations, your lochia (vaginal discharge) is no longer red, and you feel up to it. Otherwise, wait until after your postpartum visit at six weeks so your caregiver can see how you're healing. Either way, use contraception. You can get pregnant before your period returns.

Take a bath? Immediately after a vaginal delivery. If you have many stitches in your perineal area or heavy lochia, a shower might be more comfortable. If you had a c-section, wait until your sutures or staples are removed. If your wound is infected, talk to your caregiver before taking a soak.

Exercise? Generally you can start taking five- to ten-minute walks and doing simple exercises (such as leg stretches) within days of birth. Stop exercising if you're uncomfortable or your lochia increases. If you've had a c-section, wait at least six weeks (and for your caregiver's okay) to do anything beyond short walks.

Use a tampon? Not for at least six weeks after your baby's birth—using one sooner could cause an infection.

Start dieting? Wait at least six weeks. Your body needs time to recover from labor and delivery. And even then crash-dieting is out—particularly if you're breastfeeding because it can adversely affect your milk supply.

Go back to work? Six weeks is considered a normal "disability" leave following a vaginal birth, and eight weeks if you've had a c-section. If you really want to work before then, don't put in more than 20 hours a week. And if you need more time to recover, you're in good company. Many women don't feel physically or emotionally ready to work for several months (or longer) after childbirth.

while nursing, exhaustion, and stress. Women who've had back pain—either before or during pregnancy—are more likely to experience it after childbirth. (If you had an epidural, you may notice some tendness at the site for a few days after giving birth, but not back pain.)

HOW LONG IT'LL LAST: It depends on what's causing the pain. It may be short-lived or it may come and go, especially if you've suffered from back pain in the past.

HOW TO COPE:

• Take walks. This gentle form of exercise can help ease back pain, and it's safe to start almost immediately after either a vaginal birth or a c-section. (But take it slowly and keep walks short in the first few weeks.)

• Sit up straight when feeding your baby whether you're nursing or bottle-feeding. If you have lower-back pain, try using a footstool to keep your feet slightly raised off the floor. Choose a comfortable chair with armrests, and use lots of pillows to lend extra support to your back and arms. If you're nursing, bring your baby to your breast, rather than the other way around. Also, try different breastfeeding positions—if you have tense shoulders and upper-back pain, the side-lying position may be more comfortable.

• Always bend from your knees and lift objects and children from a crouching position, to minimize the stress on your back. Let someone else lift heavy objects; this isn't the time to risk throwing your back out. (If you've had a c-section, you shouldn't be lifting anything heavier than your baby for at least eight weeks.)

• Treat yourself to a massage. While massage won't address the underlying source of your back pain, it will help you relax and can temporarily soothe pulled muscles, tense shoulders, and lower-back pain. A warm bath is also a great way to ease soreness and tension.

• With your caregiver's okay, make pelvic tilts a part of your daily routine. Lie on your back with your knees bent and your feet flat on the floor. Inhale and allow your belly to expand with your breath. Exhale and lift your tailbone toward your navel while keeping your hips on the floor. At the top of the tilt, tighten your butt; then release. Repeat 8 to 10 times. (*Note:* If you've had a c-section, wait at least six to eight weeks to start exercises like this.)

• Listen to your body. If a particular position or activity causes you discomfort, stop. If your back pain is severe or you notice that you've also lost feeling in your legs, butt, groin, genital area, bladder, or anus—or you feel suddenly uncoordinated or weak—call your caregiver immediately.

Lochia

WHAT IT IS: Postpartum discharge, known as lochia, initially consists largely of blood and sloughed-off tissue from the lining of your uterus. The discharge may come out in gushes or flow more evenly, like a menstrual period. If you've been lying down for a while and blood has collected in your vagina, you may see some some small clots when you get up. After the initial bleeding slows and as you continue to heal, your lochia will turn from bright red to pink, and eventually to yellow-white.

HOW LONG IT'LL LAST: You may have lochia for as little as two to three weeks or as long as six weeks after giving birth. Your lochia will stay bright red in color for two to four days and then start turning pink. Pink lochia lasts about a week, with the flow decreasing each day. Scant pale lochia—the final stage—can last for several weeks.

HOW TO COPE:

• Use the heavy-duty sanitary pads that the hospital gives you, and stock up on more pads when you get home. As your lochia tapers off, you can switch to mini-pads.

• Don't use tampons for at least six weeks. They can introduce bacteria into your still-healing vagina and uterus and lead to infection.

• Take it easy, get as much rest as you can, and don't overdo it. If bright red spotting reappears after your lochia has already lightened, it's a sign that you need to slow down. If after resting you're still spotting, call your midwife or doctor. You should also call if your lochia is still bright red four days after your baby's birth.

• If you have abnormally heavy bleeding (saturating a sanitary pad within an hour), call your doctor or midwife *immediately*. This is a sign of a delayed postpartum hemorrhage (see below). If you're bleeding profusely and feeling faint, call 911.

Broken Blood Vessels

WHAT THEY ARE: Intense pushing during the second stage of labor can force tiny capillaries in your eyes to burst open, leaving you with a bloodshot look. Capillaries in your face and upper chest can also burst, causing pinhead-size red or purplish marks.

HOW LONG THEY'LL LAST: The blood vessels will start to heal immediately—though it can take anywhere from a few days to several weeks for your eyes to look normal again.

HOW TO COPE:

All you can do is wait for the capillaries to heal.

Constipation

WHAT IT IS: Even if you never had a problem with constipation during your pregnancy, you may now. A c-section itself or medication given in labor or prescribed for postpartum pain, can sometimes slow down your digestive system, causing that "blocked-up" feeling. If you had an enema, a long labor without food, or a bowel movement during labor, you may go a day or two without moving your bowels because there simply isn't anything in your intestines. A sore or stitched-up perineum or hemorrhoids can also cause constipation because a fear of more pain or ripping your stitches can make you hold it in.

HOW LONG IT'LL LAST: It depends. Most constipation will end within a few days if you take steps to address the problem. If you had a c-section, it can take up to three or four days for your bowels to start functioning normally again.

HOW TO COPE:

• Never ignore the urge to go, even though it might be uncomfortable the first few times. (The longer you wait, the harder your stool will get, which will only make your pain worse.)

• Eat high-fiber foods such as cereals, whole grain breads, and fresh fruits and vegetables every day.

• Drink plenty of water—at least six to eight glasses a day. (You'll need even more if you're breastfeeding.) A glass of fruit juice a day— especially prune juice if you can stomach it—can be helpful. Some people find that any warm liquid first thing in the morning helps get things moving.

• Go for a walk. It may be painful at first, especially if you're recovering from a c-section or an episiotomy, but even a short outing around the block will help kick your sluggish bowels into gear.

• Iron pills can aggravate constipation, so if you're taking iron supplements, ask your practitioner whether it makes sense to stop until constipation is no longer a problem.

• Ask your doctor or midwife if you should take a stool softener (available over the counter).

Delayed Postpartum Hemorrhage

WHAT IT IS: Some bleeding after delivery is normal. In fact, you should expect vaginal bleeding—whether you delivered vaginally or via c-section—for several days following childbirth. Sometimes, though, women have persistent bleeding or a sudden increase in bleeding. If the blood loss is extreme, it's called a late—or delayed—postpartum hemorrhage. This can happen if your uterus doesn't continue to contract and shrink as it should. This kind of hemorrhage is most commonly caused by fragments of the placenta or the amniotic sac that remain in the uterus after birth or a uterus that doesn't contract normally because of infection or other causes. Call your caregiver right away if you notice any of these signs of abnormal bleeding:

• Soaking more than one sanitary pad in an hour
• Bright red bleeding that occurs four days or more after delivery
• Blood clots that are bigger than a golf ball

HOW LONG IT'LL LAST: By definition, delayed (or late) postpartum hemorrhage is profuse bleeding that occurs between 24 hours after birth and six weeks postpartum (though it typically occurs one to two weeks postpartum). Bleeding may continue until treated and it can become life-threatening, so you'll be hospitalized until it stops.

HOW TO COPE:

You'll be treated with IV medications to help your uterus contract. In addition, you'll get a physical and a pelvic exam, and a sonogram to see if there's any retained placental tissue in your uterus. If your caregiver finds placental tissue, she'll remove it with a D & C. Once the bleeding has stopped, you'll need IV medication (usually for about 24 hours) to keep your uterus contracted. Your medical team will watch you closely for further bleeding and to see how you're recovering. You may feel weak and light-headed, and at first you shouldn't try to get out of bed on your own. Rest, fluids, a nutritious diet, and iron supplements are essential. Chances are, this is all you'll need to deal with the anemia caused by excessive blood loss. (In rare cases, a blood transfusion may be needed.)

Warning! When to Call 911

If you are bleeding profusely—*or* if you have any signs of shock, including light-headedness, weakness, rapid heartbeat or palpitations, rapid or shallow breathing, clammy skin, restlessness or confusion—call 911.

···

Perineal Pain

WHAT IT IS: Sometimes the the perineum—the area between your vagina and anus—tears or is cut during childbirth. As a result, this area can feel quite painful. (If you didn't tear or have an episiotomy, your perineum may be swollen or a little tender, but it'll likely feel fine within a day or so.)

It is possible to tear at the top of the vagina near the urethra (known as a periurethral laceration). These tears are usually small, and if you get one, you'll need only a few stitches (or none at all). Upper vaginal tears don't involve muscle, so they heal more quickly and are less painful than perineal tears. The main complaint: You might feel some burning when you pee.

HOW LONG IT'LL LAST: Healing times vary from woman to woman. But in general, the deeper the laceration, the longer the recovery. A small laceration ("first degree") doesn't involve any muscle, and it may not even require stitches. In either case, these tears generally heal quickly and cause little discomfort. A typical episiotomy or second-degree laceration usually heals in two or three weeks (the stitches dissolve on their own during this time). Some women feel little pain after a week or so, while others have discomfort for a month or two. Women with more serious lacerations (third or fourth degree) may have pain and discomfort for a month or longer. They're also at increased risk for incontinence of gas or feces and, in the first few days after birth, may have trouble urinating and having bowel movements.

HOW TO COPE:

• Right after birth ask for an ice pack (with a soft covering) to apply to your perineum. It will help decrease swelling and discomfort. It's a good idea to use ice intermittently for the next 12 hours or so.

• If you have an extensive tear and your caregiver gives you a prescription pain reliever, don't hesitate to take the pills—they'll make the pain much more bearable. Otherwise, you can take over-the-counter ibuprofen or acetaminophen. (Don't take aspirin if you're breastfeeding.) You may also want to use an anethestic spray for the first couple days.

• Change your sanitary pad each time you use the bathroom.

• Use the squirt bottle ("peri" bottle) provided by the hospital to pour warm water on your perineum while you're going to the bathroom. The water will dilute your urine so it won't burn as much when it comes in contact with your skin. Give youself another squirt afterward, using warm water (or a medicated solution if you're given one), to cleanse yourself.

• Always pat yourself dry from front to back, to avoid introducing germs from your rectum into your vaginal area.

• Limit sitting while your bottom is still very sore, and when you do sit, use an inflatable rubber "doughnut" or a small pillow.

• Take a sitz bath—soak your bottom in a small tub of warm water— for 20 minutes three times a day. Wait at least 24 hours after your baby's birth to start the sitz baths.

• Apply compresses of cotton pads soaked in witch hazel to the painful area.

• Expose the wound to air as much as possible, and keep it dry.

• Begin doing Kegel exercises the day you give birth to help restore muscle tone, stimulate circulation, and speed healing. Try doing a Kegel just before changing positions or getting up from a bed or chair—you'll feel less of a pulling sensation on your stitches.

• If you have a tear that involves your anal sphincter (third or fourth degree), start taking a stool softener right after you deliver, and continue for a week or so. (Avoid all rectal treatments, such as suppositories or enemas.)

• Consult your caregiver if you're not finding relief or if you have increased pain or swelling. Also call if you experience any fever, which can be a sign of infection.

Hemorrhoids

WHAT THEY ARE: Hemorrhoids are varicose veins—that is, blood vessels that have become unusually swollen—that show up in the rectal area. Sometimes an enlarged vein protrudes out of the anus and you'll feel a soft, swollen mass anywhere from the size of a raisin to a grape. Hemorrhoids can be merely itchy or downright painful and may sometimes even cause rectal bleeding, especially during a bowel movement. Whether or not you had hemorrhoids during your pregnancy, you're likely to have them after delivery, particularly if you had to push for a while during labor.

HOW LONG THEY'LL LAST: In most cases, hemorrhoids that developed during pregnancy or labor will get better on their own within a few days or weeks, especially if you're careful to avoid constipation.

HOW TO COPE:

• Apply an ice pack wrapped in a cloth to your rectal area on and off for the first 24 hours or more if you're still very swollen.

• Use a plastic squirt bottle filled with warm water to clean the area after a bowel movement; then wipe with witch hazel compresses, or store-bought medicated pads, instead of toilet paper.

• Take sitz baths several times a day. Use the plastic sitz bath container they gave you at the hospital (or get one at the drugstore). Fill it with warm water and position it over your toilet, and then sit down and submerge your bottom.

• Avoid constipation (page 50).

• Avoid sitting or standing for long stretches of time, to take the pressure off your rectal veins.

• If these methods don't do the trick, ask your practitioner to recommend a safe topical anesthetic or medicated suppository. (*Note:* If you had an episiotomy or a tear that extends into your rectum, it's especially important to not put anything—including suppositories—into your rectum until you're given the okay by your healthcare provider.)

• Call your practitioner if you have any rectal bleeding.

Fatigue

WHAT IT IS: Feeling tired—or just plain wiped out—is one of new moms' most common complaints. Not only has your body been through an incredible physical challenge—childbirth—but you're also caring for a newborn who needs food, diaper changes, and hands-on attention around the clock.

HOW LONG IT'LL LAST:

Unfortunately, feeling bone tired can last for months, depending on how well your baby sleeps (and how good you are at napping when you can). Most new moms report feeling noticeably better in about two to three months.

BabyCenter Buzz

How We Sleep

"We had a cradle that rocked, and I tied a rope to it so I could rock it while I lay in bed if our baby woke in the night. (I made sure the rope was out of his reach at all times!)" —*Mollie*

"On the nights that I really want undisturbed slumber, my husband and son sleep in a separate room so I don't hear them get up for feeding and changing. We also take turns sleeping in on the weekend." —*Shari*

"We've found that the best way to protect our sleep and make sure we're functional is to take our daughter in shifts. My wife usually handles the first shift (10:30 P.M. to 2:30 A.M.), while anything after that falls into my territory (2:30 A.M. to 6 A.M.)." —*Dan*

"Our daughter sleeps in our bed, which works wonderfully for me. She wakes to nurse and have a quick diaper change, and then she falls back to sleep." —*Melissa*

HOW TO COPE:

• Sleep when your baby sleeps. If you find this impossible, at least put your feet up and close your eyes. Take any opportunity you can to rest, even when you have visitors. Your family and friends will understand and can entertain themselves.

• Keep taking your prenatal vitamin, drink plenty of fluids, eat well-balanced meals as often as you can, and never skip meals. Now is not the time to crash diet. Food is your fuel.

• Take your baby out for a walk around the block. It will help you feel less tired, and the fresh air and movement will help both of you sleep better at night.

• Bring in reinforcements. Who can help do chores, cook meals, and run errands while you get some rest? Identify those people, and ask them to do specific things.

• Consider a ban on houseguests. If your mother-in-law loves cooking and cleaning, by all means invite her over, but if she expects to be entertained while she admires her new grandchild, ask her to delay her visit for a few weeks.

• If you find that you can't sleep, have lost interest in doing anything, and feel despairing, call your provider. You could be suffering from postpartum depression. Also, call your caregiver if you find you're becoming even more fatigued after about four months; you may be one of the small percentage of women who develop hypothyroidism between four and eight months after birth.

Incontinence (Urinary and Anal)

WHAT IT IS: Many postpartum women suffer a form of urinary incontinence known as stress incontinence. They find themselves leaking urine when they cough, sneeze, or exert themselves in certain ways. These surprise leaks are one of the least-talked-about side effects of pregnancy. Normally, your nerves, ligaments, and pelvic-floor muscles work together to support your bladder and keep the urethra closed so urine doesn't leak out. Overstretching or injury to these areas during pregnancy can lead to stress incontinence before you give birth. Childbirth can compound the problem, particularly if you have had a forceps or a vacuum extraction delivery, a large baby, a baby who came out face-up, an episiotomy or a deep laceration, or actively pushed for a long time. That said, some women who have c-sections (and miss labor altogether) also end up with stress incontinence.

Some women also suffer anal incontinence after childbirth, which means they have trouble controlling their gas or, less commonly, their bowel movements. You're most likely to have this problem if you've torn through your anal sphincter. This happens more often with an episiotomy than with a spontaneous tear and is more likely if you've had an assisted vaginal delivery (especially with forceps), a large baby, or a baby in the posterior position (face-up). But once again, you may still have anal incontinence after a c-section, even if you had the surgery without having gone into labor.

HOW LONG IT'LL LAST: For some women, the leaking of urine stops within a few weeks of giving birth, while in others it can persist for several months (or even years, though usually it's just a small dribble when you laugh or sneeze). Most women regain control of their bowels within a few months, though others may experience some degree of gas incontinence many years later.

HOW TO COPE:

• Use sanitary pads to protect your clothes from urine leaks or absorbent underwear if you suffer from bowel leaks.

• Go to the bathroom often so your bladder doesn't get too full.

• Do regular Kegel exercises. They can strengthen your pelvic-floor muscles, giving you better control, and increase blood flow to your perineum, which aids healing. If you're not sure you're doing them correctly, review them with your practitioner during your checkup.

• Call your caregiver if you have pain or burning when you urinate; sometimes incontinence is caused by a urinary tract infection.

• Talk to your doctor or midwife if the incontinence continues beyond a few months. In rare cases, surgery may be necessary to correct the problem.

Infections

WHAT THEY ARE: Your recovering body may be vulnerable to certain infections after childbirth. The most common postpartum infection, endometritis, happens in the endometrium, or lining of the uterus, and women who have had a c-section are at higher risk for it than women who delivered vaginally. Other infections can develop in the cervix, vagina, vulva, and urinary tract. (You're at a higher risk for a urinary tract infection if you had a catheter in your bladder.) If you had a c-section, you may develop an infection at the site of your incision. After a vaginal birth, you may have one at the site of the episiotomy or tear, though this is uncommon. Infections sometimes develop after you've already gone home, and they can be serious, so call your caregiver if you have any of the following symptoms.

• Lower abdominal pain, a fever, or foul-smelling vaginal discharge (signs of possible endometritis)

• Difficulty urinating, painful urination, or the feeling that you need to urinate, but little or nothing comes out (signs of a possible urinary tract infection).

• Redness, tenderness, and discharge around the site of a wound (such as an episiotomy or a c-section incision).

• Painful, hard, reddened area, usually only on one breast, and fever, muscle aches, fatigue, and possibly a headache (signs of a breast infection known as mastitis).

HOW LONG THEY'LL LAST:

It depends on what type of infection you have and how quickly you seek treatment. You may need to be hospitalized so you can have intravenous antibiotics; otherwise, oral antibiotics will do the job. Most likely, you'll start feeling better within a few days of starting antibiotics.

HOW TO COPE:

Take the full course of any antibiotics your practitioner prescribes, even if your symptoms disappear. If the antibiotics don't seem to be helping, let your caregiver know. You may need another drug to fight whatever you have. If you're breastfeeding, ask for medication that's safe for your newborn. Drink extra fluids, and get as much rest as possible.

Sweating

WHAT IT IS: It's common to perspire a lot in the weeks after giving birth, particularly at night. Sweating is one of the ways your body rids itself of the extra water weight you gained during pregnancy. Your kidneys are responsible for most of the purging—which means you'll be peeing more than usual for the first week postpartum—but your pores also work overtime to shed the extra water. One theory is that the dramatic drop in estrogen that occurs right after delivery may also contribute to postpartum sweats.

HOW LONG IT'LL LAST: Postpartum sweating can last anywhere from two to six weeks after birth, though it tends to last longer for breast-feeding women.

HOW TO COPE:

• Don't cut back on liquids in hopes of sweating less. Drinking lots of noncaffeinated, nonalcoholic fluids actually helps speed up the process of eliminating the extra water. It also prevents dehydration.

• Although postpartum sweating is entirely normal, if it's accompanied by a fever, your may have an infection. Check with your healthcare provider if you have a fever or you think your sweating is excessive.

Recovering from a C-Section

You may not have to contend with the perineal pain of a vaginal delivery, but a c-section is major surgery, and it comes with its own set of discomforts.

What to Expect Right after Surgery

You may feel groggy and possibly nauseated after surgery. Nausea can last up to 48 hours, but your caregiver can give you medication to minimize your discomfort. Many women whose anesthesia included narcotics experience some itchiness, sometimes all over the body, which should disappear completely within about 48 hours.

Your nurse will instruct you on how to cough or do regular breathing exercises to expand your lungs and clear them of any accumulated fluid, particularly if you've had general anesthesia. (This will decrease the risk of pneumonia.). She'll remove your IV and urinary catheter generally within 12 hours of surgery if everything is okay, and you'll be able to eat very bland, mild foods if you want them. You'll also be encouraged to get out of bed by the next day and, by the second day, to take a short walk with help from your partner or a nurse. Within three to four days, your doctor will likely remove your sutures or staples, and if all is well, you'll be discharged to go home.

When You Leave the Hospital

Expect to need help—and lots of it—once you get home. If you aren't receiving offers, ask for support from your partner, parents, in-laws, and friends. If you can afford it, hire paid help.

Don't expect to toss your pain medication as soon as you get home. You may need prescription painkillers for up to a week after surgery, gradually transitioning to over-the-counter pain relievers.

Like any woman who just delivered a baby, you'll have a vaginal discharge called lochia. For the first three or four days it will be bright red; it gradually turns pink and then yellow-white and may last up to six weeks. If menstrual-type bleeding continues after the first four days or recurs after slowing, call your healthcare provider.

Within six to eight weeks, you'll be able to start exercising moderately—but wait until your caregiver gives you the go-ahead (walking is okay immediately after surgery). It may be several months before you're back to your former fit self. You'll be able to resume sexual intercourse within four to six weeks if you're feeling comfortable enough, with your caregiver's okay.

Common Post-C-Section Complaints

Gas and Bloating

WHAT IT IS: Gas pain and bloating are common side effects of a c-section because air gets trapped in your abdomen during surgery and your intestines tend to be sluggish afterward. The gas buildup can be excruciatingly painful and often comes as a surprise to new moms. You may also have "referred" pain in your shoulder due to the buildup of air, which irritates your diaphragm.

HOW LONG IT'LL LAST: The gas should subside within a day or two.

HOW TO COPE:

• Get up and move around. Walking can help your sluggish digestive system get going again.

• The hospital nurses may give you some over-the-counter medication that contains simethicone, a substance that allows gas bubbles to come together more easily, making the gas easier to expel. Simethicone is safe to take if you're breastfeeding.

• Eat a regular diet as tolerated.

Incisional Pain

WHAT IT IS: Your doctor will sew up your internal incisions with a

Five Principles of Good Eating for All New Moms

1. Don't crash diet or skip meals.
You may be sorely tempted to start whittling off that baby weight, but the first six weeks after your baby's birth are no time for dieting. You need enough calories and nutrients to recover from childbirth, to maintain the energy to care for a newborn, and to sustain a healthy milk supply if you're breastfeeding.

2. Focus on healthy foods.
Eat whole grains and cereals, fresh fruits and vegetables, and foods that provide plenty of protein, calcium, and iron.

3. Drink plenty of water.
All new moms need to stay hydrated to stay healthy. And if you're breastfeeding, you'll be especially thirsty. Drink at least eight to 12 glasses of water a day.

4. Find out if you need a vitamin or mineral supplement.
Check with your doctor or midwife to see what she recommends. If you do continue to take vitamins, remember that they don't make up for poor eating habits. You still need a healthy, well-balanced diet.

5. Avoid irritants if you're nursing.
Cut back on or avoid caffeine because it can get into your breast milk and irritate your baby. Some nursing mothers find that eliminating cow's milk from their diet helps if the baby has colic. If your baby is unusually irritable or has eczema or hives or is wheezing, he should be seen by his doctor as soon as possible. In rare cases, a newborn can have a specific food protein allergy that makes him particularly sensitive to something you eat or drink. The doctor may recommend eliminating certain foods from your diet, such as cow's milk, nuts, eggs, fish, among others.

synthetic, absorbable material and use metal staples or some other kind of stitches to close your external incision. Shortly after the incision has been closed, you may feel numbness and soreness at the site. When they're ready to come out, the stitches or staples used to close the skin take just minutes to remove, and there may be a small pinch, but no pain. Sneezing, coughing, and other actions that exert pressure on your abdominal area can be painful at first, but you'll feel a bit better each day.

HOW LONG IT'LL LAST: The stitches or staples need to be removed by a professional, usually three to four days after your surgery and just before you leave the hospital. You may feel pain in the area for a few weeks.

HOW TO COPE:

• Take pain medication as directed by your caregiver.

• Use your hands or a pillow to support your incision when you cough (good advice for sneezing and laughing, too).

• Use the side-lying position or the football hold to nurse your baby so he's not lying directly on your incision.

The Six-Week Postpartum Checkup

This visit is the last in the long line of checkups that started with your first prenatal appointment. Although practices vary, most doctors and midwives will want to see you about six weeks after giving birth to make sure you're recovering well, physically and emotionally. If you had a c-section, you probably also saw your practitioner two weeks after delivery so she could check that your incision was healing properly.

At your postpartum checkup, your caregiver will:

Check your weight and blood pressure.

Check your abdomen and breasts. She'll feel your belly to be sure that there's no tenderness and check your breasts for lumps or abnormal nipple discharge. If you're breastfeeding, she'll make sure you don't have any clogged ducts or the beginnings of a breast infection. *Note:* Continue to give yourself monthly breast self-exams, even if you're nursing (wait until after a feeding session to do so).

Inspect your perineum and do a speculum and internal exam. During the speculum exam, she'll check to make sure any bruises, scratches, or tears to your cervix or vagina are healing properly, and she may do a Pap smear. During the internal exam, she'll feel your uterus and ovaries and check your vaginal muscle tone. She may then do a rectal exam as well.

Probably give you the green light to start having sex again. But don't worry if you don't feel up to it yet; many new moms don't feel like having sex for several months (or more!) after having a baby. Your caregiver will talk to you about birth control options during this visit, too. Remember: You can get pregnant even if you're breastfeeding and your period hasn't returned.

Talk over any concerns. You'll probably have a lot of questions about how your body has changed and may still be contending with some childbirth-related aches and pains. Make a note of your questions and concerns before your visit so you won't forget to ask them. Use this visit to talk about any emotional problems you may be having, too. It's normal to have occasional mood swings at this point, but if you think you're suffering from postpartum depression, ask for a referral to a therapist. Talk therapy can be very effective, and your therapist can help you figure out if you need an antidepressant as well. Let her know if you're breastfeeding so she can choose one that's safe for your baby.

Warning! Call Your Caregiver Right Away If . . .

- Your bleeding hasn't tapered somewhat, continues to be bright red after the first four days, resumes after slowing down, has a foul odor, or contains clots bigger than a quarter. If you're bleeding a lot and feeling faint or showing other signs of shock, call 911.

- You develop a fever, even a slight one. A low-grade fever may be something benign, but it can also be an early sign of infection, so play it safe and call.

- You have severe or persistent pain anywhere in your abdomen or pelvis, or afterpains that are getting worse instead of better.

- You're feeling extreme sadness or despair or experiencing delusions or thoughts about harming yourself or your baby.

- You have severe or worsening pain in your vagina or perineum, or swelling or discharge from an episiotomoy or a laceration site.

- You have worsening pain or soreness that persists beyond the first few weeks, redness or swelling, or any discharge at the site of your c-section incision.

- You have pain or tenderness in one area of the breast that's not relieved by warm soaks and nursing, or swelling or redness in one area, possibly accompanied by flulike symptoms or fever.

- You have pain or burning when urinating; you have the urge to pee frequently but not a lot comes out; your urine is dark and scanty; or you have any combination of these symptoms. (Stinging *after* the urine comes out and hits an abrasion or laceration is normal.)

- You have persistent or severe pain or tenderness and warmth in one area of your leg, or one leg is more swollen than the other.

- You have persistent or severe headaches.

- You have double vision, blurring or dimming of vision, or flashing spots or lights.

- You have severe or persistent vomiting.

- The site of your IV insertion becomes painful, tender, or inflamed.

Note: Call 911 if you have shortness of breath or chest pain or are coughing up blood.

YOUR EMOTIONS
AFTER THE BABY

The "Baby Blues"

Within the first two or three weeks of giving birth (though it typically starts in the first week), 60 to 80 percent of new moms experience a collection of symptoms known as the "baby blues," or "postpartum blues." You may find yourself feeling moody, weepy, exhausted, unable to sleep, or trapped or anxious. Your appetite can change (you might eat more or less), or you might feel irritable, nervous, worried about being a mother or afraid that being a mother will never feel better than it does during this down period. These feelings are hardly surprising, given the dramatic hormonal shifts that occur right after birth, the emotional adjustment involved in becoming a mother, the fatigue and discomfort you're feeling as a result of labor and birth, and the round-the-clock responsibility of caring for a newborn. It's a lot to cope with at one time.

The good news is this emotional upheaval will generally pass within two to four weeks, and you'll get through it with reassurance from your caregiver, support from family and friends, rest, and time. If your symptoms don't go away on their own within the first few weeks, or if you feel you're getting worse rather than better, it's a sign of postpartum depression, a more serious problem that requires treatment. The sooner you get help for PPD, the sooner you'll get well. And if at *any* time you think you might hurt yourself or your baby or if you feel incapable of responsibly caring for your newborn, call your caregiver right away.

Seven Ways to Feel Better

1. Share your feelings with others. Find someone you trust, and let that person know how you feel. Call a friend. Look for a new-mothers group for support. Reach out to other moms—you may be surprised at how many women experience similar feelings. It's also important to talk to your partner and make sure he knows how you're feeling and what you're worried about.

2. Take care of yourself. This starts with sleeping when your baby sleeps—day or night. You'll need to eat, too—skipping meals will only wear you down. If you won't have much help during the postpartum period, stock up on groceries and take-out menus before you have your baby. Have your partner watch your baby in the morning before he leaves for work so you can eat breakfast and take a shower. Do anything that helps you feel better. Some women find that living in their sweats for days helps. Others feel better when they put on a little makeup and clothes they like to wear. And when you're ready, go out with a friend, but use this time to talk, not run errands!

3. Get help. Part of being a good mother is knowing when to ask for help. Help can come in many forms, from friends who cook meals, bring groceries, or do the vacuuming to relatives who help entertain your other children while you recover. Consider asking someone you trust to help with your newborn, too. You don't have to change every diaper or quiet every crying spell. Let your partner, mother, or other trusted friend step in now and then. They'll love the bonding time with your baby, and you'll get a much-needed break.

4. Hire help if you can. If you don't have a good support network nearby, consider hiring a postpartum doula who will come to your home and help out with housework, cooking, errands, and child care and offer breast-feeding support. Visit the Doulas of North America Web site (www.dona.org) to learn how to find a postpartum doula near you. If you can't afford a doula, consider a local high school kid who can do odd jobs around the house for a few hours.

5. Exercise. If your caregiver has given you the okay, try to fit in some exercise. Not only will it help your body recover, but also—and perhaps more important—it can improve your mood.

6. Get out of the house. Put your baby in a stroller and take a walk around the block. Fresh air, sunshine. If even a brief excursion is too much for you right now, just go outside, take a deep breath, and sit in the sunshine for a few minutes. It will help.

7. Simplify your life. Let the chores wait. Have food delivered, or ask your partner to get takeout on the way home. Return calls only when it's

BabyCenter Buzz

How I Took Care of Myself After My Baby Was Born

"My favorite way to rejuvenate myself is to wait for the baby to go down for a nap, then pull out the latest arrival from my collection of magazine subscriptions, close the door, flop on my bed, and slowly read each and every article. It's a small but very luxurious way to spend some time by myself"   —*Myra*

"I find that just getting out of the house to run errands without the baby is a great way to have a quiet moment to myself"   —*Kelly*

"I like to go and sit on our deck for five to ten minutes and just enjoy the outdoors. It's a quick release that helps me to calm myself down if I'm frustrated or worn-out."   —*Val*

"I like to have a warm bath with candlelight, incense, and relaxing music in background"   —*Anonymous*

"We hired a doula, who got us through the first two weeks after my son was born. My partner and I had no idea what we were doing, and she made us dinner, took care of the baby, and kept the house clean. I got to nap and catch up on lots of sleep—and after she left, I was glad I had."   —*Lee*

convenient. Ask a friend to help, and set aside time—even half an hour—for you and your partner to be alone without the baby. If you're on maternity leave, banish all thoughts of the work that awaits you at the office. And don't create a monster list of things you want to get done while you're off. This leave is about you and your baby, nor reorganizing the closets.

Postpartum Depression

If your mood doesn't lift after two weeks, or you feel better but then worse again, you may have postpartum depression (PPD). About 10 to 20 percent of new mothers develop full-blown clinical depression, which can last from two weeks to a year. You're more likely to suffer postpartum depression if you've had past bouts of depression—including before your pregnancy, during your pregnancy, or earlier in the postpartum period—or, to a lesser degree, if you have a family history of depression. You're also at higher risk if you have relationship problems, are isolated and have little or no support

Just for Dad

You Can Get Blue, Too

Your partner may not be the only one feeling out of sorts. Chances are you're coping with your own set of worries, including anxiety over the loss of your freedom, financial concerns, couple time, and whether you'll be a good father. You're certainly not alone: One study found that more than two-thirds of fathers felt down at some point in the first four months following their baby's birth.

One sure way to improve your mood and keep worries from getting overwhelming is to share your anxieties with your partner, a trusted friend, or a professional. Although it may not be your style, you can benefit from talking things out. Voicing your concerns and worries can help you get a clearer perspective and the support you need to feel better. If you're keeping your feelings in for fear that sharing them will make things worse for your partner, relax. Open communication and knowing that you're in this together is often the best medicine for both of you.

If you feel fatigued and anxious, are preoccupied with finances, begin to withdraw from your family, are irritable, sleep poorly or too much, or become very angry—you could be depressed. If any of these symptoms last more than a couple of weeks, seek professional help. It can be tough to talk about your feelings, but doing so can improve every aspect of your life. Clinical depression can affect your health, your relationship with your partner and new baby, and your work. Depression is not a sign of weakness. It's a biochemical response to stress, and it can be treated with counseling and medication.

(from partners, family, and friends), or have recently experienced a stressful life event (such as a death in the family or problems with your baby). That said, postpartum depression can strike any woman.

But take heart: Help is available. Unless you've been treated before or can directly call a mental health professional you know and like, the first place to start is with your doctor or midwife, who can refer you to a specialist. Be straight with your caregiver about how you're feeling and any scary thoughts you may be having. It can be hard to admit to anyone—even yourself—that you feel despair, especially at a time when most people expect you to be thrilled about your new baby, but doing so is the only way you can get help to feel better. Feeling depressed doesn't mean you're a bad mother, so don't feel guilty about not being able to "snap out of it" or embarrassed that you can't seem to shake off the baby blues. The sooner you own up to these feelings and seek help, the better off you and your baby will be. PPD is a common and treatable problem (usually with a combination of coun-

Signs of PPD You Should Never Ignore

Call your caregiver if you have any of the following symptoms:

- Loss of interest or pleasure in most activities that you normally enjoy
- Weepiness or sadness that lasts all day, most days
- Insomnia, difficulty staying asleep, or sleeping more than usual
- Trouble concentrating
- Marked changes in appetite (eating too much or too little)
- Anxiety
- Moodiness and irritability
- Feelings of guilt, worthlessness, or hopelessness
- Panic attacks (symptoms include heart racing, dizziness, confusion, and feelings of impending doom)
- Suicidal thoughts (seek help immediately)
- Thoughts of harming your baby (seek help immediately)

seling and medication), so don't suffer any longer than you already have. If you're breastfeeding, let your caregiver know so she can take that into account when figuring out what medications are best for you. Another reason to call your caregiver sooner rather than later is to rule out a physical cause for your depression. A small—but not insignificant—percentage of women develop thyroid problems after giving birth, and out-of-whack thyroid levels are associated with depression.

Bonding with Your Baby

When experts talk about bonding, they're referring to the intense attachment you develop with your baby. It's the feeling that makes you want to shower your child with love and affection or throw yourself in front of a speeding truck to protect him. For some parents, this feeling takes hold within the first few days—or even minutes—of birth. For others, it takes weeks or months (and there's no shame in that). Like other relationships, your relationship with your baby takes time to grow.

BabyCenter Buzz

How I Felt about My Baby

"I didn't bond immediately with my son. Everything happened so fast, and before I knew it, they were taking him from me so I could get some rest. I don't think that I really bonded with him until after we got home and the haze cleared. Today I can't even imagine my life before my son. So don't worry about bonding with your baby; it will come naturally." —*Jessica*

"I wish someone had prepared me for the incredibly intense emotions I'd feel toward my baby. I never imagined I could feel such a range—from happiness and love to fear and worry" —*Bethany*

"Before I gave birth to my first child, my head was filled with thoughts of holding and cuddling my baby. However, after he was born, life was much less an oblivion of joy. I felt like the worst person alive when that bond failed to happen right away. Now he's 23 months old, and I enjoy him so much. Don't feel guilty if you're not one of those mothers you see on TV. Babies are a lot of work, and not having enough sleep and postpartum depression can put a lot of strain on you" —*Anonymous*

"I've never been especially fond of babies, so I was surprised at how quickly I fell in love with my own. The feeling is so overwhelming it can bring me to tears" —*Carrie*

There's no magic formula for bonding with your baby. A true parent-child bond is a by-product of everyday caregiving. Over time, as you get to know your baby and learn how to soothe him and enjoy his presence, your feelings will deepen. And one day—it may be the first time you see him smile—you'll look at your baby and realize you're utterly, ineffably filled with joy and love.

If after a few weeks you find that you don't feel more attached to and comfortable with your baby than you did right after he was born or if you actually feel detached and resentful of your newborn, talk to your baby's pediatrician and your own caregiver. These feelings are more common than you think, and they don't mean you're a bad mother or you don't love your child. You're just a *new* mother trying to adjust to a radical role change and enormous new responsibilities while you're sleep-deprived and fatigued. With a little help and time, you'll get the hang of it and feel closer to your child.

BREASTFEEDING: THE FIRST FEW WEEKS

Getting Started

The first time you hold your newborn, open your gown so his skin can touch yours, and put his lips to your breast. Don't panic if your newborn seems to have trouble finding or staying on your nipple—he may just lick your nipple at first. Most babies have an "alert period" for one or two hours after birth and, if given the chance, will eventually begin to nurse within the first hour or so. Don't be shy about asking your caregiver or nurse to help you get started while you're still in the birth room (or recovery room if you had a c-section).

Your milk hasn't come in yet, but your breasts are producing a substance called colostrum (often referred to as "liquid gold"), which will help protect your baby from infection. With frequent feedings, colostrum will provide all the nutrition your baby needs. But don't be surprised if your baby loses a little weight in the first three days. That's normal and expected with a breastfed baby, and he'll begin to gain weight thereafter.

Try not to get frustrated if breastfeeding isn't always easy in the early days. It's an art that requires patience and lots of practice. No one expects you to be an expert at breastfeeding your baby in the beginning. You may need to ask for help more than once until both you and your baby figure things out. Not all caregivers and nurses are equally adept at helping new moms learn to nurse, and everyone has a unique coaching style. If you've received help but are still struggling, ask if the hospital has a lactation consultant, and if one's not available, find out which postpartum nurses are especially good at helping with breastfeeding.

Getting Your Baby to Latch On

The secret to successful and pain-free breastfeeding is getting your baby to latch on to your breast correctly. How to do it:

- The best latch-on position is when your baby has more of the areola below your nipple in his mouth. To accomplish this, line up his nose with your nipple—that way his bottom gum will be far away from the base of your nipple when he opens his mouth.

- Your baby needs to take in a good mouthful of both your nipple and areola. Gently tickle his upper lip to get him to open his mouth wide; then move him to your breast with his chin (rather than nose) coming to your breast first.

- If one breastfeeding position isn't working, try another—lie side by side or hold your baby like a football (cradled under your arm with his feet behind you).

- Squeeze your breast to express a few drops of milk so your baby can taste it on your nipple. Once he realizes there's food there, he may grab on.

- If your baby is very upset, it can be hard to get him calmed down enough to correctly latch on. During these times, put your little finger (washed first, of course) nail side down in his mouth. Your baby will often suck on your finger a few times and calm down. As soon as he does, immediately move him over to your breast.

If you have a baby who initially needs special care, you may not be able to nurse him right away, but you should start pumping your milk for him. He'll get this milk through a tube or a bottle until he's strong enough to nurse. (The hospital will have an electric breast pump that you can use while you're there, and if you go home before your baby, you can rent a pump.)

For some women, breastfeeding can be uncomfortable or even painful at first. But don't suffer in silence. Pain is often an indicator that your baby isn't attached to your breast properly (known as latch-on). His mouth should cover a large part of your areola (the pigmented skin) around your nipple, and your nipple should be far back in your baby's mouth. If nursing hurts after your baby's first few sucks, break the suction by inserting your little finger between your baby's gums and your nipple—and try again until you find a position that's less painful.

Nurse your baby frequently—for his sake and yours. Breast milk is digested more quickly than formula, so your baby will get hungry more often than a formula-fed baby. Frequent feedings will also encourage your milk to

QUICK TIPS

Making Breastfeeding More Comfortable

- Because feedings can take up to 40 minutes, pick a comfortable spot for nursing. Atmosphere is important, especially in the early days of breastfeeding, when you're still learning. If you're easily distracted and disrupted by noise, go someplace quiet, or play soothing music at a low volume. Once breastfeeding is well established, you can nurse in front of the television, while talking on the phone, or any place you feel comfortable.

- Nurse your baby in a position that won't strain your arms and back. The best position is the cross-over or cross-cradle hold. If you're nursing from your right breast, use your left hand and arm to hold your baby. Rotate him so his chest and tummy are directly facing you. With your hands behind this head, guide him to your breast. Some find that lying side by side in bed works well. Others prefer the "football hold": Support your baby's head with your hand and tuck him under your arm on the same side as the breast you intend to nurse from.

- Consider buying a nursing pillow. These firm cushions, which wrap around your body, help support your baby and prevent back and arm strain.

- Put your feet on a small stool to help bring your baby closer to your breast.

- Breastfeeding makes you thirsty—so keep a large glass of water beside you.

come in more quickly and help ensure that there's plenty of milk for your baby. Plus, the more you nurse, the less likely you are to become painfully engorged. Nursing for 10 to 15 minutes per breast 8 to 12 times every 24 hours is pretty much on target. That's an average of every two or three hours, but sometimes your baby will be hungry after $1\frac{1}{2}$ hours and at other times the interval may be longer. But for the first few weeks of life, don't let your baby go any longer than three or four hours without nursing, even if you have to wake him up to eat.

You should nurse your newborn "on demand," meaning whenever he shows signs of hunger—such as increased alertness or activity, sucking motions, putting his hands in his mouth, or rooting around for your nipple. Don't wait until your baby starts crying to assume he's hungry; watch for the other cues first. Crying is a last resort for a hungry baby.

During the first few days, you may have to gently wake your baby to begin nursing, and he may fall asleep again midfeeding. If this happens, try unwrapping him and tickling his feet to get him going again. (If you feel like

Just the Facts

How to Tell if Your Baby's Getting Enough Milk

Most breastfed infants lose weight in their first few days of life—up to 7 percent of their birth weight—and that leads new moms to worry about whether they're producing enough milk. How to tell if your baby's getting enough:

- He's feeding at least eight times every 24 hours.

- He has a bowel movement at least once every 24 hours in the first few days of life, and by the third to fifth day he's passing three or four stools a day.

- By the time he's five days old, his stool looks mustard yellow and mushy, and he's having a minimum of two or three bowel movements a day.

- By the time he's three to five days old, he wets three to five diapers in a 24-hour period, and his urine is a pale yellow color.

- You hear swallowing sounds as he nurses.

- He starts gaining weight by the fifth day, putting on from a half to a full ounce per day. Your baby should be back to his birth weight by the end of week two.

Don't hesitate to call your baby's doctor if you have concerns about any of the above. Doctors who care for infants expect calls from new parents, and the American Academy of Pediatrics recommends that all breastfeeding newborns be seen by a healthcare provider at three to five days of age. The first few weeks with a newborn can be stressful, and your baby's caregiver is there to help you.

you don't have enough hands, ask your partner to help.) As your baby gets a bit older, he will (hopefully) get in the habit of feeding more often during the day and stretching things out at night.

How to Cope with Common Breastfeeding Problems

Engorgement

WHAT IT IS: As your milk production gets going in earnest (two or three days after you give birth), you may find that your breasts feel swollen, tender, throbbing, lumpy, and uncomfortably full. Increased blood and lymph fluid in your breasts that's not draining well also contributes to this problem. Sometimes the swelling can extend all the way to your armpit. You may run a low-grade fever, too, for a short time.

HOW LONG IT'LL LAST: The engorgement should subside within a day or two, and nursing your baby often is the single best thing you can do for relief. In fact, frequent nursing from the get-go can prevent engorgement. Once the engorgement passes, your breasts will be softer, although still full of milk.

HOW TO COPE:

• Nurse frequently—at least every two or three hours—even if it means waking your baby. (This is especially important because unrelieved engorgement can cause a serious drop in your milk production.) Try to get your baby to drain one breast well before offering the other side. If your baby is satisfied with just one breast, offer him the other breast at the next feeding. If not even one breast is drained well, consider pumping.

• Avoid having your baby latch on and suckle when your areola—the pigmented area around your nipple—is very firm. To reduce the possibility of nipple damage and to help your baby latch on correctly, before nursing your baby, manually express or pump a little milk until your areola softens. It may be easier to manually express milk in the shower; the warm water by itself may cause enough leakage to soften the areola. Or try placing a warm, wet washcloth on your areolas for a minute or two. (If your breasts are very engorged, a short cold treatment may work better.)

• Don't apply direct heat—such as a warm washcloth, a heating pad, or a hot-water bottle, to your engorged breasts except to soften the areola just before nursing and help your milk let down. Too much heat can make the swelling and pain worse.

• While your baby's nursing, gently massage the breast he's on. This encourages your milk to flow and will help relieve some of the tightness and discomfort you feel.

• To soothe pain and help ease swelling, apply cold packs to your breasts for about 15 to 20 minutes after your baby finishes a nursing session. Crushed ice in a plastic bag works well, though a bag of frozen vegetables or a gel pack (some are made for nursing moms) may be easier. Cover the ice pack or gel pack with a cloth to prevent ice burns on your skin.

• Some women believe that applying fresh green cabbage leaves to engorged breasts is the best way to ease symptoms (though a study comparing cabbage leaves with gel packs for the relief of engorgement found no difference between the two methods). If the cabbage leaf treatment appeals to you, here's how to do it: Strip the main vein from two large, outer leaves and cut a hole in each one for your nipple. Rinse and dry them before laying them on your breasts or sliding them into your bra cups.

• Wear a supportive—but not tight—nursing bra, even at night.

• If you're really in pain, take ibuprofen, acetaminophen, or a mild pain reliever prescribed by your healthcare provider.

• Let your caregiver know any time you have a fever during the postpartum period, even if you think it's likely just engorgement.

Leaking

WHAT IT IS: Leaking or spraying breasts are a natural, though sometimes embarrassing, part of breastfeeding. Some women never leak milk, while others leak a little from one breast during almost every feeding and when their milk lets down. Women with an especially bountiful milk supply can soak through a shirt or even emit a stream of milk that sprays across the room when their baby unlatches. Leaking tends to happen most in the mornings, when your breasts are the fullest. Some women experience leaking if they are late with or miss a feeding, think about their baby, or hear another baby cry.

HOW LONG IT'LL LAST: Many women find that the problem goes away almost completely over the first six to ten weeks of breastfeeding while others contend with it as long as they nurse their babies.

HOW TO COPE:

• Wear washable or disposable nursing pads inside your bra, but make sure you change them when they get damp, so bacteria can't breed on your nipples. Avoid pads with plastic liners; they can trap in moisture.

• When you're out and about, either with or without your baby, carry an extra top, bra, and nursing pads.

• Wear prints and fabrics (absorbent cotton versus delicate silk) that camouflage milk stains.

• If you feel your milk let down at an inopportune moment, cross your arms and hug yourself, pressing gently against your breasts. This may stop the flow of milk.

Sore or Cracked Nipples

WHAT THEY ARE: Breastfeeding can make your nipples sore, and some women even experience cracked or bleeding nipples. The main cause of cracked or bleeding nipples is positioning your baby at the wrong angle to your breast. Sometimes just the slightest correction of positioning will make a world of difference. Other possible, but less likely causes, include an easily treated yeast infection in your nipples, possibly from yeast in your baby's mouth (thrush), or incorrect use of a breast pump.

HOW LONG THEY'LL LAST: If you take steps to heal your nipples, you should start feeling better within two or three days.

HOW TO COPE:

• Check your baby's positioning. She should face your breast, tummy to tummy with you. When your baby starts suckling, your nipple should be far back in her mouth. (If you need help with proper positioning, see the latch-on tips above, or contact a lactation consultant.)

• To remove your baby from your breast, *always* break the suction by inserting your finger into the corner of your baby's mouth. Never pull her off.

• Change positions at every feeding so your baby's gums exert pressure on a different area of your breast each time.

• Offer your baby the less sore nipple first to stimulate letdown; then you can start nursing on the sorer breast.

• Nurse more frequently, but for shorter periods. The longer you go between feedings, the hungrier your baby will be—and the harder he'll nurse.

• You may want to limit comfort nursing by swaddling, rocking, or walking with your baby until the soreness has passed.

• Try rubbing a little medical-grade modified lanolin (such as Lansinoh) on your nipples. Unlike other ointments, it doesn't need to be washed off before feedings. (Note that rubbing breast milk on your nipples does not help healing and may even exacerbate the problem.)

• Don't use soap, alcohol, lotions, or perfumes on your nipples because they can be drying. And except for medical-grade lanolin, whatever you put on needs to be washed off before nursing. Frequent washing can cause further irritation. Bathing with warm water is all it takes to keep your breasts and nipples clean.

• Don't use nursing pads with plastic liners, and change them when they become moist. If a nursing pad sticks to your nipple, don't pull it. Instead, wet the pad with water until it slips off easily.

• Avoid wearing bras with seams, lace, or trim that irritates your nipples.

• Expose your nipples to the air as much as possible.

• Take pain relievers. If the pain is severe, you can take acetaminophen or ibuprofen a half-hour before nursing.

• Call a lactation consultant. These professionals are trained to help with a wide range of breastfeeding problems. If you can't afford a lactation consultant, La Leche League hosts a toll-free breastfeeding hotline at (800) 525-3243.

• Check with your or your baby's caregiver if a crack or wound on your nipple shows no sign of healing or you think yeast is the cause. Symptoms of a yeast infection include very red and cracked nipples, nipples that itch or burn, and sharp, stabbing pains when your baby suckles. If your baby has yeast, you might see white patches in his mouth (thrush) or he may have a bright red diaper rash.

Mastitis

WHAT IT IS: Mastitis is a breast infection. The usual cause is a plugged milk duct that becomes infected with bacteria (and you're even more susceptible if you have cracked nipples). That's why it's best to try to unplug a duct *before* it becomes infected. If you have a plugged duct, you'll feel a small, hard, tender lump in your breast. To drain it, feed your baby frequently from the affected breast. Before nursing, wash your hands and apply warm compresses to the lump. While your baby's feeding, massage the area. Let your baby nurse as long as he's willing. If your breast still contains milk after your baby's finished nursing, pump or manually express what's left. It's also important get plenty of rest and eat a healthy, balanced diet. The more run-down you are, the more susceptible you'll be to infection.

Mastitis can come on gradually or suddenly. If you notice any of these symptoms, call your practitioner right away.

QUICK TIPS

What to Do If You're *Not* Breastfeeding

If you've decided not to nurse your baby, it'll take a week or two for your milk to dry up. How to manage the process:

- Use a manual breast pump to extract *just* enough milk to relieve discomfort when your breasts are full. Full breasts send your body a signal to decrease milk production, whereas empty breasts stimulate more milk production.

- Wear a snug bra.

- Put cold packs on your breasts to help ease swelling. (Cover the cold packs with cloth so you don't hurt your skin.)

- Try this old folk remedy: Place clean, cold cabbage leaves over your breasts inside your bra. There's no solid evidence that cabbage leaves will decrease your milk supply, but it can't hurt to try.

- Ask your provider about taking an over-the-counter pain reliever if you need one.

- If you notice any signs of infection (pain, fever, redness), call your practitioner right away.

- Intense pain in one or both breasts
- A red, hot, or swollen breast or a hard, tender, reddened area, or red streaks on your breast (mastitis usually happens in one breast at a time)
- Flulike symptoms, such as muscle aches, headache, and fatigue
- Fever and chills

HOW LONG IT'LL LAST: If you get antibiotics right away, you should start feeling better in about 48 hours. *Note:* You need to take the full course of antibiotics—even after your symptoms go away—or the infection will recur.

HOW TO COPE:

- Call your caregiver right away if you have signs of an infection. Untreated mastitis can lead to the development of a breast abscess—a serious problem that usually requires surgery to treat.

- Ask your practitioner about using ibuprofen. It can bring down your fever and reduce pain and inflammation.

- Nurse through the pain. Your baby needs to feed frequently to keep your milk flowing and to avoid further blockage. Mastitis will not affect your baby.

- Try warm compresses on your breasts for several minutes before each feeding—this should help your letdown reflex and make nursing more tolerable.

- If your baby doesn't empty the infected breast during each feeding, finish the job yourself with a breast pump.

- If nursing is truly unbearable, try pumping your breasts and giving the milk to your baby in a bottle. But don't rely on this solely to get you through the infection because your baby can empty your breasts more effectively than any device.

• Get plenty of rest.

• Call your caregiver if your symptoms don't improve within a day or two of starting antibiotics or you notice any puslike discharge from your nipple.

PART VI

SPECIAL SITUATIONS

Your chances of having a trouble-free pregnancy are better than ever, thanks to the advances of modern medicine. Even so, an illness, an infection, or a pregnancy-related complication can pose special problems that may require extra care. In this section, you'll learn how pregnancy affects common conditions (and vice versa), how to safely manage your symptoms when a baby's on the way, and how to cope if complications arise.

Special Situation:
Tips for Coping with a Chronic Condition

If you begin pregnancy with a condition such as asthma or epilepsy, you'll need to pay special attention to your own health and the medication you're taking:

▶ Prenatal care is especially important when you have a preexisting condition—so schedule your first prenatal visit as early as possible.

▶ Make sure your regular healthcare provider (or the specialist you see for your condition) knows that you're pregnant and works closely with your midwife or doctor.

▶ Let your caregiver know about any complications you've had in past pregnancies.

▶ *Do* call your caregiver immediately to be sure any medication you're on is safe during pregnancy.

▶ *Don't* stop taking prescription meds without your health team's okay.

▶ Carefully follow any special instructions your caregiver gives you—such as tightly controlling your blood sugar if you have diabetes.

▶ Call your caregiver right away if you notice signs that your condition is getting worse.

▶ You're not alone! Online support groups (page 586) can help you cope. And if you're feeling especially fearful or overwhelmed, seek professional counseling.

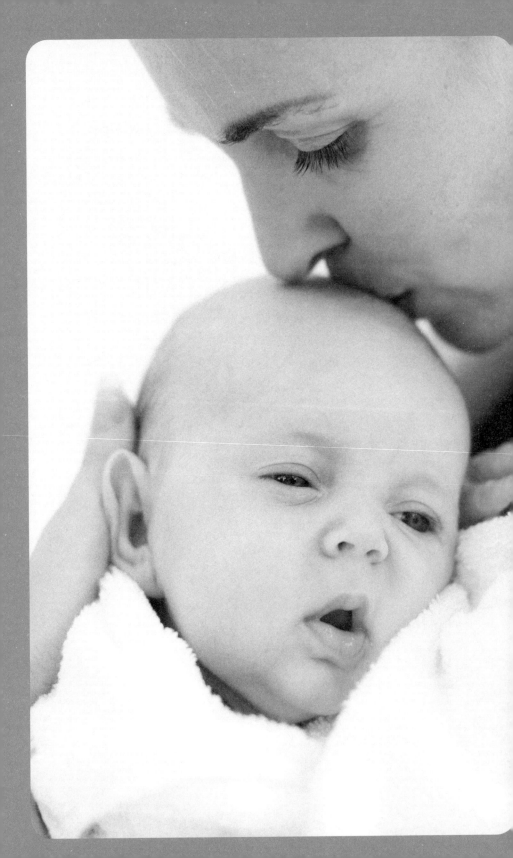

CHRONIC
CONDITIONS

If you're coping with a chronic health condition, you undoubtedly have questions and concerns about how your condition and treatment will affect your developing baby—and, in turn, how pregnancy will affect *your* health. The good news is that most chronic medical problems, when carefully managed, don't stand in the way of having a healthy baby.

Allergies

If you have allergies, work with your caregiver to identify their source (pet dander, pollen, dust, or smoke, for instance), and then avoid exposure to it whenever you can to lessen your need for medication. If you need medicine, there are some antihistamines that you can safely continue taking to relieve allergy symptoms, including runny nose, itchy eyes, and congestion. If you can't get by without antihistamines in the first trimester, many experts recommend sticking to chlorpheniramine (Chlor-Trimeton) or diphenhydramine (Benadryl) because they've been around for a long time and are generally considered safe. (Be aware, though, that unlike the newer, nonsedating antihistamines, chlorpheniramine can make you drowsy, so you'll need to plan ahead before performing activities—like driving—that require you to be alert.) Newer antihistamines such as Claritin or Allegra *may* be safe, but they haven't been around long enough for anyone to know for sure. Most experts suggest avoiding them altogether in the first trimester. If you're in your second or third trimester and have severe allergies—and chlorpheniramine isn't working for you—talk to your practitioner about the pros and cons of using these newer medications.

Asthma

Asthma is the most common lung problem in pregnancy—and one that you should continue to treat when you're expecting. Why? If you keep your asthma under control, you'll dramatically lower your risk for asthma-related problems such as premature delivery or preeclampsia, or having a low-birthweight baby. Luckily, there are a number of asthma drugs that are considered safe for you now.

Pregnancy itself affects asthma in different ways. About a third of asthmatic women find that their condition gets worse during pregnancy; another third find that it gets better; and the final third notice no change. (And some women get asthma for the first time during pregnancy.) Depending on how you're doing, your medication may need to be changed or the dosage adjusted during the course of your pregnancy. You should also get a detailed plan from your caregiver about what to do when symptoms flare up, when to call her, and when to seek immediate care at the emergency room. If you have severe asthma—whether you had a severe case before you got pregnant or it becomes severe during pregnancy—your caregiver may refer you to a high-risk pregnancy specialist.

Diabetes

Having preexisting diabetes carries increased risks for you and your baby. The good news is that diabetes is one of the best examples of how controlling a chronic disease can make a huge difference in your pregnancy's outcome. Carefully managing your diet and insulin dosage, checking your glucose levels frequently, and getting good care before and during pregnancy will maximize your chances of delivering a healthy baby.

On the whole, women with pregestational diabetes are several times more likely to give birth to babies with birth defects and are at higher risk for miscarriage. But since experts think that this is largely due to high blood sugar levels at conception and in early pregnancy, you can substantially lower your risk by making sure your blood sugar is in good control before you get pregnant—and keeping it well controlled after you conceive. (If you have type 2 diabetes and are planning pregnancy, you'll be switched to insulin while you're trying to conceive and kept on it for the duration of your pregnancy.) Uncontrolled blood sugar during pregnancy increases your risk of other problems, too—including stillbirth, too much amniotic fluid, problems associated with delivering an excessively large baby, and complications for your baby after birth.

If you have underlying diabetes-related cardiovascular or kidney disease, you're also at higher risk for developing preeclampsia. And your baby may suffer from intrauterine growth restriction if you have an advanced form of the disease.

The best thing you can do for your baby and yourself is to work closely with your medical team. Expert care, combined with closely following your doctor's plan (for instance, you'll need more insulin as your pregnancy pro-

BabyCenter Buzz

Keeping Diabetes under Control during My Pregnancy

"I've found that eating a protein snack with a low-glycemic carb keeps me full. Also, I make sure to eat regularly—every two to three hours—and never skip meals, especially breakfast. When I do eat carbs, I make sure to eat protein and fat with them and never exceed 30 grams of carbs per meal." —*Anonymous*

"I've been diabetic for ten years. I keep my proteins up and my carbs and sugars down, and exercise at least three days a week. I also try not to get too stressed, and to pamper myself more." —*Lynette*

gresses, especially in your third trimester) will give you every chance of delivering a perfectly healthy baby.

Epilepsy

First, the good news: More than 90 percent of women with epilepsy have healthy babies. Still, there are serious risks associated with this condition, and you'll need to work closely with your neurologist and your obstetrician (the two of them should be talking to each other, too) to minimize the chance of complications.

On average, women with epilepsy have a 4 to 6 percent risk of having a baby with a birth defect (about two to three times higher than normal). Experts think this is largely due to the effects of antiepileptic drugs. The risk also varies by the type of medication you're taking, the dosage needed to control your seizures, and how many different drugs you're taking (taking more than one antiepileptic drug poses a greater risk).

Ideally, you should discuss with your neurologist your desire to become a mother *before* getting pregnant so she can consider medication changes and have plenty of time to see how you adjust to them before you conceive. If your pregnancy is unplanned, though, it's absolutely vital to contact your doctor as soon as you know you're pregnant and—unless you're advised otherwise—to continue to take your medicine exactly as before. Otherwise, you risk having uncontrolled seizures, which could cause you harm and affect your baby as well.

You may have more seizures than usual when you're pregnant—25 to 33 percent of epileptic women have an increased number of seizures during pregnancy (the likelihood is highest during labor and delivery). The extent to which you're at greater risk than nonepileptic women for problems like miscarriage, high blood pressure, and preterm birth is a matter of debate, but the vast majority of epileptic women don't have any added complications.

BY THE NUMBERS

Epilepsy Stats

Women and girls with seizure disorders in the United States:
more than 1 million

Epileptic women who deliver perfectly healthy babies:
more than 9 out of 10

Source: *Epilepsy Foundation*

Because some antiepileptic drugs (AEDs) can deplete the folate in your body, you need to take a daily prenatal vitamin with folic acid to reduce the chance of birth defects such as spina bifida. You may also be advised to take vitamin K supplements after week 36 to lower the odds that your baby will get a blood-clotting disorder caused by an epilepsy-med-induced vitamin K deficiency. Finally, besides carefully following your medical team's plan for your care, do your best to avoid things, such as sleep deprivation and stress, that can trigger seizures.

Hypertension

Chronic hypertension is high blood pressure that existed before pregnancy (or, if you don't know what your blood pressure was before you got pregnant, high blood pressure that occurs before week 20). If you have chronic hypertension—particularly very high blood pressure or long-standing hypertension

BabyCenter Buzz

Managing High Blood Pressure during My Pregnancy

"My blood pressure was 160/90 when I got pregnant. I'm in week 35 now, and my BP is 125/80 without meds. I started going for a walk every day. I cut down on my salt and junk food intake and started drinking lots of water. It's working!" —*Norma*

"I was put on medication in week 8. I take 250 milligrams of Aldomet three times a day and am being watching pretty closely. Now that I'm at week 35, I'm breathing a little easier that the baby is doing well." —*Peg*

"I have hypertension and had a good pregnancy. The doctor did change my regular meds to something safer. After week 32, I had to go in every week for fetal monitoring to make sure the baby was doing well. I didn't mind that part because I could see my baby every week. I was induced about two weeks before my due date, but that was no biggie. My baby and I are doing great. I was fortunate to have good doctors taking care of me." —*Dee*

"I had hypertension prior to getting pregnant. I had a wonderful pregnancy, never developed preeclampsia, and carried my baby to term. I was scared because I never knew anyone in my situation, and I'd only read how many things can go *wrong*. But I ate a healthy diet, drank a lot of water, and followed my doctor's orders—and everything turned out fine. I'm even hoping to get pregnant again in a few months!" —*Lori*

with kidney disease or other medical conditions—you're at increased risk for a number of pregnancy complications, including preeclampsia, intrauterine growth restriction, preterm birth, placental abruption, and stillbirth.

To decrease your risk of problems, it's especially important to get *early* prenatal care (preconception care is ideal). If you have severe hypertension, you'll need to continue taking blood pressure medication during your pregnancy, though your doctor may need to switch your usual medication to one that's safer for your baby. (It's important to keep taking your medication because severe uncontrolled hypertension can be life-threatening.) But if you have only mild chronic hypertension, your caregiver probably won't recommend that you take medication to control your blood pressure while you're pregnant (unless your pressure starts to get too high) because most studies show that it's not beneficial.

It's important to keep all your prenatal appointments so your caregiver can spot any developing problems, like rising blood pressure, signs of preeclampsia, or poor fetal growth. You'll likely have extra blood and urine tests to monitor how you're doing and, on top of a routine midpregnancy ultrasound, additional ultrasounds in your third trimester to monitor your baby's growth. If he doesn't seem to be growing well or if you have severe hypertension, you'll have regular fetal testing (nonstress tests or biophysical profiles) as well, and you may be induced before your due date.

Talk to your caregiver about your diet and salt intake, and find out when you should start doing fetal kick counts. And if you're a smoker, be sure to ask her where to get help quitting; smoking is a risky habit in any case, but even more so for women with chronic hypertension—and their babies.

Lupus

Systemic lupus erythematosus (SLE) is an autoimmune disease that can range from mild to severe—affecting only a few or many parts of your body—and can cause a host of symptoms, including inflammation, achiness, swollen and tender joints, rashes, extreme fatigue, and fever. In severe cases, it can cause injury to your organs. The course of SLE is unpredictable. You can have periods when the disease is active and you have lots of symptoms (so-called flares) and other times when you're in remission and have few or no symptoms.

It's particularly dangerous for women with severe SLE (when it affects the kidneys) to get pregnant because the risks for them and their babies are too high. If you have milder SLE, you can have a successful pregnancy, though your doctors will monitor you and your baby closely because the disease increases your risk of serious pregnancy complications. If you were in remission for six months or more before conceiving, your chances of doing well are even better.

Ideally, you should be seeing a perinatologist—a high-risk pregnancy specialist—who's experienced at caring for women with lupus. (She'll confer with your rheumatologist, too.) You'll have more prenatal visits than usual and have more than the usual blood and urine tests to detect any problems. The medications you take during pregnancy will be customized according to your symptoms, what's worked for you in the past, and which drugs are safe to continue taking during your pregnancy.

Your medical team will closely monitor your baby, too. To make sure he's growing and developing the way he should, you'll have periodic ultra-

BabyCenter Buzz

Managing Lupus during My Pregnancy

"I'm in my third trimester, and so far I've only had swollen joints and muscle pain—nothing else." —*Anonymous*

"I haven't had a flare in over five years. The trick is thinking positively, getting a lot of rest, eating properly, and *no* stress." —*Anonymous*

"I'm 21 weeks pregnant with SLE. I'm scared of preterm labor. I'm also having increasing problems with pain in my pelvis and I can barely walk sometimes. I commute four hours a day to work, and I highly doubt that I can continue after this month. I've had many flares, and I don't want one during this pregnancy." —*Carol*

"Part of keeping my lupus in control is knowing when to slow down. I was going to school full-time when I was pregnant with my second child, but taking things slow and having a wonderful husband have made a world of difference for me." —*Anonymous*

"My doctors discovered that I had lupus during my first pregnancy and warned me about the risk of miscarriage or of my baby being born with a heart problem. My son is now 2 years old and as healthy and happy as can be. I'm pregnant with my second child now, and so far everything's going well." —*Edith*

BY THE NUMBERS

Lupus Stats

Women with lupus in the
United States:
more than 1 million

Women with lupus whose
pregnancies are completely
normal: **more than half**

Women with lupus who
deliver prematurely: **1 in 4**

Pregnancies that are lost due
to lupus: **fewer than 1 in 5**

Source: *Lupus Foundation of America*

sounds throughout your pregnancy and other fetal testing, such as nonstress testing and a biophysical profile in your third trimester.

It's especially important to take good care of yourself during pregnancy. Try to eat a healthy diet, avoid triggers like sunlight—which may cause skin flare-ups—take time to rest, and try to keep stress at a minimum. Exercise can also help—just be sure to talk to your practitioner about your fitness plans before you start working out.

Migraines

Migraine headaches are thought to occur when the blood vessels in your brain constrict and then dilate. Most people describe them as a severe, throbbing pain (usually on just one side of your head) that's often accompanied by nausea and vomiting. About one in five women has migraines at some point in her life, and about one in seven migraine sufferers gets them for the first time during pregnancy, usually in the first trimester.

First the good news: Up to 70 percent of migraine sufferers find that the pain improves dramatically during pregnancy—and in some cases it disappears altogether, generally in the second or third trimester. (This is more likely if you're someone whose migraines tend to be worse around your periods or started when you began menstruating.) And even if you're part of the unlucky minority whose migraines *don't* improve during pregnancy, you can at least take some solace in the fact that migraine sufferers (and their babies) are at no higher risk than other women for pregnancy complications.

Now the bad news: Many of the medications that are most effective at preventing and treating migraines are off-limits during pregnancy. So if you're taking migraine medication, you may need to stop now that you're pregnant. It's important to check with your caregiver right away about the safety of specific medications. You can take acetaminophen for pain, and ibuprofen for short periods (with your caregiver's consent, of course), though

Just the Facts

Migraine Triggers

Some women can pinpoint the things that trigger their migraines and take steps to avoid them in an effort to cut down on the number of attacks. Try keeping a headache diary to see if you can figure out your personal triggers. Include what you've eaten in the 24 hours leading up to the attack. Everyone's sensitivities are different, but some possible triggers—and prevention strategies—include:

Changes in blood sugar. Eat small, frequent meals, and avoid simple carbohydrates like refined sugars.

Specific foods. Steer clear of foods that contain monosodium glutamate (MSG), nitrites (common in processed meats like hot dogs and bacon), sulfites (used as a preservative for salads and also found in many dried fruits), and artificial sweeteners. Other foods that may provoke migraines include certain beans, nuts, aged cheese and cultured dairy products, fresh fruits (bananas, papayas, avocados, and citrus), smoked fish, chocolate and carob, and things that are fermented or pickled (like soy sauce or sauerkraut).

Fatigue. Keep to a regular sleep schedule so you get the rest you need.

Stress. Try relaxation techniques like yoga or meditation. Biofeedback may help, too. And regular exercise can decrease the frequency and severity of migraines—though you'll need to start slowly because a sudden burst of activity might trigger a migraine.

Strong sensory stimuli. Avoid glaring or flickering lights and loud noises. Excessive heat or cold or even strong odors can trigger migraines, too.

Tobacco smoke. Don't smoke, and avoid secondhand smoke whenever possible.

you'll need to avoid ibuprofen completely after 32 weeks. For severe headaches, your practitioner may prescribe acetaminophen with codeine, but use it sparingly. If you're having frequent, debilitating migraines, the benefits of medication may outweigh any possible risks to your baby, so be sure to ask your caregiver about your options.

Though most headaches during pregnancy are unpleasant but harmless, they can signal a more serious problem. If you're having a migraine for the first time ever, you'll need a full medical evaluation to be sure nothing else is going on. And in your second or third trimester, a severe or persistent headache could be a symptom of preeclampsia, so it should prompt a call to your caregiver.

Try these tips for weathering the worst of migraine symptoms when they strike:

- Apply cold compresses to the affected area. A cold shower may help, too.
- Try massaging your temples.
- Avoid strenuous activity—rest in a dark, quiet room, and try to sleep off your migraine.
- If you've vomited, sip fluids so you don't get dehydrated.

Multiple Sclerosis

Years ago, experts believed that pregnancy worsened the symptoms of multiple sclerosis (MS), a disease of the central nervous system that typically strikes women in their childbearing years. But the evidence now shows that the opposite is true. Worsening MS is *less* common during pregnancy, especially in the second and third trimesters, and being pregnant doesn't cause any increase in long-term disability from MS (and may in fact even improve your outlook).

You can also take comfort in knowing that most women with MS don't have an increased risk of any major pregnancy complications (though you may be more prone to urinary tract infections) and that the disease won't affect your developing baby.

One thing you should be aware of, though: There *is* a temporarily increased risk of MS flare-ups in the first few months after you give birth. While this doesn't seem to contribute to long-term problems, you should plan to have extra help available in case you have a relapse after your baby is born.

Many MS drugs need to be stopped before you get pregnant—in some cases a few months before. But there are other medications, like prednisone, that can safely be used if you get a flare-up during pregnancy. In any case, make sure your pregnancy practitioner and your neurologist work together to monitor your progress. And try to get plenty of rest, eat a healthy diet, keep stress in check, and get some regular, gentle exercise.

Thyroid Disease

The thyroid is a butterfly-shaped organ in your neck, under your Adam's apple. It's responsible for the production of thyroid hormone, which plays a vital role in regulating your metabolism and affects almost every system in your body.

Hypothyroidism

If your gland is underactive and you don't produce enough thyroid hormone (a condition called hy*p*othyroidism), you may experience fatigue, cold intolerance, constipation, dry skin, muscle cramps, weight gain, and other symptoms. But if your thyroid is only mildly underactive, you may not have any obvious symptoms at all. That's why experts think that women at higher risk for hypothyroidism—those whose family members have thyroid disease and those who have other autoimmune diseases like diabetes or lupus—should be tested regularly. (And some experts think all women should be tested.)

If you have hypothyroidism and it isn't properly treated, you may run a higher risk of miscarriage, preeclampsia, placental abruption, having a low-birthweight baby, or stillbirth. The good news is that hypothyroidism is easily managed with levothyroxine, a synthetic form of thyroid hormone that's totally safe for you and your baby (it's simply replacing the hormone that your body should be producing on its own). It's best to take this med-

> **BY THE NUMBERS**
>
> **Thyroid Disease Stats**
>
> Pregnant women with thyroid disorders: **1 in 50**
>
> Source: *March of Dimes*

BabyCenter Buzz

Managing My Underactive Thyroid during Pregnancy

"I took Synthroid throughout my pregnancy with no problems at all. I just gave birth to a beautiful, healthy baby girl. She's perfect!"   —*Juli*

"I was diagnosed with hypothyroidism two years ago and was able to conceive the old-fashioned way. My thyroid-stimulating hormone (TSH) levels were checked in the first month, and then every four to six weeks for the rest of my pregnancy. The goal was to keep them the same as they were before conception, so my medication dosage had to be adjusted slightly a couple of times. My pregnancy was easy, and my baby is a healthy, amazing little boy!"   —*Anonymous*

"I've had thyroid problems for six years. Once I became pregnant, my doctor told me that it was actually more dangerous to *not* take my medicine. I stuck with my meds, and my son came out fine!"   —*Lissa*

BabyCenter Buzz

Managing My Overactive Thyroid during Pregnancy

"I developed hyperthyroidism when I was six weeks pregnant. I had an endocrinologist and a cardiologist by my side for the next 34 weeks. I took medicine and was put on bed rest for my entire pregnancy. Both helped stabilize my TSH levels and lowered my heart rate." —*Anonymous*

"My TSH levels were around 19.3 when I unexpectedly got pregnant. Most of my doctors advised me to abort, but I refused. I switched doctors and started taking medication, which I was warned could cause birth defects. When my daughter was born, the doctors were amazed—she had absolutely no problems." —*Shazail*

"It's important to get your levels tested and demand treatment if you need it. During my pregnancy, I was started on a small dose of PTU, and I was careful to pay extra-close attention to my symptoms." —*Danna*

ication on an empty stomach, and you shouldn't take your prenatal vitamins (or iron or calcium supplements) until a few hours later because they'll interfere with your absorption of the levothyroxine. Your medication needs increase very early in pregnancy and you'll need to have enough hormone to ensure that your baby develops properly, so discuss your dosage with your practitioner as soon as your pregnancy is confirmed. You'll get an initial blood test that will be repeated every four to six weeks in the first half of pregnancy, and then once or twice after that.

Hyperthyroidism

If, on the other hand, your thyroid is overactive (hyperthyroidism)—meaning that it produces too much thyroid hormone—it can cause anxiety, increased heart rate and palpitations, high blood pressure, tremors, sweating and heat intolerance, and weight loss, among other symptoms.

Untreated hyperthyroidism increases your risk for preeclampsia, preterm birth, having a low-birthweight baby, and even late-term pregnancy loss. (And there's some evidence suggesting that it may increase the risk of birth defects as well.) If you need to take medication to control your condition, you'll be given an antithyroid drug like propylthiouracil (PTU)—and get blood tests on a regular basis to check your hormone levels. Your practitioner will closely monitor your baby before and after birth because the medication can temporarily shut down your baby's own thyroid function.

INFECTIONS TO WATCH OUT FOR

A run-of-the-mill cold or stomach bug is nothing to worry about, but there are some illnesses you'll want to do your best to steer clear of during your pregnancy. Your chance of contracting most of these infections is very, very small—and the chance of your baby's being harmed by them is even smaller. Still, let your caregiver know right away if you think you may have been exposed to or have symptoms of any of the following infections. In many cases, early treatment can reduce or eliminate the risk of passing the infection on to your baby.

Bacterial Vaginosis (BV)

This genital tract infection—caused by an overgrowth of certain types of bacteria that normally live in small numbers in your vagina—is the most common vaginal infection. BV increases your susceptibility to sexually transmitted infections (STIs) like chlamydia, gonorrhea, and HIV, if you're exposed to them, and has also been linked to an increased risk of preterm labor and preterm rupture of the amniotic membranes surrounding and protecting your baby.

You may or may not have symptoms with BV. If you do, you might notice a thin milky white or gray discharge with a foul or fishy smell (this odor is most apparent after sex, when the discharge mixes with semen)—though at least half of women with BV have no symptoms at all. BV is easily treated with antibiotics, but it's unclear how effective this is at preventing preterm labor. Unless you have symptoms, your healthcare practitioner won't screen you.

Avoiding BV
Because the cause of bacterial vaginosis is still a bit of a mystery (though women who have multiple sex partners, who douche, or possibly who use IUDs seem to be at higher risk), there's nothing definitive you can do to prevent the infection. Still, you can reduce your risk and prevent complications from BV by:

• Following safer-sex practices if you're not in a mutually monogamous relationship
• Not douching and not using feminine hygiene sprays or scented soaps on your genitals
• Letting your practitioner know if you have any unusual vaginal discharge or irritation

Chicken Pox

If you were raised in the United States, you're likely already immune to chicken pox because you probably had the infection as a child (you can have a quick blood test done at your first prenatal checkup if you're not sure). But if you're not immune and you come down with chicken pox in the first half of your pregnancy, you'll run a very small risk (1 to 2 percent) of miscarrying or of giving birth to a baby with scarred skin, eye problems, limb defects, or other health issues. Fortunately, the vast majority of babies whose mothers have chicken pox during pregnancy escape these problems.

If you get chicken pox in the second half of your pregnancy (but more than five days before giving birth) your baby will likely be fine. Here's why: About five days after coming down with the virus that causes chicken pox, your body develops antibodies to it and passes them on to your baby, providing protection that his own immature immune system can't. He might get chicken pox shortly after birth, but it's much less likely to be serious.

If you get chicken pox within five days before giving birth (or within two days after delivery), though, your baby won't have time to get antibodies from you. If this happens, there's a chance that he'll develop a severe case of newborn chicken pox, which can be very serious. Fortunately, the danger can be greatly reduced by giving your baby, shortly after birth, a shot of varicella-zoster immune globulin (VZIG), which contains chicken pox antibodies.

Avoiding Chicken Pox

If you're not already immune, here's how to protect yourself:

- Stay away from anyone who has flulike symptoms (people are contagious up to 48 hours before they get the telltale rash) or who has chicken pox sores that haven't yet crusted over, and anyone who's never had chicken pox but has been exposed to the infection within the past three weeks.

- If you've been exposed to chicken pox, let your doctor or midwife know right away. Getting a shot of VZIG within four days will decrease your risk of a severe infection and dangerous complications like chicken pox pneumonia (though, unfortunately, it may not decrease your baby's risk of infection).

- Steer clear of anyone with shingles (a severe, reactivated form of chicken pox). Shingles usually affects older adults and people with weakened immune systems. You can't catch shingles from them, but you can catch chicken pox.

- Ask your caregiver if she thinks the healthy members of your household who aren't already immune should get vaccinated against chicken pox, especially if they've recently been exposed, because this will lower the odds of their catching the infection and then passing it along to you.

BY THE NUMBERS

Chicken Pox Stats

Women who are already immune to chicken pox:
as many as 9 in 10

Women who contract chicken pox during pregnancy:
fewer than 1 in 1,000

Source: *March of Dimes*

Cytomegalovirus (CMV)

CMV is a member of the herpes virus family. CMV can be spread by contact with an infected person's bodily fluids, such as saliva, urine, feces, semen, vaginal secretions, blood, tears, and breast milk. You can get it from direct contact like mouth-to-mouth kissing or sharing eating utensils, by touching an infected fluid and then touching your mouth or nose, or by having sex with an infected person. An infected woman can transmit the virus to her baby in several ways: through the placenta during pregnancy, when her baby comes in contact with infected fluids at birth, or through infected breast milk after delivery. (Fortunately, most babies who contract CMV during birth or from breast milk develop few or no symptoms, so vaginal delivery and breastfeeding aren't considered risky for women with CMV.)

Like other herpes viruses, CMV remains dormant in your body after your initial infection. So despite the presence of CMV antibodies, the virus can periodically become reactivated, resulting in what's known as a recurrent CMV infection. Fortunately, the risk of passing the virus to your baby during a recurrent infection is very low, and the risk of serious complications is even lower. If you already had the virus before you conceived (one-half to four-fifths of all pregnant women have), CMV poses only a very small risk to you and your baby.

If you get CMV for the first time while you're pregnant, though, your chance of passing the infection to your baby is much higher, and your baby, in turn, has a much higher chance of developing serious complications. The most severely affected babies (5 to 18 percent) have physical abnormalities that are apparent at birth, and later these babies may also suffer from hearing loss, mental retardation, and other developmental problems. Even infected babies who seem healthy at birth can develop problems later—most commonly hearing loss, which affects 10 to 15 percent of these babies.

A new CMV infection is hard to recognize because most people don't develop any symptoms. Those who do tend to notice flulike symptoms such as fever, chills, swollen glands, fatigue, and achiness. If you suspect you've recently been exposed to CMV, though, let your practitioner know so you can get a series of blood tests to make the diagnosis. If the tests show that you've had a recent infection, you'll get a thorough sonogram to look for problems in your developing baby. You may also have amniocentesis to see if your baby is infected, though the test doesn't pick up all cases of congenital CMV and won't be able to tell if your baby is mildly or severely infected. Unfortunately, there's no treatment for CMV (though a vaccine is in the works).

Avoiding CMV

• Be careful when handling items such as diapers or tissues that may contain others' bodily fluids, and wash your hands thoroughly after disposing of them. (Daycare workers are at especially high risk for CMV and should use disposable latex gloves when changing diapers and be sure to wash their hands immediately afterward.)

• Don't share food, eating utensils, or drinking glasses.

• Practice safer sex if you aren't in a mutually monogamous relationship; use latex condoms, and avoid oral sex.

Fifth Disease

Chances are 50-50 that you've already had fifth disease (caused by parvovirus B19), also known as "slapped cheek disease," and are immune to the virus that causes it. But even if you're not immune and contract it while you're pregnant, your baby will most likely be fine. Still, the virus can be transmitted to your baby and in a relatively small number of cases results in severe fetal anemia, miscarriage, or fetal death. (The risk is higher if you get the virus in the first half of your pregnancy.)

In otherwise healthy people, an infection usually causes a low-grade fever, achiness, headache, fatigue, or sometimes coldlike symptoms. Children with fifth disease usually get a fiery red facial rash (which looks like "slapped cheeks") a few days to a week later, followed by a lacy (and sometimes itchy) rash on their torso and limbs. By the time the telltale rash appears, most people are no longer contagious. Adults don't usually get the characteristic rash, though women in particular might notice some joint pain. About a quarter of those infected have no symptoms at all.

If you think you've been exposed to fifth disease, your caregiver can do blood tests to see if you're infected. If so, you'll get regular ultrasounds for the next couple of months to look for potential problems caused by fetal anemia. And if your baby continues to look fine, don't worry—the virus doesn't appear to cause birth defects or developmental problems.

Hepatitis B

The hepatitis B virus (HBV) is an infection you can get from exposure to blood, semen, or other bodily fluids of an infected person. Transmission can happen during sex, from a dirty needle (or from unsterilized tattooing or body piercing equipment), and even from sharing a toothbrush or razor that has trace amounts of infected blood on it.

If you contract hep B, you may feel very tired or have abdominal pain, nausea and vomiting, a loss of appetite, joint pain, or jaundice (your eyes and skin take on a yellow tinge). But many people have no symptoms and never even know they've been infected. What's more, 5 to 10 percent of the people who are over age 5 when they contract HBV end up as hepatitis B carriers—meaning that they have a chronic HBV infection. About a quarter of those with a chronic infection will eventually end up with a life-threatening liver disease, and everyone with a chronic infection can pass the disease on to anyone who has contact with their body fluids.

If you're a carrier, you could pass HBV on to your baby at birth. That's why your provider should test your blood for HBV at your first prenatal checkup. The good news is that if you know you carry the virus, your baby will get two injections—hepatitis B immune globulin and the hepatitis B vaccine—right after he's born, to help prevent transmission. (For complete protection, the hep B vaccine requires three injections—so your baby will also need to get a second shot at 1 to 2 months old and another six months later.)

If you test negative and haven't received the hep B vaccine, your practitioner may advise you to get immunized if you're at high risk for the disease. (The most vulnerable women include healthcare workers, housemates and sexual partners of HBV carriers, women with multiple sexual partners, and IV drug users.) The shot is safe and won't affect your developing baby.

Rubella (German Measles)

Though rubella is normally a mild and (thanks to a successful vaccination program) increasingly unheard-of illness in the United States, coming down with it when you're pregnant can lead to miscarriage, stillbirth, or birth defects. A baby born with congenital rubella syndrome (CRS) may have deafness, blindness, heart defects, mental retardation, growth deficits, and a host of other problems. Fortunately, most women of childbearing age who were raised in the United States are immune (a routine blood test at your first prenatal checkup will let you know for sure), either from childhood vaccinations or from a previous bout with rubella. The risk to a developing baby from rubella depends on when her mother gets it. In the first trimester, a baby is at high risk for CRS—but in the second and third trimesters, infection-related defects are rare.

> ### BY THE NUMBERS
>
> **Rubella: Before the Vaccine and Now**
>
> Reported number of cases in 1969: **12.5 million**
>
> Reported number of cases in 2002: **18**
>
> Source: *Centers for Disease Control and Prevention*

Avoiding Rubella

Fortunately, rubella outbreaks are exceedingly rare. But if you think you're not immune:

- Steer clear of any infected person and wash your hands often.
- Make sure your children are up-to-date on their vaccines, and that anyone else in the house who isn't immune gets vaccinated.
- Avoid travel to developing countries, where rubella may still be common.

Sexually Transmitted Infections (STIs)

STIs are infections that you can get from genital, oral, or anal sex with an infected partner, and they can have serious health consequences for you and your baby. Not only that, but having one untreated STI can increase your risk of contracting another (and potentially more dangerous) one like HIV if you're exposed. An untreated STI can also lead to pelvic inflammatory disease, which can scar your fallopian tubes, increase your risk of ectopic pregnancy, and possibly result in future infertility.

Because it's so important to spot and treat STIs during pregnancy, your practitioner will screen for many of these infections during your first prenatal visit. (Be sure to let her know if you've ever had any STIs in the past, too, or if you or your mate has more than one sexual partner.) If you're at high risk for STIs, you'll be screened again in your third trimester—or sooner if you develop any STI symptoms during the course of your pregnancy. (If your caregiver doesn't routinely offer tests for chlamydia, gonorrhea, hepatitis, HIV, and syphilis, ask for them—though you may not be in a high-risk relationship now, some STIs can lurk in your body for years without symptoms.) And if there's any chance that you've been exposed to an STI during your pregnancy, or if you have any unusual symptoms, let her know right away so you can be re-tested. If you do have an STI, you'll want to learn all you can about the risks and treatment options.

Chlamydia

If left untreated, this relatively common bacterial infection can raise the odds of miscarriage, preterm birth, or a postpartum uterine infection. What's more, there's a chance you could pass chlamydia on to your baby during delivery, leading to problems ranging from serious eye infections to life-threatening pneumonia. Unfortunately, without testing it can be tricky to figure out if you have chlamydia, especially since most infected women don't have any symptoms. Because of this, you can carry the infection for years without realizing you have it. When symptoms do show up, they include burning during urination, abnormal vaginal discharge, or

---

QUICK TIPS

Avoiding STIs

- The only surefire way to avoid getting an STI is to abstain from sex completely (including vaginal, oral, and anal sex) or to have sex only with a partner you're absolutely sure is monogamous and who's recently been tested and given a clean bill of health.

- Avoid sex with anyone who has sores or symptoms of an STI—including a partner you otherwise believe to be faithful. If you're in a nonmonogamous relationship, be sure to use latex condoms every time you have sex, which will reduce the risk of transmission of most STIs.

- With a few exceptions, if you're being treated for an STI, your partner also needs to be treated, and you should abstain from sex until you've both completed treatment and are symptom-free. Otherwise, you'll just keep passing the infection back and forth.

- If you're at high risk for STIs, get vaccinated against hepatitis B (page 502).

lower abdominal pain. Once it's caught, chlamydia is simple to cure with antibiotics—and the sooner you start treatment, the better your chances of having a healthy baby. (Your partner will need treatment, too, to avoid re-infecting you.)

Genital Herpes

Genital herpes is most often caused by the herpes simplex virus type 2 (HSV-2) and is spread by sexual contact (including oral sex). Let your caregiver know at your first prenatal visit if you think you or your partner has ever had a herpes outbreak. The main concern is that you might transmit the disease to your baby during delivery. Though newborn herpes is relatively rare, it can be devastating.

If you get genital herpes for the first time (called a "primary infection") when you're pregnant, it's also possible—though highly unlikely—for the virus to infect your baby in the womb, which can cause serious birth defects. A few studies have found that a primary infection during the first trimester can even increase the risk of miscarriage, though other studies have found no connection. Finally, if you have a primary infection during your second or third trimester, you may be at increased risk for preterm delivery.

You may not notice any symptoms from a primary infection. Possible symptoms include red bumps on your vagina or vulva, which turn into blisters that eventually rupture and become painful sores. There may be just a few, or there may be a large cluster, and they can last up to three weeks. You may also feel itchy or have a burning, painful, or tingling sensation in your genital area, as well as vaginal discharge; tender, swollen lymph nodes near your groin; pain when you urinate; and flulike symptoms, including fever, headache, and muscle aches.

If you've already had oral herpes (cold sores) when you get your first genital herpes infection, it's called a "nonprimary first episode," and your symptoms will probably be less severe because the antibodies your immune system has made against HSV-1 (the virus that usually causes oral herpes) will offer some protection against HSV-2. You're less likely to get severe flu-like symptoms, and you'll generally have fewer sores and less pain for a shorter time than with a primary infection.

Herpes is not curable. Once you're infected, the virus stays in your body and may surface from time to time. Outbreaks that occur after a primary infection (or a nonprimary first episode) are called "recurrent infections." With a recurrent infection, there's generally less pain and fewer sores than with either of the infections above, and they tend to clear up faster. You can also have outbreaks in which you're contagious because the virus is present in your genital area, though you don't have any symptoms.

If you have a primary infection in the first half of your pregnancy or if you had herpes before you got pregnant, you should be able to have a normal vaginal delivery (as long as you don't have any active genital lesions when your water breaks or your labor starts) because the risk of your baby's contracting the disease is minimal. To increase the chances of a woman's being able to deliver vaginally, some experts recommend taking the antiviral medication acyclovir from week 36 until delivery, to lower the risk of an outbreak. If a woman first gets genital herpes in her third trimester, on the other hand, some experts recommend having a c-section—even if she doesn't have symptoms when she goes into labor—because the risk of transmission to the baby is high.

When Your Partner Has Herpes

Even if your partner has had herpes for years without passing the infection to you, it's important to take extra care to stay herpes-free now.

- Abstain from sex (including oral sex if your partner has oral herpes) or even skin-to-skin contact near your partner's genitals or mouth when he has an active outbreak or feels one coming on (some people notice a tingling or painful sensation before sores actually appear).
- Even when your partner is outbreak-free, be sure to use latex condoms when you make love; they don't always prevent transmission, but they'll reduce your risk.
- Some experts recommend that your partner take an antiviral medication for the duration of your pregnancy because preliminary research has shown that this lowers the risk of his passing the infection along to you. Ask your caregiver about this option.
- To avoid contracting herpes close to your due date, you'll need to skip intercourse altogether in your third trimester (you'll also need to pass on getting oral sex in your third trimester if your partner has ever had oral herpes).

Genital HPV (Genital Warts)

Genital human papillomavirus (HPV) is a common STI that usually has no symptoms, though it may cause genital warts. In most cases, the virus clears up on its own, though it may persist for life. (HPV includes more than 100 different strains, over a third of which infect the genital tract. Some strains are called "high risk" because they increase a woman's chances of developing genital cancers, but most genital warts are caused by the "low-risk" HPV strains.)

Genital warts usually show up in or around the vagina, near the anus and in the rectum, and on the cervix. (You can also get warts in your mouth and throat from performing oral sex on an infected partner, but it's less common.) The warts are skin-colored or a little lighter and can be small or large, single or multiple, sometimes growing in clusters with a cauliflower-like appearance. Your practitioner can usually diagnose genital warts simply by looking at them.

The warts are often painless (though they may occasionally itch, burn, or bleed), and in most cases they won't pose any problems for mother or baby. They do tend to grow during pregnancy, though, possibly from the extra vaginal discharge that provides the virus with a moist growing environment. In certain cases, your practitioner may offer to remove them with a mild acid solution. But unless your warts are so large or numerous that they block your birth canal or there's a concern that they'll bleed excessively, you can still have a normal vaginal birth whether they're treated or not. (What's more, they often improve on their own or even disappear altogether after delivery.)

Though HPV can be transmitted to your baby during birth and lead to a serious condition characterized by warts on his vocal cords and other areas, this is extremely rare. Having a c-section doesn't seem to offer a baby complete protection

BY THE NUMBERS

HPV Stats

Women who acquire one of the many strains of HPV at some point in their lives: **about 1 in 2**

Women currently infected with HPV: **about 3 in 20**

Women who have genital warts: **about 1 in 100**

Babies who contract HPV during birth and develop warts: **about 1 in 100,000**

Source: *Centers for Disease Control and Prevention*

BY THE NUMBERS

Gonorrhea Stats

Number of pregnant
women who contract
gonorrhea each year:
about 40,000

Source: *Centers for Disease
Control and Prevention*

from the virus, anyway, so your birth won't be managed any differently than it would have been if you were HPV-free.

Gonorrhea

Gonorrhea is a serious bacterial infection that, if left untreated, can cause health problems for you and increase your risk for miscarriage, preterm birth, premature rupture of the membranes, and postpartum infection. During pregnancy the infection is usually limited to the cervix, urethra, and vagina, although—depending on a woman's sexual practices—it can also infect the throat and anus. A woman can pass gonorrhea on to her baby during delivery, which can lead to health problems such as meningitis and joint, blood, or serious eye infections that can eventually cause blindness. (This is why most states require that all newborns be treated with antibiotic eyedrops.)

Gonorrhea may not cause symptoms, but if symptoms do show up (usually two to ten days after sex with an infected partner), they can include increased vaginal discharge, burning during urination, and bleeding during intercourse. Fortunately, gonorrhea can be treated with antibiotics that are safe to take during pregnancy. Your partner will need medication as well.

HIV/AIDS

Human immunodeficiency virus (HIV) is the infection that causes acquired immune deficiency syndrome (AIDS). If you're HIV positive, you can pass the virus on to your baby during pregnancy, birth, or breastfeeding, so it's vital to diagnose and treat this potentially deadly disease as soon as possible. Because it can take 15 years or more to develop symptoms, you may not even know if you're HIV positive. That's why you should be offered an HIV test at your first prenatal visit. And if there's any chance that you've been exposed to the virus after that by a nonmonogamous or new sexual partner (or one who's been sharing drug needles), you'll need to be tested again.

Fortunately, even if you test positive, the odds of having a healthy baby are in your favor. By taking special antiviral drugs, having a scheduled c-section if that's deemed necessary, getting preventive treatment for your newborn, and avoiding breastfeeding, you can drastically cut the risk of transmission.

If you're HIV positive, try to find a practitioner who has experience in treating pregnant women with HIV. If that's impossible, at least make sure the practitioner who treats and manages your HIV works closely with your pregnancy caregiver.

> **BY THE NUMBERS**
>
> **HIV Stats**
>
> Number of HIV-positive pregnant women each year:
> **about 8,000**
>
> Babies who contract HIV from untreated mothers who deliver vaginally: **about 1 in 4**
>
> Babies who contract HIV from infected mothers who get all appropriate interventions:
> **fewer than 1 in 50**
>
> Source: *Centers for Disease Control and Prevention*

Syphilis

Syphilis is a very serious but relatively rare bacterial infection. It can infect your baby in the womb or at delivery, leading to miscarriage, stillbirth, or debilitating health problems.

The first symptom of syphilis is a hard, painless, and highly infectious sore (or sores) called a chancre that shows up at the site of infection. Because the chancre may be located inside your vagina or on your cervix, you might never see it. This is followed, weeks or months later, by symptoms that may include a rash (typically on your palms and the soles of your feet); flat, wart-like sores on your vulva or on the skin between your vagina and anus; sores around your mouth; and flulike symptoms. Though these symptoms clear up on their own, the infection stays in your body and can cause very serious problems years later. In its late stages, untreated syphilis can cause serious heart abnormalities; mental disorders, blindness, and other neurologic problems; and death.

Unless you're tested during your first prenatal checkup, you might never even know you have the disease. Syphilis is treated with penicillin injections, and the earlier in your pregnancy you receive them, the better the outcome for you and your baby. Your partner will also need to be tested and treated.

Trichomoniasis

"Trich" is a fairly common STI caused by a microscopic parasite that can bring on unpleasant vaginal discharge and discomfort—or no symptoms at all. You may notice yellowish, greenish, or grayish vaginal discharge with a frothy appearance and an unpleasant odor. Your vagina and vulva might get red, irritated, or itchy, and you might experience some discomfort during intercourse or while urinating. Less commonly, you may notice some lower abdominal discomfort. A trich infection during pregnancy can increase your risk of preterm birth and premature rupture of the membranes.

The only drug that cures trich is oral metronidazole. But because treatment doesn't seem to lower the odds for preterm birth, prenatal screening and treatment aren't routine. That said, if you have symptoms of trich, let your practitioner know so you can be tested and treated accordingly.

Toxoplasmosis

Toxoplasmosis is an infection caused by a parasite, and though most women aren't immune to the disease, the chances of getting it during pregnancy are relatively small. Still, getting infected during pregnancy (or even a couple of months before conception) can have serious consequences: miscarriage, stillbirth, or a host of health and developmental problems for your baby.

The parasite that causes toxoplasmosis reproduces in cats' intestines, and you can get the disease from a variety of sources, including cat feces, garden soil, unwashed produce, raw or undercooked meat or eggs, unpasteurized milk, and contaminated water. Infection is hard to spot because in most cases either you have no symptoms or the symptoms—such as fever, achiness, swollen glands, and possibly a rash—mimic a mild flu. Even so, if there's a chance that you've been infected with toxoplasmosis, let your practitioner know right away so you can be tested. If you're diagnosed with a recent infection, antibiotic treatment will lower your odds of passing the disease along to your baby. If further testing shows that your baby is already infected, continued antibiotic treatment will improve your baby's chances for a healthy outcome.

Avoiding Toxoplasmosis

For the most part, practicing good hygiene and simple food safety techniques is all you need to do to keep toxoplasmosis at bay:

- Cook your meat well. Use a food thermometer to test the internal temperature; most meat should be cooked to a temperature of 160°F (180°F in the thigh for whole poultry). If you're not measuring the temperature, cook meat until it's no longer pink. (And be sure not to sample meat before it's done cooking!)
- Wash or peel fruits and vegetables before eating them.
- Avoid eating raw eggs and unpasteurized milk.
- Don't touch your mouth, nose, or eyes while you're preparing food.
- Wash counters, cutting boards, and utensils with hot, soapy water after food preparation.
- Keep flies and cockroaches away from your food.
- Drink only bottled water when you're camping or when you're traveling to developing countries.
- If you own a cat, have someone else empty the litter box every day. (Changing it daily decreases the risk of infection because the parasite eggs in cats' feces are dormant for the first 24 hours.) If you must do the job yourself, wear rubber gloves. Some experts even suggest wearing a mask in case any particles become airborne when the litter is stirred up.
- Don't get too cuddly with kitty if he prowls outdoors, and don't let him sleep on your bed.
- Don't feed your cat raw or undercooked meat, and keep him from hunting small animals (like mice or birds) outdoors by keeping him inside.
- Don't play with strays (even kittens), and don't get a new kitten or cat while you're pregnant.
- Wear waterproof gloves when you're gardening.
- Cover your child's sandbox when it's not in use, and stay away from public sandboxes. (Toxoplasmosis isn't likely to harm your child and you can't catch it from him, but you do need to keep your distance from sand that might contain infected cat feces.)
- Wash your hands well before eating and after handling raw meat, soil, sand, cats, or litter.

Urinary Tract Infections

Pain or burning when you pee can signal a urinary tract infection (UTI), the most common bacterial infection in pregnancy. Higher levels of progesterone during pregnancy are probably partly to blame—the hormone relaxes your urinary tract and bladder, causing urine to stay in your system longer, giving bacteria more time to accumulate and multiply. Later in pregnancy, your growing uterus can contribute to the problem by further compressing part of your urinary tract.

UTIs may be symptomatic or asymptomatic. Typically, bacteria from your rectum enters your urethra (the short tube that carries urine from your bladder to the outside) and makes its way up to your bladder, where it continues to multiply, sometimes leading to a bladder infection called cystitis. This type of UTI is marked by pain, discomfort, or burning during urination, plus pelvic discomfort or lower abdominal pain. Your urine may look cloudy and have a foul smell, and you may have an uncontrollable or frequent urge to pee, even when there's little urine in your bladder. See your practitioner right away so you can be tested and treated.

Bacteria can also multiply in your urinary tract without symptoms (a condition called asymptomatic bacteriuria), which is why your practitioner will take a urine sample at your first prenatal visit. If your urine culture is positive, you'll be treated with antibiotics.

An untreated UTI is much more likely to lead to a kidney infection—which in turn can make you seriously ill and increase your risk for preterm labor. Symptoms of a kidney infection may include fever, chills, pain (on one or both sides, or in your back or abdomen), nausea or vomiting, general malaise, and cloudy or bloody urine.

Avoiding UTIs

- Drink plenty of water—at least eight 8-ounce glasses a day.
- Drink cranberry juice. It won't cure an existing infection, but it may discourage new bacteria from taking hold.

- Don't ignore the urge to pee—and empty your bladder completely when you urinate.
- After a bowel movement, wipe yourself from front to back so you don't drag bacteria from your rectum to your urethra.
- Keep your genital area clean with mild soap and water. Avoid scented soaps and feminine hygiene sprays or powders, which can irritate your urethra and genitals and make them a better breeding ground for bacteria.
- Don't douche.

PREGNANCY COMPLICATIONS

Sometimes even the best prenatal care isn't enough to guarantee a problem-free pregnancy. And though experts know more than ever about what causes some complications, they're still a long way from fully understanding others.

One important thing to know is that there's no way to prevent most of these problems and that almost nothing you do (or don't do) is to blame for them. Still, getting early and regular prenatal care is the best way to keep yourself and your baby safe and to manage any complications that come up.

Keep in mind that while most pregnancy complications are worrisome—and some are devastating—many (like gestational diabetes) are manageable as long as you get proper treatment. And others (like expecting twins or more)—while undeniably "complicated" from a medical point of view—can actually be cause for celebration. Whatever the particulars of your pregnancy situation, there are many resources for helping you get through it.

Amniotic Fluid Problems

Amniotic fluid fills the sac surrounding your developing baby and plays several important roles: It has a cushioning effect that protects your baby from trauma (if you take a tumble, for instance); it prevents the umbilical cord from being compressed and reducing your baby's oxygen supply; it helps maintain a constant temperature in the womb; it protects against infection; and it allows your baby to move around so that his muscles and bones develop properly. Also, your baby both swallows amniotic fluid and "inhales" and "exhales" it from his lungs. The fluid and the special factors it contains help his digestive and respiratory systems develop normally.

Early in the second trimester, your baby starts to swallow the fluid, pass it through his kidneys, and excrete it as urine—which he then swallows again, recycling the full volume of amniotic fluid every few hours. (Yes, this means that most of the fluid is eventually your baby's urine!) So your baby plays an important role in keeping just the right amount of fluid in the amniotic sac. Sometimes, though, this system breaks down, resulting in either too much or too little fluid—both of which can present problems.

Too Much Fluid (Hydramnios or Polyhydramnios)

Your healthcare provider may suspect that there's too much amniotic fluid— a condition that occurs in one out of 100 pregnancies—if your uterus is growing more rapidly than it should. You may also have unusual abdominal discomfort, increased back pain, shortness of breath, and extreme swelling in your feet and ankles. Your practitioner will do an ultrasound to confirm or rule out the condition.

Experts don't know what causes many cases of hydramnios, particularly mild ones. Some of the common causes of moderate to severe cases, however, include maternal diabetes, carrying twins or multiples, and having a baby with fetal anemia or certain abnormalities. If you're diagnosed with hydramnios, your practitioner will order a high-resolution ultrasound to check for abnormalities, and possibly amniocentesis to test for a genetic defect. You'll also need to have regular nonstress tests and ultrasounds for the rest of your pregnancy to closely monitor your baby's development, and you'll be watched closely for signs of preterm labor. And if you haven't yet been tested for gestational diabetes, you'll be tested now.

You'll be monitored carefully during labor as well. Because of all of the extra amniotic fluid, you have an increased risk of an umbilical cord prolapse

Just the Facts

Amniotic Fluid Volume

Under normal circumstances, the amount of amniotic fluid you have increases until the beginning of your third trimester and generally peaks in week 34, at which point you may carry about a quart of the stuff. After that, it gradually decreases until you give birth.

(when the cord falls though the cervical opening) or a placental abruption when your water breaks. Either occurrence requires an immediate c-section. That's why your caregiver will have you come to the hospital early in labor (or immediately if your water breaks before you go into labor). You're also at increased risk for postpartum hemorrhage, since your overdistended uterus may have a hard time contracting—so you'll be watched closely after you give birth, too.

Too Little Fluid (Oligohydramnios)

Your practitioner may suspect this problem if you're leaking fluid, measuring small for your stage of pregnancy, or not feeling your baby move very much. She'll also be on the lookout for it if you've had a previous baby whose growth was restricted; if you have chronic high blood pressure, preeclampsia, diabetes, or lupus; or if you're past your due date. To find out what's going on, she'll send you for an ultrasound.

The consequences for your baby depend on what's causing the problem, how far along you are, and how little fluid you have. Oligohydramnios can be caused by a leaking or ruptured amniotic sac, by placental problems (such as a partial abruption), by fetal problems (such as poor growth or a genetic abnormality), by chronic health conditions like high blood pressure, or by preeclampsia. And sometimes no apparent cause is found. It's most common late in the third trimester, particularly if a woman is overdue. The later in pregnancy the condition develops, the better the outlook for your baby.

If you have low amniotic fluid, your caregiver will follow your baby closely to be sure he continues to grow normally. How your pregnancy will be managed depends on how far along you are, how your baby is doing, and whether you have other complications as well. If you're near term, your

BabyCenter Buzz

I Was Diagnosed with Too Little Amniotic Fluid

"Since my diagnosis, my OB has had me drinking 100 ounces of water a day for a week. I'll go back for another ultrasound in a few days to see if all this water guzzling has made a difference." —*Laura*

"In week 36, I found out that I had low amniotic fluid, which my doctors thought was brought on by high blood pressure. The next day, I delivered a healthy baby girl by c-section." —*Michelle*

labor will be induced. If you're earlier in pregnancy, the decision will be based on how you and your baby are doing. In some cases—for instance, if you have severe preeclampsia or your baby isn't thriving inside the womb—you'll need to have your baby early. In other situations it may be considered safe to wait until your baby's more mature, although you still may end up delivering early. In this case, your baby will be monitored very closely with frequent ultrasounds and nonstress tests to make sure he's thriving. You'll be asked to drink plenty of fluids, do fetal kick counts, and let your caregiver know immediately if you notice any decrease in your baby's movements.

Low fluid can increase your risk of complications during labor. The main concern is that the fluid level will get so low that your baby's movements or your contractions will compress the umbilical cord. During labor, your practitioner may pass a flexible catheter through your cervix and pump a steady supply of warm saline solution into the amniotic sac to reduce the risk of cord compression. If your baby can't safely tolerate labor, your doctor or midwife will recommend a c-section (page 426).

Breech Baby

By about the eighth month, your baby has settled into position in your uterus after months of floating blissfully free. By this time there's not much room, and most babies maximize their limited quarters by settling into a head-down position.

If your baby is still bottom-down, or breech, in week 37, though, your doctor may try to turn her by applying pressure to your abdomen and manually manipulating her into a head-down position. If you're seeing a midwife, she can refer you to an OB for this procedure. This process is called an external cephalic version (ECV), and if it works, it will dramatically reduce your chances of needing a c-section. Sometimes, though, the baby refuses to budge—or even rotates back into a breech position after a successful version.

BY THE NUMBERS

Breech Babies

Term babies in the head-down position at the beginning of labor: **96%**

Term babies who are breech when labor starts: **4%**

Success rate of external cephalic version: **about 58%**

Source: *American College of Obstetricians and Gynecologists*

BabyCenter Buzz

My Baby Was Breech

"I was scheduled for a version in week 37. The night before the procedure, my husband got down and talked to the baby in my belly, joking around and saying things like 'Come on down here, little guy!' I felt the baby move, but didn't think it was anything other than the normal squirming. The next morning, when they turned on the ultrasound before the version, we realized that the baby had flipped on his own—and the whole thing was called off." —*Leah*

"I had a successful ECV. My baby's now head-down, and I'm waiting for labor to begin. I'm extremely grateful to the doctors who were able to perform this procedure so I could avoid a c-section." —*Paige*

"I had a version, which I found very painful and uncomfortable. Mine was unsuccessful—the stubborn little one is comfortable right where he is. We're scheduled for a c-section near my due date." —*Linda*

The procedure isn't entirely risk-free, so discuss the pros and cons with your caregiver. To be safe, your baby should be monitored continuously by ultrasound during the procedure, and you should have the procedure done in the hospital with facilities and staff available for an emergency c-section in case any complications arise. Some studies show higher success rates of ECV when uterine-relaxing drugs are used. (And moms who are Rh negative should get an injection of Rh immune globulin for the procedure.) If the ECV doesn't work and your baby doesn't turn on her own before you go into labor, you'll need to deliver by c-section.

Turning a Breech Baby

While the scientific jury is still out on whether the following techniques are effective, there's no danger in trying them if you want to—*after* having an ultrasound to make sure your baby's position isn't due to a short umbilical cord or other problem.

Assume a baby-flipping position. Get into one of the following positions twice a day for a few weeks, starting around week 32. The idea is to employ gravity to help your baby somersault into a head-down position. (Do this on an empty stomach so your lunch doesn't come back up. And if you find these positions uncomfortable, stop doing them.) Lie down flat on your back, and then raise your pelvis so that it's 9 to 12 inches above your head. Support your hips with a pillow, and stay in this position for five to 15 minutes. Alternatively, get on your knees with your forearms in front of you on the floor so that your bottom sticks up in the air. Stay in this position for five to 15 minutes.

Ask your caregiver about moxibustion. This ancient Chinese technique uses burning herbs to stimulate key acupressure points. To help turn a breech baby, an acupuncturist or other practitioner burns the herb mugwort near the acupressure point of your pinky toes, which—theoretically, at least—stimulates your baby's activity enough that she may change positions on her own. Even if you don't particularly subscribe to alternative medicine practices, it's interesting to know that one study found that a higher percentage of babies turned when their mothers had moxibustion—and, even if it doesn't work for you, there's certainly no harm in it. To find a licensed practitioner who uses moxibustion, contact your state acupuncture or Chinese medicine association.

Try hypnosis. One study found that women who were hypnotized into a state of deep relaxation were more likely to have their babies turn than women who weren't hypnotized. If you're willing to try this technique, ask your caregiver if she can recommend a skilled hypnotherapist.

Cervical Insufficiency (Incompetent Cervix)

If your cervix is softer and weaker than normal or is unusually short to begin with, it may painlessly start to efface and open as the weight of your growing baby puts increasing pressure on it. Cervical insufficiency (sometimes called

BabyCenter Buzz

I Have Cervical Insufficiency

"I've been diagnosed with cervical insufficiency for the third time in as many pregnancies. This time, I really believe the cerclage is helping. I'm still working five days a week and I feel fine—besides the normal backaches and foot swelling." —Loretta

"I've been seeing a high-risk specialist since week 18. At my 17-week ultrasound, my cervix was measuring 2.8 centimeters—but still firm, which was a good sign. Then I went in at week 23, and my cervix had softened and shortened. I'm on modified bed rest now and am really hoping that I'll make it to week 33, at least." —Gigi

"incompetent cervix") can result in second-trimester miscarriage, premature rupture of the membranes, or preterm delivery.

If you've had a second-trimester miscarriage with no known cause or a preterm delivery in a previous pregnancy, you may have cervical insufficiency. You're also at risk if you've had a procedure such as a cone biopsy, if you were exposed prenatally to the drug DES (used decades ago to prevent miscarriage and no longer recommended for pregnant women), or if your cervix was injured during a previous birth or dilation and curettage (D & C).

In the past, cervical insufficiency was diagnosed only after a woman had had several second-trimester miscarriages or very early preterm births (before week 32). Now if you're at risk for this condition, your practitioner will do regular ultrasounds beginning in midpregnancy to measure the length of your cervix and to check for signs of early dilation. But diagnosing this condition is still tricky, and there's no solid evidence that treatment strategies will prevent preterm delivery. (Even so, having early warning that your cervix is changing gives your caregiver enough time to administer corticosteroids, which help minimize health problems in premature babies.) Call your practitioner immediately if you have any of these symptoms: increased vaginal discharge, spotting, pelvic pressure, or menstrual-like cramping or "heaviness."

If you have cervical insufficiency, your practitioner may recommend a cerclage—a purse-string type stitch around your cervix to hold it closed—though recent research has called into question the effectiveness of this procedure in preventing miscarriage or preterm birth. And it's not without risks: Cerclage increases the risk of uterine infection and of preterm premature rupture of the membranes.

Though there is considerable controversy (and ongoing research) about the benefits of cerclage, if you've had three or more unexplained second-trimester losses or preterm births, your practitioner might recommend this procedure between weeks 13 and 16, before you have any changes in your cervix. If you get a cerclage, the stitch is usually removed a few weeks before your due date. Once you reach this point, you can relax and wait for labor to begin.

Gestational Diabetes

Most women who develop diabetes during pregnancy go on to have healthy babies—as long as they get good prenatal care and follow their healthcare provider's advice. If you're diagnosed with gestational diabetes mellitus (GDM), your practitioner will monitor you closely, and you'll need to keep your blood sugar levels under control with diet and exercise and perhaps with insulin shots or oral medication. Because GDM usually has no symptoms, almost all pregnant women are given a glucose screening to test for it between weeks 24 and 28. But if you're at high risk for diabetes or are showing signs of it before then, your caregiver will recommend glucose testing at your first prenatal visit and then again at the normal time if the result is negative. If the result is positive, it doesn't mean that you *have* GDM, but you will need to take the longer glucose tolerance test. Only a small percentage of women with GDM remain diabetic after pregnancy. But once

BY THE NUMBERS

Gestational Diabetes Stats

Pregnant women
with GDM: **about 1 in 25**

Women with GDM who
need insulin: **about 1 in 7**

Chance that GDM sufferers
will develop GDM in a
future pregnancy and/or
diabetes later in life: **1 in 2**

Sources: *American Diabetes Association; March of Dimes*

Just the Facts

Risk Factors for Gestational Diabetes

Your chances of developing GDM are higher if:

- You're obese (that is, your body mass index is over 30)
- You had GDM in a previous pregnancy
- You have a family history of diabetes

Some practitioners will also screen you early if:

- You've previously given birth to a big baby (some use 8 pounds, 13 ounces as the cutoff; others use 9 pounds, 14 ounces)
- You've had an unexplained stillbirth
- You've had a baby with a birth defect
- You have high blood pressure
- A routine urine test shows you have sugar in your urine (which is tested at each prenatal visit)

QUICK TIPS

Controlling Gestational Diabetes

- Keep diligent track of your glucose levels, using a home glucose meter or strips.

- Exercise. Moderate activity improves your ability to process glucose and keep your blood sugar levels in check. Many women with GDM benefit from 30 minutes a day of aerobic activity, such as walking or swimming. Exercise isn't advisable for everyone, though, so ask your practitioner what makes sense for you.

- Take insulin shots if your practitioner recommends them. Injecting yourself with a substance may sound scary, but the insulin shots are safe for your baby.

- Eat a well-planned diet to keep your glucose levels where they should be. A registered dietitian can help you develop very specific meal and snack plans based on your height, weight, and activity level.

you've had it, you have a 50 to 80 percent risk of getting GDM again in a future pregnancy and of developing diabetes later in life. (Losing weight after your baby is born can help reduce this risk.)

Having GDM doubles your odds for developing preeclampsia, and poorly controlled diabetes can have serious consequences for you and your baby. Your baby can put on too much weight, particularly in his upper body. The result: His shoulders may be too broad to pass through your birth canal without extra help from your medical team. Because of this risk, you may have to deliver by c-section (page 426). Fortunately, though, only a small percentage of women with well-controlled GDM end up with overly large babies.

At birth, your baby may also have low blood sugar and be at higher risk for jaundice, overproduction of red blood cells, and low blood calcium—all of which can be treated. If *your* blood sugar is especially out of control, your baby's heart function may be affected.

Finally, some studies have found a link between poorly controlled GDM and an increased risk for stillbirth. Because of this, your practitioner may want to monitor your baby more intensively during your last trimester, depending on the severity of your diabetes and whether you have any other pregnancy-related problems. She'll explain how you should begin counting your baby's movements so you can alert her right away if you sense a decrease. If you're unable to keep your blood sugar under control or it's high enough that you need insulin (or if you have any other risk factors), you'll likely begin periodic nonstress tests or biophysical profiles around week 32 to check on your baby's well-being. If you can keep your diabetes under control without insulin—and if you have no

BabyCenter Buzz

How I Cope with Gestational Diabetes

"Luckily, I've been able to control my diabetes with exercise and a good diet. I used to be hungry all the time, but I've found that drinking extra water and having more veggies helps." —*Blanca*

"A few quick suggestions that I find helpful: Keep a food diary detailing your meals. That way, if you have a good glucose reading, you can repeat a similar meal—or avoid a bad meal again if the reading is high. Also, walk for 20 minutes, if possible, after each meal." —*Jennifer*

"Eating a protein snack with a low-glycemic carb keeps me full. I also make sure to eat every two to three hours, and I never skip meals." —*Anonymous*

"I'm taking insulin shots four times a day. I hardly remember how it was to eat without taking shots!" —*Shalini*

other problems—you may not begin this testing until close to your due date.

Your practitioner may also order an ultrasound at the beginning of your third trimester to measure your baby and estimate his weight. She may order another one closer to your due date if she suspects your baby is large then, but an ultrasound isn't usually very accurate at calculating your baby's size this late in the game. Depending on your circumstances, you might be induced (page 436) before your due date or have your baby via c-section.

Diet for Diabetics

Good nutrition is especially important if you have GDM because if large amounts of glucose accumulate in your blood, it means that your cells aren't getting the fuel they need. One way to keep your blood sugar levels under control is to follow a specific meal plan. (*Note:* If dietary changes aren't enough to keep your blood sugar in a healthy range, you'll need to take insulin as well. If your practitioner prescribes insulin shots, you'll need to meet again with your dietitian to reassess your diet.)

A dietitian will start by figuring out how many calories you need each day. Then she'll teach you how to measure portion sizes and how to balance your meals with just the right amounts of protein, carbohydrates, and fat. She'll also scrutinize your current eating habits to make sure you're getting enough vitamins and minerals. It's hard to make dietary changes, but take comfort in knowing that you're doing what's best for yourself and your baby. Get the rest of your family on board with your new eating plan, too—it'll make mealtimes easier on you and healthier for them!

Managing Gestational Diabetes with Smart Food Choices

Eat a variety of foods. Distribute your calories and carbohydrates evenly throughout the day, and make sure that your meals and snacks are well-balanced. The American Diabetes Association recommends eating three small-to-moderate-size meals and two to four snacks—including an after-dinner snack—a day.

Don't skip meals. Your blood sugar will be more stable if your food is distributed evenly throughout the day and consistently from day to day, so be consistent in the amount of food you eat at each meal and when you eat.

Eat a good breakfast. Your blood glucose levels are most likely to be out of whack in the morning. To keep them in a healthy range, you may have to limit carbohydrates (breads, cereal, fruit, and milk), boost your protein intake, and possibly avoid fruit or juice altogether in the A.M.

Include high-fiber foods. Fresh fruits and vegetables, whole grain breads and cereals, dried peas and beans, and other legumes are broken down and absorbed more slowly than simple carbohydrates, so they may help moderate your blood sugar levels after meals.

Limit simple sugars. Soda, fruit juice, flavored teas, and most desserts will quickly elevate your blood sugar. Ask your practitioner about using foods sweetened with an artificial sweetener whenever you need a sweet fix.

Gestational Hypertension (Pregnancy-Induced High Blood Pressure)

If you had normal blood pressure before conception or in early pregnancy and then develop high blood pressure (generally a reading of 140/90 or higher) after week 20—but have no protein in your urine—you have what's known as gestational hypertension. About a quarter of the time, it progresses to preeclampsia, meaning that your initial rise in blood pressure is later accompanied by protein in your urine and perhaps other symptoms as well. Because of this risk—and because high blood pressure in itself can be risky

BabyCenter Buzz

How I Managed My High Blood Pressure

"After week 32, I had to go in every week for fetal monitoring. I didn't mind because I could see my baby. I was induced about two weeks before my due date. My baby and I are doing great. I was fortunate to have good doctors taking care of me." —Dee

"During my pregnancy, my blood pressure became slightly elevated. Luckily, I gave birth to a healthy baby boy with no complications." —Anonymous

during pregnancy—your caregiver will monitor you carefully and keep a close watch on your baby as well. What to expect if you develop gestational hypertension depends on how high your blood pressure is, how your baby's doing, and how far along you are in your pregnancy.

If you develop mild gestational hypertension at week 37 or beyond, you'll likely be induced (page 436) or possibly delivered by c-section (if your baby can't tolerate labor or there are other reasons you can't have a vaginal birth). If you haven't yet reached week 37, you may be hospitalized for a day or two of monitoring. After that, if you and your baby are doing well, you might be sent home and told to take it easy (or possibly put on bed rest), and you'll be closely watched for changes in your condition. Your baby will be closely monitored as well—with nonstress tests, ultrasounds, and daily kick counts.

If you're diagnosed with *severe* gestational hypertension, on the other hand, you'll be hospitalized until you have your baby. If you're at week 34 or beyond, you'll be induced or—if necessary—deliver by c-section (page 426). If you're earlier in your pregnancy, you'll be given corticosteroids (to speed the development of your baby's lungs and help prevent other problems). How soon you give birth after that will depend on your condition and your baby's. If your condition is worsening or he isn't thriving inside your womb, you'll deliver even though he is still premature. If you don't need to deliver right away, you'll remain in the hospital so both you and your baby can be monitored very closely while he's given more time to mature.

Intrauterine Growth Restriction

Your practitioner will check the size of your uterus by measuring your belly at every prenatal visit in your second and third trimesters. If the measurement is smaller than your due date would indicate (a condition known as "small for dates"), she'll follow up with an ultrasound to pinpoint your baby's size and weight. (If you're in the first half of pregnancy and haven't yet had an ultrasound, measuring small may simply mean that your due date is off.)

A baby whose estimated weight is below the 10th percentile for his gestational age may be suffering from intrauterine growth restriction (IUGR). A variety of factors can cause this condition, including placental problems; maternal medical conditions (such as kidney, heart, or serious lung disease; advanced diabetes; or lupus); birth defects and genetic disorders; carrying twins or higher-order multiples; smoking, drinking, or abusing drugs; certain infections (such as toxoplasmosis); certain medications; and severe malnutrition. Sometimes, though, nothing is wrong—it is just that the baby is naturally smaller.

Babies with IUGR are at risk for a host of health problems at birth, though the eventual outcome partly depends on what caused the growth problem in the first place. Also, research suggests that problems are much more likely in babies whose birth weights are below the 5th percentile, and particularly if they're below the 3rd percentile.

If IUGR is diagnosed in your second trimester or if anatomical defects are seen on an ultrasound, you may also be offered an amniocentesis to check for chromosomal abnormalities. And depending on your individual situation, your caregiver may offer you blood tests to check for infection or blood-clotting abnormalities. You'll have an ultrasound every two to four weeks so your practitioner can see how your baby's growing and estimate the amount of amniotic fluid in your womb. Your baby's well-being will also be monitored with nonstress tests, biophysical profiles, and possibly Doppler sonography. Finally, your practitioner may want you to do daily fetal kick counts.

Generally, if you're at or near term when IUGR is diagnosed, you'll be induced (page 436) or—if your baby can't tolerate the stress of labor— scheduled for a c-section (page 426). If you're not near term, what your doctor does will depend on your condition and your baby's. Sometimes,

BabyCenter Buzz

My Baby Doesn't Seem to Be Growing Well

"At week 34, I measured 28 weeks. At week 36, I measured 29 weeks. After a couple of ultrasounds, the baby was measuring only two weeks behind. We had our son in week 38. He was 5 pounds, 12 ounces. Very healthy—just small." —*Anonymous*

when a baby simply isn't doing well in his mother's womb (or his mother is very sick, such as with severe preeclampsia), early delivery may be necessary.

Iron Deficiency Anemia

One easily controlled condition that may show up in your second trimester is iron deficiency anemia. Iron is a mineral essential for producing hemoglobin, the substance that carries oxygen in your blood. When you're pregnant, you need 50 percent more iron than before to keep up with the increased amount of blood circulating in your body, your baby's, and the placenta.

Signs of anemia include fatigue, sallow skin, dizziness, labored breathing, rapid heartbeat, and hair loss. But often, the condition is symptomless and is discovered only through routine prenatal blood tests in early pregnancy and again between weeks 24 and 28. If you're low in iron, you should get a prescription for iron supplements. (You're probably already getting extra iron from a prenatal vitamin, but you may need even more if you're anemic.) For some women, these supplements can cause constipation, but drinking lots of fluids, exercising moderately, and including plenty of fiber in your diet should help. Your healthcare provider may also recommend a stool softener.

Though iron deficiency is the most common cause of anemia, it's possible to

> ## BY THE NUMBERS
>
> ### Anemia in Pregnancy
>
> Pregnant women who develop iron deficiency anemia: **1 in 12**
>
> Source: *National Anemia Action Council*

BabyCenter Buzz

How I Manage My Anemia

"I find that eating fiber-rich foods helps prevent the constipation that iron supplements cause. A small packet of raisins or a fruit smoothie a day does the trick for me." *—Anonymous*

"When I entered my third trimester, I was constantly tired. I practically slept through a whole month! Then I had a routine hemoglobin check that signaled a borderline deficiency. I started taking an iron and folic acid supplement, and a few weeks later my levels had climbed and I wasn't tired anymore. I was amazed that such a mild deficiency could cause such intense fatigue." *—Anonymous*

"When my iron level dropped, my doctor told me to take an iron supplement with a stool softener built right into it. I feel so much better now." *—Anonymous*

develop anemia from a lack of folic acid or vitamin B_{12} as well. Anemia can also be caused by blood loss, by certain diseases, or by inherited blood disorders such as sickle-cell disease or thalassemia.

Placental Abruption

A placental abruption is a serious condition in which the placenta partially or completely separates from your uterus before your baby is born. No one knows for sure what causes most cases of placental abruption, but the condition is more common in mothers-to-be who've had an abruption in a previous pregnancy or who have chronic hypertension, gestational hypertension, or preeclampsia; who have blood-clotting disorders; who have preterm premature rupture of the membranes; who have polyhydramnios; or who had bleeding earlier in pregnancy. You're also at greater risk if you're pregnant with multiples, especially

BY THE NUMBERS

Placental Abruption Stats

Pregnant women who experience placental abruption: **1 in 200**

Source: *Williams Obstetrics, 21st edition*

Warning! Signs of Placental Abruption

Sometimes a placental abruption can cause a sudden hemorrhage, but in some cases there may not be any bleeding at first. Call your practitioner immediately if you have:

- Vaginal bleeding (if you have a significant amount of bleeding or if you have any signs of shock—you feel weak, faint, pale, sweaty, disoriented, or have a pounding heart—call 911)
- Cramping (with or without back pain)
- Uterine tenderness or abdominal pain
- Frequent contractions or a contraction that doesn't end
- A decrease in fetal movement

after the delivery of the first baby; if you're involved in an accident or have other trauma to your abdomen; if you smoke or use cocaine; if you've had many babies; or if you have a uterine abnormality.

Placenta Previa

If your placenta lies unusually low in your uterus, you may have a condition called placenta previa. The placenta may cover your cervix completely (total previa), or it may be very close to the edge of your cervix but not overlap it (marginal previa).

No one knows exactly what causes placenta previa, but several factors increase your risk (though many women who develop it have *no* apparent risk factors): placenta previa in a previous pregnancy, previous c-section(s) (your risk increases with each c-section) or other uterine surgery (such as a D & C or to remove uterine fibroids), carrying twins or more, being older, smoking, or having had many babies.

BY THE NUMBERS

Placenta Previa Stats

Pregnant women with placenta previa at birth:
4 in 1,000

Source: *National Institutes of Health*

BabyCenter Buzz

I Was Diagnosed with Placenta Previa

"I had a placenta previa. I was spotting and cramping until about 6 months. It eventually corrected itself, and I was able to deliver normally."   —Amber

"At my 20-week ultrasound I had placenta previa. My doctor told me to prepare to have a c-section at week 37 and possible bed rest if I had spotting. Yesterday I went in for my 28-week ultrasound, and the placenta had completely moved—it's not even considered low-lying now."   —Beth

In early pregnancy, placenta previa isn't a problem because the location of the placenta in relation to your cervix will likely change as your pregnancy progresses—as your uterus expands, the placenta "travels" farther away from the cervix. So don't panic if your placenta is low early on; only a small percentage of placenta previas seen on ultrasound in the first half of pregnancy will persist. You'll get a follow-up ultrasound later in pregnancy—usually late in your second or early in your third trimester—to check on the placenta's location. (If you have any vaginal bleeding in the interim, you'll get an ultrasound then to find out what's going on.)

If the previa persists, though, it's cause for concern since it can lead to a hemorrhage—which is dangerous for you and requires your baby to be delivered early. That's why you'll be monitored carefully, have regular ultrasounds, and need to watch for any vaginal bleeding. You'll be put on "pelvic rest"—meaning that *nothing* should go into your vagina—so you'll have to refrain from vaginal sex for the remainder of your pregnancy. You'll also be advised to take it easy and avoid activities (like strenuous housework or heavy lifting) or exercise that might provoke bleeding.

Bleeding from placenta previa can start without any warning and can range from spotting to profuse hemorrhaging (sometimes requiring a blood transfusion). In most cases, the bleeding doesn't happen until the second half of pregnancy, and about half the time it doesn't start until you're near term. The bleeding will often stop on its own, but it's likely to occur again. (If you're Rh negative, you'll need a shot of Rh immune globulin.)

If you have bleeding, you'll need to be hospitalized. What happens then will depend on how far along you are in your pregnancy, how heavy the bleeding is, and your baby's condition. If you're near term, you'll have your baby by c-section—since the placenta covers your cervix, it blocks his way out.

If your baby is still premature, he'll be delivered only if his condition warrants it or if you have heavy bleeding that doesn't stop. Otherwise, you'll be watched in the hospital until the bleeding stops. (You may be given corticosteriods to speed up your baby's lung development and to prevent other complications.) At that point—assuming both you and your baby are in good condition—you'll probably be sent home. If your bleeding recurs, return to the hospital *immediately*. Even if you don't have any bleeding at all, you'll be scheduled for a c-section in week 37 or 38.

Preeclampsia

Preeclampsia (also known as "toxemia") is a complex disorder that strikes in the second half of pregnancy. It's characterized by high blood pressure and protein in your urine, though there may be other signs as well. Preeclampsia can range from mild to severe, and it can progress slowly or rapidly. Some women sail through pregnancy with normal blood pressure, and then become preeclamptic during labor, and in others it might not even show up until *after* delivery.

Preeclampsia causes your blood vessels to constrict, decreasing blood flow to many of your organs. This can lead to a host of symptoms (page 177) and—in severe cases—serious complications, including seizures, stroke, and renal failure. The only "cure" is to deliver your baby.

Ask the Experts

Will Taking Extra Calcium Prevent Preeclampsia?

Dr. George Mussalli, maternal-fetal medicine specialist: Some small studies suggest that extra calcium may benefit women who are at increased risk for developing preeclampsia. But if your pregnancy is healthy and you're at low risk for preeclampsia, there doesn't seem to be any benefit to taking more than the recommended 1,000 milligrams of calcium a day. Your doctor or midwife is the best person to ask if extra calcium is right for you.

What to expect if you develop preeclampsia depends primarily on the severity of the disease, how your baby's doing, and how far along you are in your pregnancy. The effects of preeclampsia vary widely from woman to woman, but those who develop mild preeclampsia near their due dates generally do just fine.

If you're diagnosed with mild preeclampsia, if your baby is in good condition and if you're at week 37 or beyond, you'll likely be induced (page 436), or have a c-section (page 426) if it looks like your baby can't tolerate labor. If you're not yet at week 37, you may be temporarily hospitalized for monitoring. After that, you'll need to take it easy and be closely watched for signs of worsening preeclampsia. Your baby will be watched closely as well (with nonstress tests, periodic ultrasounds, and daily kick counts).

If you're diagnosed with severe preeclampsia, you'll have to spend the rest of your pregnancy in the hospital. You'll be given an IV medication called magnesium sulfate to prevent seizures and possibly another medica-

Just the Facts

Risk Factors for Preeclampsia

Despite extensive research, the cause of preeclampsia remains a bit of a medical mystery. It's likely that there are many factors responsible for the disorder. For reasons that still aren't totally understood, preeclampsia is more common in first pregnancies. Other risk factors include:

- Having chronic high blood pressure
- Having had preeclampsia in a previous pregnancy
- Being obese
- Having a close relative who had preeclampsia
- Carrying multiples
- Being over 40 or under 20
- Having diabetes
- Having certain blood-clotting disorders
- Having kidney disease
- Having an autoimmune disease like lupus

BabyCenter Buzz

I Was Diagnosed with Preeclampsia

"At my 36-week checkup today, they found signs of preeclampsia. I have high blood pressure (154/90), extreme swelling in my feet and ankles, and protein in my urine. Now I'm terrified that something will go wrong. My doctor says they may have to induce me tonight. I'm so scared." —*Kerry*

"I had preeclampsia with my first pregnancy and was induced three weeks early. With my second pregnancy, I was hospitalized for two weeks. After the doctors tried for five days to induce labor, I had a c-section. After the delivery, I needed heart monitoring for four days. It was a very scary situation, but I'm happy to say that both my baby and I are fine and I'm very happy it's all over now!" —*Eve*

tion to lower your blood pressure. If you're at week 34 or more, you'll be induced or deliver by c-section. If you haven't yet reached week 34, you'll get corticosteroids to speed the development of your baby's lungs and other organs. How quickly you deliver after that will depend on your and your baby's condition—it's a delicate balancing act between protecting your health and giving your baby as much time as possible to develop inside your womb. If you don't deliver right away, both you and your baby will be monitored very closely, and your baby will be delivered at the first sign of worsening preeclampsia, regardless of where you are in your pregnancy.

Because of changes in the placenta and decreased blood flow brought on by preeclampsia, there are risks for your baby as well—including poor growth, decreased amniotic fluid, placental abruption, and, in rare cases, death. These risks are increased when preeclampsia is more severe and occurs earlier in pregnancy. And because women with severe or worsening preeclampsia are induced early, their babies can also suffer the effects of prematurity.

Preterm Labor and Birth

More than one in eight babies in the United States (and nearly one in five African American babies) is born prematurely (or "preterm"), meaning that they're delivered before week 37. About a quarter of these preterm deliveries are planned. (For instance, your medical team decides to induce labor early or perform a c-section because you have a serious medical condition, such as severe or worsening preeclampsia, or because your baby has stopped growing.) The rest are known as spontaneous preterm births. You may end up having a spontaneous preterm birth if you go into labor prematurely, if your water breaks early (this is called preterm premature rupture of the

Just the Facts

Risk Factors for Spontaneous Preterm Birth

In many cases, no one knows what causes a baby to be born prematurely. Still, the following factors may increase your likelihood of having a preterm birth:

- Having a previous preterm birth (the earlier the birth, the higher the risk)
- Uterine or cervical abnormalities, such as cervical insufficiency
- An overly large uterus (often the case if you're pregnant with multiples or have too much amniotic fluid)
- Placental problems, such as placenta previa or placental abruption, or having had vaginal bleeding in more than one trimester even if the cause wasn't known
- Chronic maternal illnesses such as diabetes, sickle-cell anemia, severe asthma, lupus, inflammatory bowel disease, or hepatitis; nonuterine infections, such as kidney infection; abdominal surgery; abdominal trauma; and periodontitis, a serious gum infection
- Certain genital tract infections, such as chlamydia, bacterial vaginosis, and tri-chomoniasis (Substances produced by the bacterium that causes the infection can weaken the amniotic sac and cause it to rupture early. Even when the sac remains intact, bacteria can get inside and bring on preterm labor.)
- Smoking, abusing alcohol, or using illicit drugs (especially cocaine) during pregnancy

Other factors associated with an increased risk for preterm birth include being under 17 or over 35, African American, short, or underweight, as well as getting little or no prenatal care, and getting pregnant within 18 months of a previous delivery (particularly if you gave birth less than six months before getting pregnant again).

Some research also suggests that there might be a link between high levels of stress and preterm birth. One study showed that women who had to stand for long periods (more than 40 hours a week) or had extremely tiring jobs were more likely to deliver prematurely. Researchers are also studying the possible effect of genetic factors because preterm birth seems to be more common in some families and among certain ethnicities.

BabyCenter Buzz

I Went into Labor Too Soon

"I delivered my baby girl at 25 weeks. She was 1 pound, 7 ounces, and about a week after she was born, she caught pneumonia. I was so scared that she wasn't going to survive. Since then she's had other problems, and we're basically taking it day by day." —*Anonymous*

"My daughter was born at 26 weeks, weighing 2 pounds, 1 ounce. She spent 69 days in the NICU, which was very emotional and stressful. Thankfully, she has no complications now." —*Anonymous*

"I was admitted to the hospital for strict bed rest in week 29. I was given two steroid shots to mature my baby's lungs. Luckily, she made it to week 32 before being delivered via emergency c-section due to low amniotic fluid and IUGR. Jasmine came out hollering (thanks to those steroid shots!) weighing 2 pounds, 4 ounces. She spent 29 days in the NICU, and the only complication so far has been a brain bleed that's self-resolving." —*Nicole*

membranes, or PPROM), or if your cervix dilates prematurely with no contractions (cervical insufficiency).

Some premature babies do very well and adjust to life outside the womb with little or no medical help. Others may need lots of special care for days, weeks, or even months after birth. Later, some premature babies need a little extra time to catch up with their full-term peers, but unfortunately others—particularly those born very early—end up with lasting health or developmental problems, and some babies don't survive. In general, the more mature your baby is at birth, the more likely he is to survive and the less likely he is to have short- and long-term health problems.

If you start having contractions or other signs of preterm labor (page 297) or you think you're leaking amniotic fluid before you reach week 37, call your practitioner right away. She'll likely meet you at the hospital, where she'll monitor your contractions and your baby's heart rate, do an exam to see if your water has broken, and check your urine for signs of infection. She may also swab your vagina for fetal fibronectin (fFN) to get more information about your risk of giving birth soon.

If your water hasn't broken, your practitioner will do a vaginal exam to find out if your cervix has started to dilate and efface. You might also

Just the Facts

Fetal Fibronectin Screening

If you're having early contractions, you may have this test to determine if you're really at risk for preterm delivery. The test analyzes your cervical and vaginal fluid for the presence of fetal fibronectin (fFN), a protein that helps bind the amniotic sac to the lining of your uterus. Between weeks 24 and 34, elevated levels of fFN mean that this "glue" is disintegrating ahead of schedule (due to contractions or injury to the amniotic sac surrounding your baby), and signal a higher risk of preterm birth. The test itself is simple, involving a vaginal swab similar to getting a Pap smear and a wait of six to eight hours for results.

The fFN test isn't as accurate at predicting who'll deliver shortly as it is at predicting who *won't*: If you get a negative result, the likelihood that you'll deliver in the next two weeks is less than 5 percent. If your caregiver is trying to decide whether you should be hospitalized or need immediate treatment, for instance, a negative result may reassure her (and you!) that these interventions aren't needed.

If you're having contractions and you get a positive fFN result, on the other hand, you'll likely stay in the hospital, and your caregiver will administer labor-suppressing drugs. These can often hold off delivery for a few days so corticosteroids—which reduce your baby's chance of respiratory and other problems—have a chance to work.

Because the fFN test is relatively new, it's still not widely available. What's more, researchers are still debating whether it makes sense to screen women who have significant risk factors for—but no symptoms of—preterm labor. For now, most experts feel that with a few exceptions, the test should be reserved for women who are having contractions.

have an ultrasound to check on your baby and further evaluate your cervix. If all tests are negative, you and your baby appear healthy, your water hasn't broken, and your cervix isn't dilating or effacing, your caregiver will most likely send you home.

If it turns out that you're in preterm labor, what happens next depends on how far along you are in your pregnancy, whether your water has broken, whether there are signs of infection or other problems, and how your baby is faring. If your water hasn't broken and there are no other problems, your practitioner will generally try to hold off delivery as long as possible to give your baby time to mature. She may give you medication to stop your contractions, antibiotics in case you have a Group B strep infection, and corticosteroids to speed up your baby's lung development and lower the risk of certain other complications.

If your water breaks before week 37 but you're not having contractions (a condition called preterm premature rupture of the membranes, or PPROM), you'll be hospitalized and treated with antibiotics. Your practitioner may decide to wait for the onset of labor, to induce labor, or to try to delay labor. It's a difficult balancing act: Waiting buys your baby more time to mature but increases the risk of a dangerous infection, so experts don't always agree on how to proceed. Of course, if you develop symptoms of infection or your baby's condition isn't reassuring, you'll need to deliver right away.

In most cases, if you're in labor after week 34, you'll be allowed to deliver your baby. Babies born between weeks 34 and 37—and who have no other health problems—may need a short stay in the neonatal nursery and may have short-term health issues, but in the long run they generally do as well as full-term babies.

Rh Sensitization

Here's how sensitization occurs: If you're an Rh-negative woman carrying an Rh-positive child (your baby having inherited that blood-protein characteristic from an Rh-positive father), your blood types are considered Rh incompatible. Rh incompatiblity itself isn't a problem. Difficulties arise if you become what's called Rh-sensitized.

Here's how it works: If some of your baby's red blood cells leak into your bloodstream (which can happen at certain times during pregnancy and birth), your immune system may react to the Rh factor on the surface of your baby's cells by making antibodies against it. The next time you're pregnant with an Rh-positive child, these antibodies will cross the placenta and possibly attack your baby's blood, leading to anemia and other serious problems. The good news is that getting shots of a substance called Rh immune globulin when you need them can prevent you from becoming Rh-sensitized. If you're Rh negative, your caregiver will do a blood test at your first prenatal visit and again later during your pregnancy to be sure you aren't sensitized.

Unless you're already sensitized, you'll get a shot of Rh immune globulin in week 28 to protect you in case any of your baby's blood gets into yours during your third trimester. (Note: If your baby's biological father is also Rh-negative, this shot isn't necessary.) And because the shot offers protection for only about 12 weeks, you'll need another one within 72 hours of delivery (unless your baby turns out to be Rh negative as well). You'll also need the shot at any other time that there's a possibility of your baby's blood mixing with yours, including:

- After an abortion
- After a miscarriage
- After a molar pregnancy
- After an ectopic pregnancy
- After an invasive procedure, such as chorionic villus sampling or amniocentesis
- After a stillbirth
- After an external cephalic version
- After a trauma to your abdomen
- After bleeding in your second or third trimester

You may also need an injection if you have any unexplained bleeding during your pregnancy. If you find yourself in any of these situations, remind your caregiver that you're Rh negative, and make sure you get the shot. The regular use of Rh immune globulin has had a major impact on preventing Rh disease and its serious consequences for your baby.

BY THE NUMBERS

Twins or More

Average chance of bearing twins: **about 1 in 32**

Chance of bearing identical twins: **about 1 in 250**

Average chance of bearing triplets or higher-order multiples: **about 1 in 540**

Rise in the rate of twins born in the United States between 1980 and 2002 (largely due to increased use of fertility treatments): **65%**

Rise in the rate of triplets and higher-order multiples born in the United States between 1980 and 2002: **nearly 400%**

Source: *National Center for Health Statistics*

Twins, Triplets, and Higher-Order Multiples

Discovering that you're carrying more than one baby is shocking, but it can also be thrilling. Still, as with other complex prenatal health situations, you'll need special care because you're at higher risk for complications such as preterm labor, preeclampsia, and gestational diabetes. So expect more prenatal appointments, usually every two to three weeks in your first and second trimesters and weekly in your third trimester. Your provider will also want to keep close tabs on your babies'

BabyCenter Buzz

I'm Having Twins (or More)!

"I'm in week 7 and just found out—via an early ultrasound—that I'm pregnant with triplets. I'm very nervous." —*Anonymous*

"At week 9 I told my doctor that I was already wearing maternity clothes and felt huge. We did an ultrasound just to see, and surprise . . . two heartbeats!" —*Laurie*

"When I was 20 weeks, I measured 28 weeks. That's when I found out I was having twins." —*Anonymous*

growth, so you'll probably have frequent ultrasounds to make sure they're developing properly. Finally, starting in your late second or early third trimester, you'll begin having nonstress tests or biophysical profiles to make sure your babies are continuing to thrive.

You can also expect normal pregnancy aches and pains to be more intense than they are for women carrying just one baby. Women pregnant with twins, triplets, or more are especially likely to have severe early-pregnancy symptoms—particularly a bad case of morning sickness—and these symptoms tend to last longer. Other common complaints include heightened fatigue, discomfort, water retention and swelling, and—as your pregnancy progresses and your belly grows ever bigger—trouble sleeping, shortness of breath, and more difficulty getting around comfortably. At some point in your pregnancy, your practitioner may recommend that you restrict your activity or even go on bed rest—though there's no good evidence that bed rest helps prevent complications. You'll probably need to take an iron supplement as well because your body's producing more blood than ever.

All About Bed Rest

Whether you've been sent to bed for two weeks or six months, take some comfort in knowing you're not alone: Each year, hundreds of thousands of pregnant women—perhaps as many as one in five—are put on bed rest at some point in their pregnancy. If you're one of them, chances are you're at risk for preterm labor (perhaps you've had a previous preterm birth or are carrying twins) or you have another pregnancy complication.

For some women, bed rest means 24 hours a day in bed and getting up only to use the bathroom. In this situation, you'll usually need to lie on your side most of the day (this position takes the pressure of your heavy uterus off the vena cava, a large vein that returns blood from your lower body to your heart). For others, bed rest is less limiting: You may need frequent rest periods in bed, but you can still have occasional outings in the car (usually to see your caregiver) and get up to make yourself lunch or to take a shower.

While extended bed rest might sound like heaven if you're feeling exhausted, it's not as great as it sounds. As a treatment method, bed rest is controversial, and medical experts disagree about its benefits. It's often recommended in an effort to prolong pregnancy, the idea being that it may help "quiet" your uterus or keep the weight of your baby off a weak cervix. But there's no clear scientific evidence that it has any real value in prolonging pregnancy.

Bed rest is also often prescribed for intrauterine growth restriction, gestational hypertension, or preeclampsia in the hope that it will improve blood flow to your uterus, increasing the supply of nutrients and oxygen to your developing baby—but again, there's no proof that it helps.

The reason caregivers prescribe bed rest so often is that it seems harmless and worth a try when there's no proven treatment for a problem. But there are downsides to bed rest: Besides being emotionally trying for you (and often for your entire family), it can have negative health effects as well. Being on complete bed rest for an extended period boosts your odds of blood clots and also leads to muscle atrophy, leaving you weak and causing enormous fatigue when your bed rest order is eventually lifted—or worse, when you have a newborn to care for. Bottom line: If you have a pregnancy complication and your caregiver prescribes bed rest, ask her to discuss the pros and cons with you.

Sleeping Well When You're on Bed Rest

Spending weeks or months in bed can wreak havoc on your natural sleep-wake cycle and on your sense of time. A few steps you can take to sleep better on bed rest:

BabyCenter Buzz

How I Survived Bed Rest

"My days have been filled with working from home, reading books, watching movies, and taking naps. Visits from friends have helped pass the time, and my mother was able to come and stay with us for a month to help with chores and meals." —*Anonymous*

"I have all my activities organized into baskets and Tupperware containers right next to my bed. It keeps them easy to find." —*Jami*

"Some things I've found helpful: calling volunteer organizations to see if they need help with mailings and callings, working on my cross-stitch, getting a book on learning how to draw, getting simple craft projects to do with my son, and writing long-overdue letters." —*Kelly*

Stick to a normal day-and-night routine. Even though you'll be spending most or all of your time in bed, try to keep up with regular daytime activities such as taking a shower in the morning (if your practitioner gives you the go-ahead) and wearing something other than PJs. And keep yourself busy doing things you like so you won't be tempted to sleep the day away.

Get some sunlight. If you can, move your bed or a couch close to a window so you can enjoy the daytime light. It will boost your spirits and help keep your internal clock on track, too.

Nap, but not too much. You're on bed rest because you need to *rest*. Go ahead and nap, preferably at a scheduled time. If you snooze too late in the day, though, you may find yourself having a hard time falling asleep at bedtime.

Eat meals at roughly the same time every day. Ask a friend or relative to drop by and join you for a breakfast or lunch (or, better yet, to *bring* you lunch). Having meals at the same time will help keep your body on a schedule.

Ask your caregiver if it's okay to exercise. Doing some simple stretching and isometric exercises with your arms and legs will be good for your muscles—and perhaps your mood as well.

Genetic Problems and Other Birth Defects

When you daydream about your baby-to-be, you undoubtedly picture a child in perfect health. Sadly, not every baby can escape genetic disorders and other health problems. These problems may be inherited, or they may be caused by environmental factors, such as drug or alcohol abuse or exposure to certain infections, medications, or chemicals. Most of the time, though, no one knows what's caused a particular defect. Some birth defects are fatal, while others are mild and easily treatable. If prenatal testing signals a severe defect, you'll have a difficult decision to make about whether or not to keep the pregnancy. Either way, it's normal to feel a host of different emotions, including denial, grief, guilt, and anger. If you find you're having difficulty coping, talk to your caregiver about getting help.

BabyCenter Buzz

What We Did When We Got Bad News About Our Baby

"Take your time figuring out what's best for you, your baby, and your family because the shock and grief need to subside a little." —Amee

"If your baby's problem is treatable, count your blessings. You won't have the 'perfect' child you envisioned, so do allow yourself time before the baby is born to grieve. Get it out of your system so you're open and ready to welcome this baby with all your heart. You'll love your child no matter what—because he's yours." —Anonymous

"Via an early ultrasound, we discovered that one of the twins I was carrying had defects that would lead to (at worst) miscarriage of the entire pregnancy or stillbirth of one of the babies or (at best) bringing a child with zero quality of life into the world. After untold tears, raging, and grief, we decided to have a 'selective reduction' to give our healthy daughter the best chance for life and to get through the worst of our grieving before we had a newborn who needed us 100 percent. There was nothing we could do to help the baby we lost, but the choice we made—as heartbreaking as it was—was the best one for us, and for our surviving child." —Anonymous

"When I was pregnant with my daughter Celine, we discovered that she had serious heart defects. I was given the option to terminate, but rejected that course. Since her birth, Celine has had three heart surgeries. I understand what it's like to come to terms with uncertainty, and to bank on hope and faith—and, in our case, on the talent of doctors who wanted to give my child the best possible chance at life." —Monica

Ask the Experts

What Does It Mean When a Baby Has an Extra Chromosome?

Dr. Russell Turk, obstetrician: It means the baby has a chromosomal abnormality. Normally, we inherit 23 chromosomes from each parent, for a total of 46. Each chromosome matches the corresponding chromosome from the other parent, forming a numbered set. Because of biological errors that happen during the early stages of cell division, some fetuses develop with 47 chromosomes, which means that instead of 23 pairs, they have 22 pairs plus one set of three, a condition called trisomy. Most fetuses with trisomy miscarry during the first trimester; those that survive often have Down syndrome (also known as trisomy 21, since it's the 21st set of chromosomes that's affected). The risk of having a baby with trisomy increases with age, which is why healthcare providers suggest genetic testing for women who will be 35 or older on their due date.

Pregnancy Loss: Miscarriage and Ectopic Pregnancy

It's not uncommon to lose a pregnancy in the early months, but that doesn't make it any less heartbreaking. There are a number of culprits responsible for the unexpected end of a pregnancy, but the reason for most will never be known. Here's a look at the two most common forms of pregnancy loss—miscarriage and ectopic pregnancy—plus warning signs to watch out for:

Miscarriage

About one in five known pregnancies ends in a miscarriage, and more than 80 percent of these losses happen before week 12. Most miscarriages are caused by chromosomal abnormalities that prevent the fertilized egg from developing normally. An example of this is the so-called blighted ovum, in which a placenta and a gestational sac begin to develop but there's no baby inside because the embryo either failed to develop or stopped developing very early. In other cases, an embryo does grow for a little while but has abnormalities that make survival impossible, and development stops before the heart starts beating. Once your baby has a heartbeat—usually visible on ultrasound around week 6—the odds of your having a miscarriage drop significantly.

Just the Facts

Who's at Risk for Miscarriage

Most first miscarriages are considered random events, and fertility experts don't consider a single early-pregnancy loss a sign that there's anything wrong with you or your partner. In most cases, your risk for future pregnancy loss after one miscarriage is close to the same as it was before. After two miscarriages in a row, some practitioners will order special blood and genetic tests to try to find out what's going wrong, particularly if you're older than 35 or have certain medical problems. (Others will wait until you've had three consecutive losses.) Though any woman can miscarry, pregnancy loss is more likely for women with these risk factors:

Age. Older women are more likely to conceive babies with chromosomal abnormalities, and to miscarry as a result. In fact, 40-year-olds are twice as likely to miscarry as 20-year-olds.

A history of miscarriages. Women who've had two or more miscarriage in a row are more likely than other women to miscarry again.

Certain diseases or disorders. Poorly controlled diabetes, blood clotting problems, autoimmune diseases, and hormonal disorders can make it harder to carry a baby.

Uterine or cervical problems. Having a uterine abnormality or a weak or unusually short cervix (called cervical insufficiency) can increase your risk of pregnancy loss.

A history of birth defects or genetic problems. Having another child with a birth defect or having a family history (or a partner with a family history) of genetic problems can also boost the odds of miscarriage.

Certain infections. Rarely, some foodborne infections, childhood diseases, and sexually transmitted infections can increase your risk for miscarriage.

Smoking, drinking, and using drugs. Cigarettes, alcohol, and drugs like cocaine and ecstasy can all increase your risk of miscarriage. Even drinking more than four cups of coffee a day has been associated with a higher risk of pregnancy loss.

Taking certain medications. Some medications have been linked to a heightened chance of miscarriage, so it's important to ask your caregiver about the safety of any medications you're taking while you're trying to conceive. This goes for both prescription and over-the-counter drugs, including nonsteroidal anti-inflammatory drugs (NSAIDs) like ibuprofen or aspirin.

Exposure to environmental toxins. Environmental factors that might increase your miscarriage risk include lead, arsenic, and some chemicals like formaldehyde, benzene, ethylene oxide, and large doses of radiation or anesthetic gases.

Family size and spacing. Your risk of miscarriage increases with each additional child you bear, and when you get pregnant again within three months of giving birth.

Paternal factors. Little is known about how your partner's condition can contribute to your risk for miscarriage. Older fathers may face an increased risk, as may those who've been exposed to mercury, lead, and some industrial pesticides and chemicals.

BabyCenter Buzz

I Had a Miscarriage

"I started spotting in week 11 and called my doctor. He had me come in and found that there was no longer a heartbeat. I'm having trouble knowing what's normal to be feeling now." —*Anonymous*

"At my 12-week ultrasound, there was no heartbeat. I had a D & C the next day. The actual surgery and physical recovery wasn't bad, but the emotional healing is harder. Be sure to give yourself time to grieve." —*Kari*

"I miscarried and am doing well now, but the sadness still hits me at times. I have a 20-month-old daughter, and I've found a great deal of comfort in her. I think it's made me appreciate her more than I did before . . . realizing how fragile life is and how lucky we are to have her. I know I will never forget the baby I lost, but I hope to try again soon." —*Alicia*

Vaginal spotting or bleeding sometimes signals an impending miscarriage. Spotting (that is, finding spots of red or brownish blood on your underpants or toilet tissue) is relatively common in early pregnancy and doesn't always mean there's a problem. Abdominal pain (which may feel crampy or persistent, and mild or sharp), lower-back pain, or pelvic pressure may also be signs of a miscarriage. If you have any of these symptoms, call your doctor or midwife right away so she can figure out what's going on. Some miscarriages are discovered only during a routine prenatal visit, when your practitioner can't hear the baby's heartbeat or notices that your uterus isn't growing as it should.

If an ultrasound confirms that your pregnancy has stopped developing but there's no threat to your health, you may choose to let the miscarriage happen on its own timeline. (More than half of women spontaneously miscarry within a week of finding out that their pregnancy is no longer viable.) On the other hand, if you find that it's too emotionally trying or physically painful to wait for nature to take its course—or if you're bleeding a lot—you may be be offered medication to speed up the process, or have a suction curettage (or a dilation and curettage—a D & C) to remove the pregnancy tissue. If you're Rh negative, you'll need to get a shot of Rh immune globulin.

Ectopic Pregnancy

If a fertilized egg implants outside your uterus, usually in one of your fallopian tubes, it's called an ectopic pregnancy, and one in 50 pregnancies ends this way. After conception, the fertilized egg travels down your fallopian tube on its way to your uterus. If your tube is damaged or blocked—or fails for whatever reason to propel the egg toward your womb—the egg may implant itself in your tube and continue to develop there. (That's why ectopic pregnancies are often called "tubal" pregnancies.) Much less commonly, an egg implants in another part of your abdomen, in an ovary, or in your cervix.

There's no way to transplant an ectopic (literally, "out of place") pregnancy into your uterus, so ending the pregnancy is the only option. In fact, if an ectopic pregnancy isn't recognized and treated, the embryo may grow until your fallopian tube ruptures. Treatment usually involves surgery or sometimes medication. Luckily, the vast majority of ectopic pregnancies are caught in time.

Just the Facts

Who's at Risk for Ectopic Pregnancy

If you're at high risk for having an ectopic pregnancy, see your practitioner as soon as you know (or suspect) that you might be pregnant. Your odds of having an ectopic pregnancy are higher if:

- You got pregnant despite having had your tubes tied.
- You've had pelvic or abdominal surgery.
- You've had a previous ectopic pregnancy.
- You got pregnant with an intrauterine device (IUD) in place. (An IUD doesn't cause ectopic pregnancy, it just doesn't prevent it the way it does a normal pregnancy.)
- Your mother took the drug DES while she was pregnant with you.
- You're being evaluated or treated for infertility.
- You've had pelvic inflammatory disease or a sexually transmitted infection such as gonorrhea or chlamydia.
- You smoke.

Call Your Caregiver If . . .

Ectopic pregnancies are usually discovered in week 6 or 7. If left untreated, an ectopic pregnancy can be life-threatening, so call your practitioner right away if you have:

- **Abdominal or pelvic pain or tenderness.** It can be sudden, persistent, and severe—but may also be mild and intermittent early on. You may feel it only on one side, but the pain can be anywhere in your abdomen or pelvis and is sometimes accompanied by nausea and vomiting.
- **Vaginal spotting or bleeding** that's red or brown, copious or scant, and continuous or intermittent.
- **Pain that gets worse** when you're active or while you're moving your bowels or coughing.
- **Shoulder pain.** Cramping and bleeding can mean many things, but pain in your shoulder, particularly when you lie down, is a red flag for a ruptured ectopic pregnancy. The cause of the pain is internal bleeding, which irritates nerves that go to your shoulder area.
- **Signs of shock,** such as a weak, racing pulse; pale, clammy skin; and dizziness or fainting. This may mean a fallopian tube has ruptured. Get immediate medical attention.

Dealing with Grief

It's normal to feel shock, grief, depression, guilt, anger, and a sense of failure and vulnerabilty when you lose a pregnancy, decide to terminate for medical reasons, or learn that you're expecting a baby with major health or developmental problems. The days, weeks, and even months following a loss or a diagnosis of serious trouble can be incredibly difficult—even more so if this wasn't your first pregnancy loss or if you carefully planned this pregnancy and thought you'd done everything "right." Or you may simply feel withdrawn and moody and unable to concentrate or sleep. If you told people you were pregnant, you'll probably worry about announcing this news—and you may find even the sincerest expressions of sympathy difficult to take. A few things to keep in mind as you work through this troubled time:

Understand that it's not your fault. Pregnancy loss or complications can strike anyone. Talk openly and honestly with your partner about what's happened and how you feel about it, and allow time to mourn, to heal, and to move on.

Give it time. Depending on your circumstances, getting over the loss may not come quickly. Grief comes in waves, even when you think you've cried all you can, especially around your due date or other milestones.

Consider taking time off from work. Even if you feel physically fine, you may find taking some time away from work helpful. You need a chance to process what's happened, and jumping right back into your regular routine as if nothing were amiss won't aid your long-term emotional recovery.

Don't expect those around you to grieve in the same way. Someone who hasn't gone through what you're going through really *can't* know what it's like. Even your partner may brush off your loss without truly understanding how deeply you're hurting (it was his baby, too, of course—but he didn't have the same visceral, physical connection that you did). Everyone grieves differently, so don't misread his stoicism as not caring about you or your loss. As off-the-mark as they are, do your best not to let well-meaning but insensitive comments like "It was God's will" or "You can try again" rattle you. Remind yourself that grief is something most people are uncomfortable with and unaccustomed to expressing their feelings about, especially when it's a pregnancy loss. Try not to take it personally if they say the wrong thing or nothing at all. If someone says something that strikes you the wrong way, let them know you appreciate their concern—just not the way it was communicated.

Don't close yourself off. At the same time, you may be surprised by how many previously unknown stories of loss and healing you'll hear from mothers, cousins, coworkers, neighbors, and friends. You may find understanding and support from unexpected people—which can help make up for the fact that some of those you *expected* to understand don't seem to get how much you're hurting.

Get support. Ask your doctor or midwife about pregnancy-loss support groups in your community. It may take a while to find one that suits you best, so don't get discouraged if you don't like the first one you try. You may also want to seek out a professional counselor to help you grapple with the difficult emotions you're experiencing right now and, ultimately, to come to terms with your grief.

BabyCenter Buzz

How I Coped with Pregnancy Loss

"It's gotten easier with time, but it still hits me—usually when I'm reminded that I should be pregnant right now. I think cycling between being fairly okay and being very sad is a pretty normal way of handling a very sad event. It does get better, and it helps to know that there are others who understand."   —*Alicia*

"At 12 weeks, I learned that my baby had stopped growing and didn't have a heartbeat. I was shocked, sad, and overwhelmed: I had a breakdown and couldn't stop sobbing. Yesterday I cried on and off all day. This morning I'm feeling better. Hopefully, I'll continue to feel that way. I'm trying to stay positive now and looking forward to getting pregnant again. We'll get through this. We are all tough and brave."   —*Anonymous*

"I lost my daughter Annabelle. I delivered three days before my due date, but she was tangled in her umbilical cord. Time does help to heal. I found it good to do things that helped me remember my daughter, even something as small as wearing earrings with her birthstone. I also attend a monthly support group with people who've had similar experiences. It's hard to believe now, but there does come a time when you can think of your loss without tears."   —*Anonymous*

Trying Again
Pregnancy After a Loss

You'll likely get your period four to six weeks after losing—or ending—a pregnancy. Though you may be *physically* ready to get pregnant again at that point, you're probably not emotionally ready. Every woman deals with the grief of pregnancy loss in her own way. Some cope best by turning their attention toward trying for a new pregnancy as soon as possible. Others find that months or more go by before they're interested in trying again. Take time to examine your feelings, and do what feels right for you and your partner. If you do become pregnant, it will help to blunt your grief—but it can never fully replace your loss because each pregnancy is unique and special.

Once you *have* conceived again, it's normal to be especially anxious about this new pregnancy and to feel uneasy until you're safely past the time when you miscarried before. But remember, too, that unless your caregiver tells you otherwise, you have every chance of having a normal pregnancy

BabyCenter Buzz

My Previous Miscarriage Is Making Me Nervous

"I'm seeing a therapist who's really helping me. It's nice to have a neutral party put my fears into perspective." —*Karen*

"Staying busy is always better than sitting and worrying about possible problems. If you really feel that something isn't right, call your doctor or midwife rather than allowing your fears to get the best of you." —*Annie*

"If you're religious, trust in God. Pray for your baby's health and safety and for your own emotional well-being." —*Tess*

this time around. After a first miscarriage, your odds of having another are almost no higher than they were before, and even after two miscarriages, your risk of a third increases only slightly. If you've had two or more miscarriages, talk to your caregiver to make sure that any diagnosable problems that may have led to your losses are identified and treated before you try to conceive again.

While you can't stop yourself from worrying, you *can* do your best to stay well-rested and as stress-free as possible during these fretful early months. You can also ask your pregnancy caregiver to do an early sonogram to help ease your mind. Once you see your developing baby and hear the reassuring gallop of his or her heartbeat, you'll probably worry less. Ask your caregiver if you can have an additional ultrasound or be seen more often if it helps ease your mind. Finally, whatever you do, resist the urge to stoically hide your fears: Talking to your partner, your close friends, and your healthcare provider about your anxieties will help you feel less frightened and alone. (Let your caregiver know as soon as possible if your anxiety or worry is so overwhelming that it's affecting your daily life. She can put you in touch with a counseling professional who can help.)

IS IT SAFE?

Health and Medicine Guide: What's Safe, What's Not

When you're newly pregnant and trying to cope with the bothersome symptoms that crop up in your first trimester, your first thought may be to head to the medicine cabinet. In some cases that's totally fine, but in other, even seemingly safe remedies are suddenly off-limits. What's more, things that you never gave a second thought to before—donating blood, getting dental X-rays, cleaning the litter box, going to a rock concert—may suddenly seem iffy. Here, we've sorted out which treatments and situations you should avoid, which ones you can stop worrying about, and everything in between. Always talk to your pregnancy practitioner before taking *any* prescription or over-the-counter medication, herb, or nutritional supplement—and be sure to tell anyone prescribing medication for you or performing any medical procedure (including your dentist) that you're pregnant.

Drugs and Other Remedies: Is It Safe?

. . . To Take Acetaminophen?

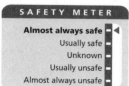

Ronald Ruggiero, pharmacist clinical specialist: Acetaminophen (Tylenol) is safe, but be careful not to take more than the amount recommended on the label. If you take too much, it can cause liver failure, and in a small number of cases, pregnant women who overdosed on acetaminophen had babies with birth defects.

. . . To Take Antibiotics?

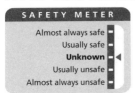

Gerald Briggs, pharmacist clinical specialist: It depends. Some antibiotics are safe throughout pregnancy, some pose known risks to a developing baby, and a host of others fall in between—either there's not enough safety information or the potential risk of the antibiotic needs to be carefully weighed against the harmful effects of the condition it's being used to treat. Plus, the safety of a particular antibiotic (like *any* medication) depends not only on characteristics of the drug itself, but on factors such as how much you take, how long you take it for, and when in pregnancy you take it.

With so many antibiotics available, it isn't possible to list all of them here. But common antibiotics that are considered safe during pregnancy—provided you're not allergic to them—include penicillins (including amoxicillin and ampicillin), cephalosporins (cephalexin), and erythromycin. All are used to treat a wide range of infections.

Antibiotics to *avoid* include streptomycin (used to treat tuberculosis), which can cause hearing loss in your baby, and tetracycline (including minocycline, oxytetracycline, and doxycycline, used to treat acne and respiratory infections). If you take tetracycline in your first trimester, you may run a small risk of birth defects, but most experts now believe it's unlikely; what's more likely is that if you take tetracycline in your second or third trimester, it may discolor your developing baby's teeth.

Trimethoprim, a common ingredient in drugs used to treat urinary tract infections (such as Bactrim or Septra), is another drug to be cautious about because it can block the effects of folic acid (page 64). If you have no other choice but to take it, be sure to take your daily prenatal vitamin as well.

. . . To Take Antidepressants?

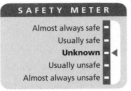

Diane Sanford, psychologist, and Gerald Briggs, pharmacist clinical specialist: You should always consult a psychiatrist or your pregnancy practitioner about treatment for depression, as well as about the specifics of your particular situation. Most of the evidence to date suggests that the preferred treatment for depression—a class of antidepressant drugs called selective serotonin reuptake inhibitors (SSRIs), including fluoxetine (Prozac), paroxetine (Paxil), and sertraline (Zoloft)—is relatively safe during pregnancy. Although recent research suggests that SSRI exposure in the womb may affect a baby's motor development and control, there's no significant difference in the rate of major birth defects, miscarriages, stillbirth, and premature births between women who take these drugs and women who don't. As with most medications taken in pregnancy, you and your practitioner will need to carefully weigh the pros and cons before making a final decision about treatment with SSRIs.

. . . To Take Aspirin?

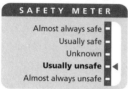

Ann Linden, certified nurse-midwife: In most cases, no. While it's highly unlikely that taking a single dose of aspirin while you're pregnant will cause problems, the drug could harm your baby if you regularly take it in normal doses, so it's best to avoid it altogether. That's because aspirin has been linked to miscarriage (page 543), growth problems (page 526), placental abruption (page 528), delayed labor, heart and lung problems for your baby, and bleeding complications.

Check the labels of all over-the-counter medications (or better yet, check with your caregiver or pharmacist) before taking them to make sure they don't contain NSAIDs. (Some products list aspirin as "salicylate" or "acetylsalicylic acid.")

If you're already taking a prescribed dose of aspirin for a specific health condition, though, be sure to check with your practitioner before discontinuing it. There are also circumstances in which your caregiver might advise you to take a small daily dose of low-strength aspirin, and most experts say this low-dose aspirin therapy is safe. In women with a condition called antiphospholipid syndrome, for instance, low-dose aspirin therapy (plus a blood thinner called heparin) may actually *prevent* miscarriage and other problems. Also, in some women at high risk for preeclampsia (page 531)—including those with chronic hypertension (page 589), severe diabetes (page 525), or kidney disease, or who had severe preeclampsia in a previous pregnancy— low-dose aspirin therapy may lower the risk for this pregnancy complication.

. . . To Take Ibuprofen?

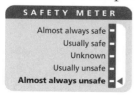

Dr. Kay Daniels, obstetrician: It's best to avoid it in your first trimester as well as in your last. That's because this painkiller, like all nonsteroidal anti-inflammatory drugs (NSAIDs), has been linked to miscarriage when it's taken regularly in the weeks before conception or during the first 12 weeks of pregnancy. And after 32 weeks, NSAIDs can cause the opening between the major arteries in your baby's heart to close prematurely or lead to damage to your baby's kidneys.

. . . To Take Medicine That Contains Alcohol?

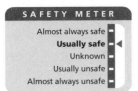

Christina Chambers, epidemiologist: There's no reason to believe that taking a few doses would put your baby at risk if you're using the medicine as prescribed and for a short period of time. In that case, it's unlikely that you'd be getting enough alcohol to cause the kinds of problems associated with regular alcohol consumption. Still, medicines like Nyquil contain other ingredients that aren't always recommended during pregnancy, so ask your practitioner about an alternative.

. . . To Take Cold Medications?

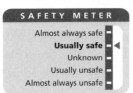

Dr. Joyce and Dr. Marshall Gottesfeld, obstetricians: Using plain acetaminophen as directed on the bottle to relieve aches and pains is fine. Many antihistamines (such as Chlor-Trimeton) are safe to take during pregnancy, but because some cold preparations contain active ingredients that aren't known to be completely safe during pregnancy, it's best to talk to your doctor or midwife before taking these or any other over-the-counter medication.

In the meantime, try sitting in a steamy bathroom, using saline nasal drops, or using a steam vaporizer to provide some relief from nasal and chest congestion, and get plenty of rest and drink lots of liquids to help you feel less miserable overall. If you have a fever, let your practitioner know so she can rule out problems like bronchitis or pneumonia.

. . . To Take Motion Sickness Medications?

Ronald Ruggiero, pharmacist clinical specialist: Stick to over-the-counter drugs that contain dimenhydrinate (Dramamine) or diphenhydramine (Be-

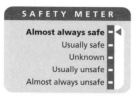

nadryl). But avoid prescription drugs like scopolamine; they're not dangerous for your baby, but they can cause side effects such as dizziness, tremors, fatigue, and confusion that are uncomfortable for you.

. . . To Use Nasal Decongestant Sprays?

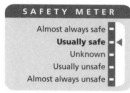

Ronald Ruggiero, pharmacist clinical specialist: Nasal decongestant sprays are probably safe to use in pregnancy, but they're not a good idea in general. That's because, after using them for two or three days, you start to get rebound congestion, which makes you worse off than when you began. If you can't treat your congestion with a plain saline nose spray, then try rubbing a camphorated ointment, such as Vicks VapoRub, at the bottom of each nostril, taking a doctor-recommended decongestant, or even eating a spicy meal.

. . . To Take Echinacea?

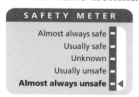

Ronald Ruggiero, pharmacist clinical specialist: Echinacea isn't recommended during pregnancy because it could stimulate your uterus and cause premature labor. And because your immune system changes when you're pregnant to give you extra protection against illness, you don't want to take anything that could interfere with that process. The one published study on echinacea in pregnancy didn't find any increased risk for birth defects, but it was too limited to be definitive.

. . . To Take Homeopathic Remedies?

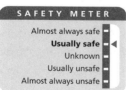

Morgan Martin, naturopathic midwife: Homeopathy is safe when you're in the hands of a skilled licensed practitioner. One remedy you *should* steer clear of is caulophyllum, a homeopathic form of the herb blue cohosh, which is used to stimulate uterine contractions.

. . . To Get a Flu Shot?

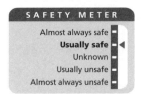

Ann Linden, certified nurse-midwife: Yes, in fact, it's recommended unless you're allergic to eggs or have had a previous severe reaction to a flu shot. (If you've ever had a rare condition called Guillain-Barré syndrome, let your caregiver know—she may advise holding off on the flu vaccine in that case as well.) The Centers for Disease Control and Prevention (CDC) recommends the flu shot for all other pregnant women during flu season (November through March). That's because if you get the flu while you're pregnant, you're more likely to have complications, such as pneumonia, that might put you and your baby at risk. And if you have a chronic illness—such as asthma, diabetes, or heart disease—that makes getting the flu particularly risky, you should get the flu shot *before* the flu season starts (September or October).

The flu shot is considered safe because it's made from inactivated (killed) virus (unlike the nasal-spray vaccine, which is made with live virus and which you should *not* get during pregnancy). Though flu shots contain the controversial preservative thimerosal (a mercury compound), the CDC has concluded that the benefits of the shot outweigh any potential risks. If you're concerned about this, ask your caregiver about getting a dose of the preservative-free version of the flu shot, which contains only trace amounts of thimerosal.

Treatments and Procedures: Is It Safe?

. . . To Donate Blood?

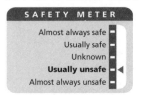

Dr. Craig Winkel, obstetrician: No. Your blood volume increases by nearly 50 percent when you're pregnant because you need more of it circulating to your placenta and baby. When you give blood, you reduce the amount of oxygen that your blood can carry to your baby. No blood bank would even consider drawing blood from a pregnant woman. (Don't worry if you gave blood before you knew you were pregnant, though. Your caregiver will check your blood for anemia—page 162—and recommend iron supplements if needed.)

. . . To Get an X-Ray?

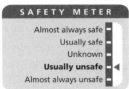

Kristina Kahl, genetic counselor: It's best to avoid X-rays while you're pregnant. That's because recent research has found that getting numerous dental X-rays may increase your odds of delivering a low-birthweight baby. While the exact reason for this is still unclear, researchers theorize that the radiation from the X-rays may damage your thyroid, pituitary, or hypothalamus gland; these glands regulate key hormone levels that influence your baby's growth. If your dentist thinks that X-rays can't wait, be sure she knows you're pregnant and provides you with both an abdominal and a thyroid shield. (Whatever you do, though, continue to visit your dentist and to take good care of your teeth and gums while you're pregnant. Poor dental hygiene can also increase the risk of preterm delivery and of poor fetal growth.)

While it's best to avoid X-rays during your pregnancy, if your dentist or doctor feels they're necessary for your health, you can minimize any risk they may pose to your baby by taking the proper precautions.

. . . To Get Vaccinated?

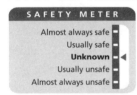

Kristina Kahl, genetic counselor: It depends on the type of vaccine. In general, avoid any vaccines that use live, attenuated (weakened) viruses, such as the MMR (measles, mumps, and rubella) and chicken pox shots. In theory, the weakened virus could give you a mild case of the infection it's designed to protect against, which you could then pass on to your baby. (Don't panic if you did receive the MMR vaccine after you became pregnant. It's highly unlikely that it affected your baby.) Vaccines that contain inactivated (or killed) viruses, such as the flu shot, are generally considered safe during pregnancy. Before getting any particular vaccine, be sure to discuss the pros and cons with your practitioner.

. . . To Have Mercury Fillings?

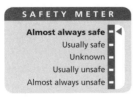

Michael Ignelzi, pediatric dentist: An extensive review by the U.S. Department of Health and Human Services concluded that amalgam fillings containing mercury pose no health risk, except in the rare case that you're allergic to them. And while some women continue to worry that these fillings may be harmful to their developing babies, no reliable studies have contradicted the government's conclusion.

The substance most often used in dental fillings is an amalgam (or mixture) of silver, mercury, tin, and copper. Amalgam fillings have been used for more than 150 years and are widely considered to be safe, more effective than plastic (the tooth-colored option now available), and more economical than gold or porcelain.

. . . To Sit in a Vibrating Massage Chair?

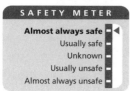

Dr. Cornelia Graves, maternal-fetal medicine specialist: That's fine. The electro-magnetic frequencies aren't a problem, and your baby probably gets more vibrations from your walking around all day than from your sitting in one of these chairs.

. . . To Get Acupuncture?

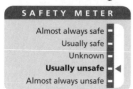

Wendy Page-Echols, osteopath: Some practitioners feel it's safe to do ear points (in which acupuncture needles are inserted into your ear) when you're pregnant, but not body points, which have more systemic effects. Because pregnancy causes so many changes in metabolism and circulation, there could be an interaction from an acupuncture point that you didn't intend and that might affect your uterus. I don't like to use accupuncture early in pregnancy, for instance, for fear it will bring on contractions. In general, American practitioners only use acupuncture in the last month to turn a breech baby, to help women who are past their due dates, to control labor pain, and to prevent postpartum bleeding. It's different in Europe: In Germany, about half of all deliveries use acupuncture anesthesia; it's about as widespread there as epidurals are here.

. . . To Use a Heating Pad?

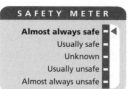

Tekoa King, certified nurse-midwife: A heating pad applied to sore muscles won't harm your baby because moderate heat applied to one area of your body won't raise your overall blood temperature.

And there's no evidence that EMFs (electromagnetic fields) pose any danger to developing babies.

Household Chores: Is It Safe?

... To Use Cleaning Solutions?

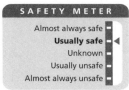

Kristina Kahl, genetic counselor: Just make sure you have good ventilation, and use gloves to avoid getting the products on your skin. Skip cleaning the oven unless you're using something nontoxic, like baking soda, because it's hard to get good ventilation in such a tight space. If any fumes make you feel nauseated, have someone else do the cleaning, or use "chemical-free" supplies such as vinegar or baking soda (health-food stores and some mainstream supermarkets sell "environmentally safe" cleaning products, too). Finally, remember never to mix different products, such as ammonia and bleach, because the resulting fumes could be very dangerous.

... To Change Cat Litter?

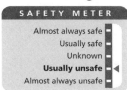

Dr. Deborah Ehrenthal, internist: No—at least not with bare hands. The danger is toxoplasmosis (page 510), a parasitic infection carried by cats and transmitted in cat feces. If you get toxoplasmosis for the first time when you're pregnant—especially when you're newly pregnant—it can cause significant neurologic damage in your baby. If you've never had toxoplasmosis, don't change the litter box yourself (if you have no other choice, wear gloves and a mask, and make sure it gets done daily).

... To Fertilize Your Yard?

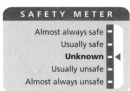

Christina Chambers, epidemiologist: There's almost no information on how most kinds of chemicals used in the house or garden might affect the fetus. So we just don't know if using fertilizer is safe or unsafe—though there's no data suggesting that any particular fertilizer causes birth defects. If you garden, take a "better safe than sorry" approach.

... To Live in a Home with Lead Paint?

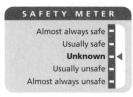

Dr. Lewis Holmes, teratogen specialist: If you have lead paint in your home (and almost every building erected before 1960 does, as do many built before 1978), lead dust is a legitimate concern—and something you'll need to take steps to avoid. Paint chips, peeling paint, and renovations that include sanding down wood and paint can produce inhalable lead dust. That kind of exposure can increase the amount of lead in your blood and the amount that reaches your developing baby. It's not clear whether lead exposure has a lasting effect on a fetus or what specific level you need to be worried about, but it's pretty clear that high levels of lead can affect development and IQ. Unfortunately, I wouldn't recommend getting your blood levels tested because the tests vary in quality and their accuracy is often questionable. Instead, contact your county health department to find out how to get the lead risk in your home assessed and how to minimize your exposure to lead dust.

. . . To Paint or Refinish Furniture?

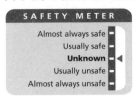

Kristina Kahl, genetic counselor: We don't know exactly how the chemicals and solvents used in paints, furniture strippers, and stains affect a fetus. The simplest and safest answer is to let someone else do the work or to save this project until after the baby's born.

Painting can expose you to oils, resins, solvents, driers, extenders, vinyl, latex, and acrylic. Paint can include potentially toxic substances such as lead, zinc, and aluminum. Stripping and refinishing furniture exposes you to potentially dangerous solvents and other chemicals. Because these projects involve so many chemicals, and because it's so difficult to measure how much of the various substances your body actually absorbs, it's difficult to know the exact risks. (If you've already done some painting or furniture stripping but haven't felt ill, don't worry. The chance that your baby will be affected is tiny.)

Some evidence suggests that exposure to chemical solvents during pregnancy may increase the risk of having a baby with birth defects. Of course, the degree of chemical exposure is much higher for someone inhaling solvents on a regular basis. Researchers don't know what the effects are on a pregnant woman who just wants to paint the nursery or refinish an heirloom cradle.

Painting Precautions

Though the CDC recommends avoiding paint fumes altogether, if you must tackle tasks such as painting or furniture refinishing, take these steps to limit your exposure to potentially harmful substances:

- Limit the amount of time you spend on the project. (Because it's hard to say exactly how much exposure is safe, you'll have to use your best judgment.)

- Don't scrape or sand paint off, because old paint often contains lead.
- Brush or roll on paint rather than using spray paints, which disperse chemicals into the air.
- Keep the windows open to avoid inhaling fumes, and make sure to wear a mask or ventilator to screen out harmful particles.
- Wear gloves, long pants, and a long-sleeved shirt to protect your skin.
- Don't eat or drink where you work, so you won't accidentally ingest any chemicals.
- Avoid oil paints, paint thinner, and latex paints that contain ethylene, glycol, ethers, and biocides.

. . . To Use a Microwave?

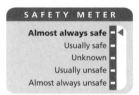

Dr. Lewis Holmes, teratogen specialist: There's no substantive research to support any concerns about using microwave ovens during pregnancy. Heating something in a microwave doesn't expose you to any significant radiation.

. . . To Use an Exterminator for Termites?

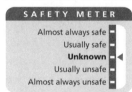

Julie Daniels, epidemiologist: The evidence is inconclusive, so it's hard to say for sure. I personally advocate avoiding extermination or other use of pesticides during pregnancy. If that's not possible—because you have an infestation of pests that also could pose risks—then I recommend the following safety precautions: Stay away from the house or yard for at least the designated period of time recommended by the exterminator to avoid inhaling the chemicals. Afterward, wipe down cabinets, floors, and furniture with a wet cloth to avoid pesticide contact with your skin.

. . . To Use Ant and Roach Spray?

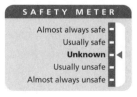

Christina Chambers, epidemiologist: The most toxic pesticides we know about are no longer in use (though it's possible that you still have an old can or two in your garage)—but we know very little about the ones that are out there now. My advice is that if you *have* to use one of these newer products, then double the "stay away" time recommended by the manufacturer or professional applicator. If you're told to stay out for four hours, for instance, then don't go home for eight. Also, look for products that aren't sprayed in the air, like "roach motels," ant traps, or garden stakes. To prevent pests without chemicals:

- Keep standing water covered and fix leaky plumbing.
- Store food in containers with tight lids, empty your garbage frequently, and keep your kitchen clean.
- Make sure shrubs, mulch, and woodpiles are at least 18 inches from the house.
- Caulk cracks and crevices.
- Wash and brush your pets often.
- Use screens on windows, and seal openings in your walls or floors.

. . . To Use Bug Repellents?

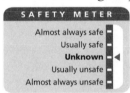

SAFETY METER
Almost always safe
Usually safe
Unknown ◀
Usually unsafe
Almost always unsafe

Kristina Kahl, genetic counselor: Most insect repellents contain diethyltoluamide, commonly known as DEET, which can be absorbed into your bloodstream through your skin. Although there's no evidence that using DEET as directed puts your baby at risk for birth defects, it's best to minimize your exposure by wearing long sleeves and pants and applying the repellent to your *clothes* instead of your skin. (If you must travel to an area where malaria, Lyme disease, West Nile virus, yellow fever, or dengue fever is a problem, you'll want to be extra sure to apply a DEET-based insect repellent to avoid getting one of these mosquito- or tick-borne illnesses.)

Many experts consider products with citronella oil—an essential oil used to ward off bugs—to be a safer alternative to DEET-based repellents. While the safety of citronella oil in pregnancy hasn't been well studied, experts say there's no potential harm from applying small amounts of citronella products to your clothes (rather than your skin) to keep bugs at bay.

Other Dangers: Is It Safe?

. . . To Be Around a Recently Vaccinated Child?

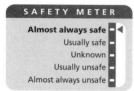

Gerald Briggs, pharmacist clinical specialist: A recently vaccinated child generally poses no risk. True, it's dangerous for a *nonimmune* pregnant woman to be exposed to certain viruses that vaccines protect against, such as chicken pox and rubella. But as long as you've been vaccinated or have otherwise become immune to these diseases yourself, there's no evidence that the usual vaccines given to another person with whom you come into contact can harm your developing baby.

. . . To Go to a Rock Concert?

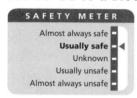

Lisa Lamson, pediatric audiologist: Going to an occasional rock concert is fine, but I wouldn't recommend it every night. It's hard to measure exactly how much noise can affect a developing baby. One study showed that women who work eight hours a day around very loud noise (at levels so loud that hearing protection is needed) run a higher risk of delivering babies with hearing loss. Another study looked at whether amniotic fluid buffered or amplified sound. It turns out that low-pitched sounds (like bass guitar) are slightly *amplified* by amniotic fluid. As the pitch gets higher, though, the fluid dampens the sound. (This study also found that amniotic fluid enhances a mother's voice by about 5 decibels, but dampens other voices.)

. . . To Run a Fever?

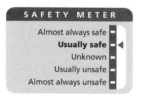

Dr. Thomas Easterling, obstetrician: It depends. Running a high fever in the first trimester—when your baby is still forming—increases the risk for neural tube defects. After the first trimester, having a fever can stress your baby; you're both burning up both calories and oxygen faster, so it's like your baby has a fever, too. But it's not dangerous unless your pregnancy is already complicated. If you have cystic fibrosis or heart disease, for instance, a fever could lead to more serious complications. But if you're healthy, a routine cold with a low-grade fever isn't going to have much effect.

. . . To Smoke Cigarettes?

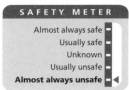

SAFETY METER
Almost always safe
Usually safe
Unknown
Usually unsafe
Almost always unsafe ◀

Kristina Kahl, genetic counselor: Absolutely not. Smoking during pregnancy increases your risk of delivering a low-birthweight baby. On average, babies born to women who smoke are almost ½ pound lighter than those born to women who don't smoke. Low birthweight is one of the leading causes of infant illness, disability, and death. Smoking is also linked to ectopic pregnancy (page 546), miscarriage (page 543), placental problems (page 529), premature delivery (page 440), and stillbirth.

What's more, some research has found that smoking when you're pregnant could hurt your child's mental development and behavior, leading to a short attention span and hyperactivity. Other research suggests that smoking may increase the likelihood of certain birth defects in some women's babies. One study found that pregnant women who smoke a pack a day are more than twice as likely to have babies with these problems. Smoking may also increase the risk of clubfoot and certain skull malformations.

Finally, the further into your pregnancy you continue to smoke, the greater your risk of problems. If you stop smoking before your pregnancy hits the midway mark, for instance, your baby will most likely be a normal weight. So if you haven't quit yet, giving up cigarettes *now*—or at least cutting down on the number you smoke—will benefit both you and your baby. If you need help, ask your practitioner about enrolling in a smoking-cessation program.

. . . To Inhale Secondhand Smoke?

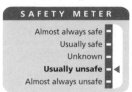

SAFETY METER
Almost always safe
Usually safe
Unknown
Usually unsafe ◀
Almost always unsafe

Christina Chambers, epidemiologist: Avoid it as much as possible. Some of the contaminants from the smoke will get into your blood. The more often you're around someone who's smoking, the more of these contaminants you can absorb. Studies have shown that when pregnant women are exposed to someone else's tobacco smoke, they give birth to babies who weigh less than the babies of women who aren't exposed.

. . . To Inhale Wood Smoke?

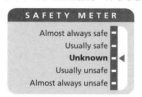

Christina Chambers, epidemiologist: It hasn't really been studied, but one potential problem might be that wood treated with harmful chemicals would send those chemicals into the air, where they could be inhaled. Also, theoretically, breathing smoke could reduce the amount of oxygen in your bloodstream—and therefore the amount of oxygen that's available to the baby.

. . . To Sleep with an Electric Blanket?

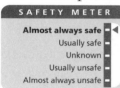

Dr. Carol Archie, obstetrician: Yes, unless you're really baking. You don't want to raise your core body temperature above 103°F or so because that could cause physical abnormalities in your developing baby. So as long as you're comfortable and not too hot, you're okay. What's more, there's no evidence that being exposed to electromagnetic fields can harm your baby in any way.

. . . To Sleep on Your Stomach?

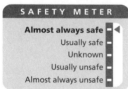

Dr. Catherine Lynch, obstetrician: There's no problem lying on your stomach in early pregnancy. At this point, your uterus is still nestled behind your pubic bone, so it's totally protected. Later in your pregnancy, stomach sleeping just isn't going to be comfortable; you'd be uncomfortable long before you could ever hurt your baby.

. . . To Sleep on Your Back?

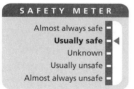

Dr. Craig Winkel, obstetrician: Back sleeping is safe during your first trimester, especially if you're healthy and your pregnancy is normal. But once you hit about 20 weeks, lying on your back can cause your uterus to press on the inferior vena cava (a major vein that returns blood from your lower body to your heart), resulting in dizziness, blood pressure changes, and a possible reduction in blood flow to your uterus. As your pregnancy progresses, try to lie on one side or the other, and support your hip with a pillow. This allows for better blood flow to your developing baby.

. . . To Take Sleeping Pills?

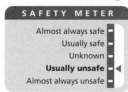

Ronald Ruggiero, pharmacist clinical specialist: I would never recommend any of the new generation of sleeping pills, such as Ambien and Sonata, because there's no data on their safety during pregnancy. The only sleeping pills I recommend are those containing the antihistamine doxylamine (like Unisom SleepTabs). Doxylamine has strong sedative effects, and there's no evidence that it causes any harm when taken as advised during the first trimester.

. . . To Take Herbal Sleep Remedies?

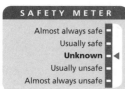

Dr. Mary O'Malley, sleep medicine specialist: It's easy to assume that because herbs are "natural," they're always safe. Yet some herbs can be just as powerful as prescription drugs—and just as toxic, too. Consult your caregiver before taking *any* herbal remedy (even herbal tea). If your practitioner gives the go-ahead to try a particular herbal sleep remedy, be sure to ask her or your pharmacist to recommend a brand name because the quality of herbs varies by manufacturer.

Nutrition: Is It Safe?

. . . To Drink Milk from Cows Given Hormones?

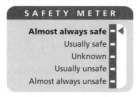

Jeff Hampl, registered dietitian: The Food and Drug Administration says bovine growth hormone is safe, but the issue is controversial. Some consumer advocates and environmental groups are concerned that milk from cows given this hormone may contain substances that are harmful to humans. (No one's claiming that the hormone *itself* is dangerous, but it may have side effects for the cow, which could lead to other substances turning up in the milk you drink.) Even though some of the hormone given to cows does get into the milk, it turns into a protein that's broken down in your digestive system and doesn't pose a risk to you or your baby.

. . . To Eat Meat from Livestock Given Antibiotics?

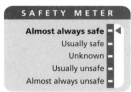

Dr. Cornelia Graves, maternal-fetal medicine specialist: There's no reason to worry about eating meat that contains antibiotics, since the amount that gets to your baby is extremely small. Most livestock in the United States is treated with antibiotics, so buying organic meat is the only way to avoid it. The main concern about eating antibiotic-laced meat is that it could contribute to antibiotic-resistant bacteria, but there's no research showing that eating meat from animals treated with antibiotics causes this problem. (The major culprit for antibiotic-resistant bacteria is people taking antibiotics for the common cold or flu—for which they're useless.)

. . . To Eat Fish and Other Seafood?

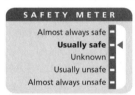

Edward Groth, environmental health expert: Most seafood is an excellent source of the protein, vitamins, and minerals you need now—but certain types are off-limits during pregnancy. The reason: Pollutants such as mercury, dioxins, PCBs, and pesticides are absorbed by some fish as they swim and feed in tainted waters. Eating large doses of these contaminants has been linked to miscarriage, preterm birth, and physical and developmental delays in babies who were exposed to them in the womb.

Fortunately, only some fish contain harmful amounts of pollutants. When it comes to mercury, for instance, it's typically shark, king mackerel, swordfish, and tilefish that carry the highest concentrations, so steer clear of them completely while you're pregnant and nursing. Tuna also contains moderately high levels of mercury, so limit your consumption to no more than 6 ounces of "light" tuna a week. Albacore (or "white") tuna and tuna steaks have *three times* as much mercury as light tuna, so it's probably safest to lay off those for now.

Salmon can also be problematic, but for different reasons. Although it's low in mercury, some research has found that compared with wild salmon, farmed salmon has high levels of PCBs, dioxins, and other contaminants. And because it can be difficult to tell for sure where the salmon at your local supermarket comes from, consider taking it off your prenatal menu for now.

If you enjoy seafood and tend to eat a lot of it (12 ounces or more a week), choose varieties that are relatively pollutant-free: shrimp, scallops, flounder, sole, clams, oysters, tilapia, catfish, whitefish, sardines, crayfish, king crab, and croaker. Also vary the types of fish you eat from this list so that you have no more than one serving of any particular kind of fish or seafood during a week.

Finally, because pollution levels vary from one body of water to the next, never eat sport-caught fish without first checking your state or local health department's "fish safety advisory" (listed in the "local government" section of your phone book).

. . . To Eat Sushi?

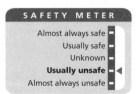

Jill Stovsky, registered dietitian: Some types of cooked sushi, such as California roll or unagi (which, respectively, contain steamed crab and broiled eel), are fine. But it's best to avoid the kinds that contain raw seafood. That's because fresh, raw seafood can harbor parasites such as tapeworm, which could rob your body of nutrients that your growing baby needs. And be sure to stick with cooked fish selections that aren't contaminated with mercury and other chemicals.

. . . To Eat Raw Oysters?

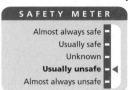

Robert Price, seafood safety expert: You can get pretty sick—and even die—from eating a contaminated oyster. Raw oysters (as well as clams and mussels) are probably the biggest cause of illness from seafood in this country, due to all the bacteria, toxins, and viruses they can carry. Once oysters are harvested, bacteria grow rapidly in them if they're not stored at a low enough temperature. If you just can't live without oysters, steam them first, which should kill any bacteria and viruses. You might also want to try pasteurized oysters, which are very similar in flavor and texture to raw oysters but which have been processed under high pressure or a mild heat treatment and are free of illness-causing bacteria.

. . . To Eat a Lot of Chocolate?

Dr. Cornelia Graves, maternal-fetal medicine specialist: Yes, except for the fact that eating too much might make you sick to your stomach. While chocolate

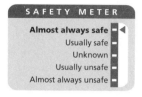

does contain some caffeine, there's no evidence that moderate amounts of caffeine are dangerous for pregnant women. On the other hand, there *is* evidence that chocolate works on the neurotransmitters in your brain to give you a feeling of well-being.

. . . To Eat Blackened Foods?

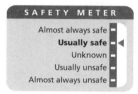

Pennie Morrison Bosarge, nurse-practitioner: There's no danger in having an occasional piece of grilled steak or blackened fish. Theoretically, anyone who eats a lot of blackened or grilled meats could have a problem because of potentially carcinogenic (cancer-causing) compounds that form on the surface of the food, but you'd have to eat an awful lot of burned, blackened food over a long period of time for that to happen.

. . . To Drink Diet Shakes?

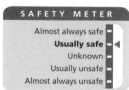

Dr. Thomas Bader, obstetrician: There's certainly no reason you couldn't, as long as they're not *all* you're consuming. But because you need about 2,500 calories a day when you're pregnant—and because you're more prone to low blood sugar now—don't rely on diet shakes as the major source of your calories. If one shake is all you're having for lunch, for instance, you're likely to get low blood sugar by midafternoon, and you might feel dizzy and faint. But since many pregnant women end up eating four or five small meals over the course of a day, it's fine if one of these meals consists of a diet shake or drink. In fact, it's probably a good source of protein and vitamins.

. . . To Drink Diet Sodas?

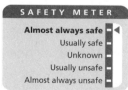

Jeff Hampl, registered dietitian: Most diet sodas are made with aspartame (sold under the brand names NutraSweet, Equal, NatraTaste, and others). Aspartame is considered safe for pregnant women with one exception: Women with the disease phenylketonuria (PKU) shouldn't have aspartame because they can't metabolize it. Remember, too, that most diet sodas have caffeine and that all are nutritional losers, so drink them sparingly.

. . . To Eat Foods with MSG?

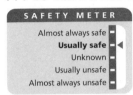

Jill Stovsky, registered dietitian: MSG (monosodium glutamate) is a natural component of many foods. Some restaurants, home cooks, and food manufacturers also use it as a flavor enhancer. The FDA has been testing MSG for years and rates it "generally recognized as safe"—though it also requires that all foods containing MSG say so on their labels because of the negative side effects the additive can have, including headaches, nausea, vomiting, dizziness, and sleep disturbances. So while there's no evidence that MSG can harm your developing baby, you may want to avoid it during pregnancy—when you probably already have your fair share of the above problems!

. . . To Eat Salty Foods?

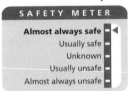

Jill Stovsky, registered dietitian: You probably don't need to hide the salt shaker unless you have chronic high blood pressure. In the old days, some experts suggested limiting sodium during pregnancy because they thought it contributed to water retention and bloating and that limiting it might help to prevent preeclampsia. Now most experts believe that some increase in body fluids is necessary and normal and that a moderate amount of salt can help maintain adequate fluid levels. What's more, some degree of water retention in pregnancy is perfectly normal, and restricting salt neither prevents nor lessens the severity of preeclampsia. So unless your practitioner recommends that you limit sodium because of chronic hypertension or other concerns, salt is fine to eat—in moderation, of course.

. . . To Eat Spicy Foods?

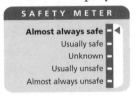

Dr. Kay Daniels, obstetrician: Spicy foods won't hurt your baby, but you may get more heartburn after eating them. That's because the pregnancy hormone progestin relaxes the muscles that normally keep digestive acids in your stomach. Plus, your growing baby is pushing against your stomach. Add spicy food, and it can be a recipe for discomfort.

. . . To Drink Unpasteurized Juice?

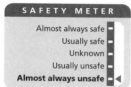

Larry Pickering, infectious disease specialist: No. Unpasteurized juice may contain dangerous germs, such as salmonella or *E. coli*. *E. coli* can produce toxins in your digestive tract that could cause severe diarrhea, which in turn could lead to serious dehydration. You could also develop kidney failure, anemia, or blood-clotting problems. Finally, these germs or the toxins they produce could cause an illness severe enough to bring on miscarriage.

. . . To Use Artificial Sweeteners?

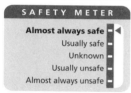

Kristina Kahl, genetic counselor: Consuming moderate amounts of aspartame, the artificial sweetener found in NutraSweet, Equal, and most sugar-free treats, is considered safe during pregnancy. (Women with the genetic disease phenylketonuria [PKU], however, should avoid aspartame at all times.)

Saccharin, on the other hand, is more controversial. Though there's no evidence that saccharin causes cancer in humans, it has been linked to bladder cancer in animal studies. Because of this concern, it's probably best to ban saccharin from your diet while you're pregnant. Luckily, saccharin is much less common today than in years past, so avoiding it shouldn't be too difficult.

Fitness: Is It Safe?

. . . To Go Bowling?

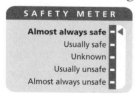

Dr. Raul Artal, obstetrician: Bowling should be fine. It's true that your joints and ligaments relax during pregnancy, but how much they relax varies from woman to woman. Most expectant mothers don't experience that relaxation to such an extent that they'd injure themselves while bowling. I do have one caution, though: Once you hit your third trimester, lift your bowling ball in a way that won't strain your back muscles. That means making sure to bend at your knees and to keep your back straight.

... To Take a Dance Class?

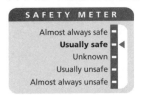

Jill Stovsky, fitness expert: Yes, as long as you were doing it before you got pregnant and you take some extra precautions now. For starters, reduce the intensity of your dancing to a level okayed by your caregiver. Also, keep your moves low impact by keeping one foot planted on the floor at all times, skip any jumping or fast side-to-side steps, use fewer arm movements, and avoid quick turns that might cause jarring.

... To Go Downhill Skiing?

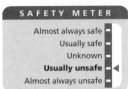

Dr. Jeanne-Marie Guise, obstetrician: It's best to avoid sports, such as downhill skiing, with a high likelihood of impact or falling. That said, if you are used to skiing and you ski well (and if you're willing to accept some degree of risk), then it's probably okay during your first two trimesters. But I'd definitely stop by the time you get to your third trimester because your center of gravity will shift and there's more risk of falling. A fall could lead to premature delivery by causing the placenta to tear away from the wall of your uterus (called a placental abruption) or by bringing on preterm contractions.

... To Get My Heart Rate over 140 Beats per Minute?

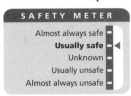

Dr. Raul Artal, obstetrician: The 140-beats-per-minute guideline is outdated; instead, we now recommend that during the first four to six weeks of pregnancy, you shouldn't engage in strenuous activities that could raise your core body temperature over 103°F, because a very high body temperature early in pregnancy could theoretically cause birth defects. Later in pregnancy, being poorly hydrated or having an elevated body temperature puts you at risk for premature labor. If you're exercising to keep your heart and lungs in shape, moderate exercise is all you need.

... To Use a Hot Tub or Sauna after a Workout?

Dr. Jeanne-Marie Guise, obstetrician: It's not a good idea unless you can control the temperature and set it at no more than 100°F. Soaking in hot

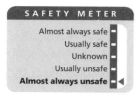

water or sitting in a hot, steamy room can make you overheat, which raises your heart rate and reduces blood flow to your uterus, potentially putting your baby under stress or interfering with normal development. And because pregnant women have a hard time cooling down, you're more likely to pass out if you get overheated in a hot tub or sauna—an especially dangerous proposition in either setting.

. . . To Ice-Skate or Inline-Skate

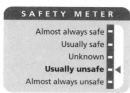

Dr. Jeanne-Marie Guise, obstetrician: Only if you're an experienced skater, but even then, I'd tell you to stop before your third trimester. You don't want to risk falling, which could bring on contractions or cause the placenta to tear away from your uterus, either of which puts you at risk for preterm delivery. In general, pregnancy's not a good time to take up *any* new sport or to overexert yourself, because you're more likely to get hurt. That's why it makes sense to avoid sports that put you at risk for rough contact or falling, including hockey, soccer, basketball, gymnastics, horseback riding, downhill skiing, and racquetball.

. . . To Get Really Hot during a Workout?

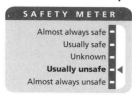

Dr. Jeanne-Marie Guise, obstetrician: You don't want to exercise so hard that you get overheated in your first trimester. If you do, there's some concern that it can affect your baby's development— there's a slightly increased risk of the baby's abdominal wall's not closing all the way, for instance. Also, as your body diverts blood to your skin to help you cool off, it's taking some of that blood flow away from your baby. It's harder to cool down when you're pregnant, so if you get overheated, you're more likely to pass out. You'll know you've gotten too hot if you break a sweat and *keep* sweating. To prevent this from happening, avoid exercising in very hot weather or in overheated rooms, take frequent breaks, and drink plenty of water.

. . . To Go Mountain Biking?

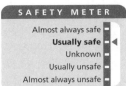

Dr. Raul Artal, obstetrician: Yes, but remember that mountain biking has a certain amount of inherent risk whether you're pregnant or not. And the further along you are in your pregnancy, the greater the risk to your baby should you fall off the bike. A fall could cause trauma to your abdomen, and that could lead to premature separation of the placenta, premature labor, or, in the worst case, fetal death.

. . . To Run?

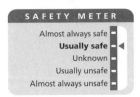

Dr. Raul Artal, obstetrician: Yes, as long as you don't have any complications. If you're at risk for premature labor, have had bleeding, or have preeclampsia, then activities like running can aggravate your condition.

. . . To Do Sit-ups or Crunches?

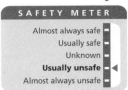

Dr. Jeanne-Marie Guise, obstetrician: Sit-ups and crunches are fine in your first trimester, but by your second trimester you'll need to avoid lying flat on your back. As your uterus grows, its weight can compress the blood vessels leading to your heart, potentially depriving your developing baby of oxygen. Of course, by that time you'll most likely find that sit-ups are almost impossible to do, anyway.

. . . To Swim in a Chlorinated Pool?

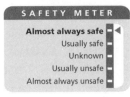

Dr. Catherine Lynch, obstetrician: As long as the chemicals are appropriately monitored, swimming in a chlorinated pool isn't a problem at all. It might actually make you feel good to float in the water—especially later in your pregnancy.

. . . To Play Tennis?

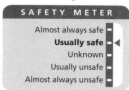

Dr. Mary Lake Polan, obstetrician: It depends. Anything you've been doing, you can generally continue to do. But if you haven't played tennis before, don't start now because you won't be in shape for it. If you want to stand on the court and bat balls around, that's probably okay. If you want to play five sets and spend three hours sweating, on the other hand, that's probably *not* okay.

Beauty: Is It Safe?
. . . To Take a Bath?

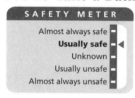

Dr. Catherine Lynch, obstetrician: Yes, as long as the water temperature isn't over 100°F. If you have to ease your foot into the tub, it's too hot. If you're comfortable getting into the water, the temperature is close to your own body temperature, which is where you want it to be. Anything hotter can damage your baby's developing cells, and though you can cool off by sweating, your baby can't. It's also fine to use bath oils or bubble bath; your cervix is closed, so there's no danger that these products could reach the baby.

. . . To Get a Belly Button Piercing or Wear a Belly Button Ring?

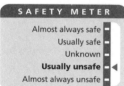

M.J. Hanafin, certified nurse-midwife: Yes and no. As your belly stretches, having a belly button ring can be very painful. Some women remove their ring and put in a sleeper—a little plastic stud that holds the hole open—while others go through their whole pregnancy without taking theirs out. It just depends on how big your baby gets and how your body reacts to pregnancy. Actually *getting* your belly button pierced when you're pregnant isn't advisable, though, because of the risk of infection. Besides, your navel has more blood vessels than some other areas, so it takes belly button piercings longer than other kinds to settle down and stop being irritated.

. . . To Get a Bikini Wax?

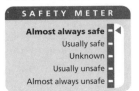

Dr. Cornelia Graves, maternal-fetal medicine specialist: There's no reason you can't. But because you have more blood flowing to your skin now—especially in your pubic area—you'll probably be more sensitive to anything that tugs or pulls, so that bikini wax is likely to be even more painful than usual. You're also more likely to see some broken blood vessels after the waxing.

. . . To Bleach Body Hair or Use Chemical Hair Removers?

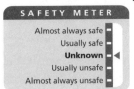

Christina Chambers, epidemiologist: To my knowledge, there's no evidence that the use of topically applied bleach or depilatories increases the risk of birth defects, though this issue hasn't been well-studied. Most likely, very little of the chemical would seep into your bloodstream and get to your baby. If you choose to bleach or chemically remove facial or body hair, you can minimize your potential risk by rinsing your skin with cold water beforehand (to keep your pores small), working in a well-ventilated area, and limiting the amount of time the products stay on your skin.

. . . To Bleach Your Teeth?

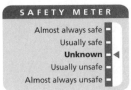

Yiming Li, professor of dentistry: We don't have any evidence that tooth bleaching poses any significant risk to your baby, but we don't have enough data to say that it's *safe*, either. The peroxide used in bleaching causes an oxidative process, and we know that oxidation can be harmful to tissues and cells. But we don't know whether that can affect your baby. There's another whitening process, called microabrasion, that uses acidic components to remove stains, but we have even less data on the safety of that in pregnancy. To be on the safe side, wait until after you've given birth and you're done nursing to have your teeth bleached. And though there are various whitening products you can get over the counter, it's best to seek your dentist's advice first because tooth discoloration can be a sign of a larger dental or health problem.

. . . To Get a Body Wrap or Mud Bath?

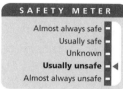

Dr. Catherine Lynch, obstetrician: A body wrap or a mud bath usually involves heat, so I wouldn't recommend them because they can raise your core body temperature. A raised internal temperature, especially early in pregnancy, can cause birth defects.

. . . To Get Botox Treatments?

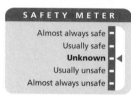

Dr. Lewis Holmes, teratogen specialist: Botox use by pregnant women hasn't been studied, although it's unlikely that an injection of Botox in your face would end up circulating throughout your body at a high enough level to hurt your baby.

. . . To Color Your Hair?

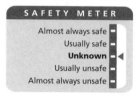

Ann Linden, certified nurse-midwife: Though the evidence is limited, coloring your hair during pregnancy is probably safe. The chemicals used in hair dyes have been around a long time, and no research shows that low-level exposure causes birth defects. Plus, very little is actually absorbed into your system. Still, no one has enough information to absolutely guarantee that using chemical dyes during pregnancy is safe. To err on the side of caution, I suggest at least waiting until after your first trimester to color your hair.

Some experts recommend vegetable dyes as a good alternative to synthetic coloring products. But buyer beware: In addition to various "natural" substances listed as ingredients, many of these dyes contain the same chemical compounds (such as p-phenylenediamine, dihydroxybenzene, and aminophenol) that the major cosmetic companies put in their dyes. Pure henna, which comes in a number of colors, is the exception. Henna is considered safe.

Another alternative is highlighting, painting, or frosting your hair. You absorb hair-coloring agents into your system through your skin, not through your hair shaft. So any process that puts less of the chemical in contact with your scalp, such as streaking, reduces your exposure. One final note: If you choose to color your hair, be sure to do it in a well-ventilated area—and if you're doing it yourself, don't forget to wear gloves.

. . . To Get a Facial?

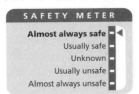

Dr. Cornelia Graves, maternal-fetal medicine specialist: Absolutely. But since your skin is more sensitive now, you should be more careful about pulling and tugging on your face—so ask the facialist to go easy. Pregnancy can also cause skin discolorations and increased visibility of blood vessels, so even if your facialist is gentle, you may be disappointed with the results.

. . . To Take Isotretinoin (Accutane)?

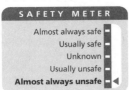

Kristina Kahl, genetic counselor: No. Isotretinoin (Accutane or retinoic acid), which is used to treat acne, can cause miscarriage and multiple serious birth defects, such as mental retardation, brain malformations, blindness, heart defects, and facial abnormalities. If you think you might be pregnant, stop taking the drug immediately and be sure to let your practitioner know about it. Fortunately, recent studies show little to no increased risk for birth defects if women stop taking the drug within two weeks after conceiving.

. . . To Have Your Nails Done?

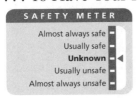

Dr. Kay Daniels, obstetrician: Although there's no evidence that getting your nails done is dangerous, I'd err on the side of caution and avoid nail salons during your first trimester, when your baby is most vulnerable. That's because organic solvents like toluene in nail polish or acetone in polish remover pose a theoretical risk.

. . . To Get a Perm or Use Chemical Hair-Straightening Products?

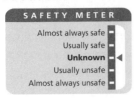

Dr. Lewis Holmes, teratogen specialist: It's not something anyone has studied much, but what little evidence there is indicates that perming or chemically straightening your hair is no cause for concern. The fumes might be annoying, but the exposure probably isn't significant enough to have any effect on your baby. It's possible that solvents are used in hair-processing solutions, and while there is concern about the effects of solvents on a developing baby, that's most likely an issue only for women who work around them all day and develop symptoms from the exposure.

. . . To Use a Salt Scrub?

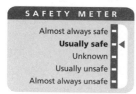

Dr. Cornelia Graves, maternal-fetal medicine specialist: Your skin is more sensitive during pregnancy because there's more blood flowing to it, so a salt scrub is more likely than usual to break blood vessels if the skin is stressed. But there's no risk that salt on the outside of your body would do anything on the inside because it isn't absorbed through your skin.

. . . To Use Self-Tanning Lotions?

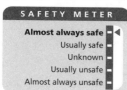

Dr. Sandra Johnson, dermatologist: If you're not feeling so attractive during your pregnancy, the look of sun-kissed skin that a self-tanner provides can do wonders for your self-esteem. The good news is that the ingredients in self-tanners are harmless, so it's fine to use them during pregnancy. These lotions and sprays are basically dyes that stay on the surface of your skin and won't harm your developing baby. Best of all, self-tanners have improved dramatically during the past few years, so you don't have to worry about looking like an orange-skinned Oompa Loompa from *Willy Wonka and the Chocolate Factory.*

. . . To Use a Tanning Bed?

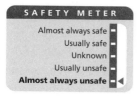

Dr. Sandra Johnson, dermatologist: There's no conclusive evidence that tanning beds are harmful to a developing baby, but there's plenty of proof that they're dangerous to *you.* Tanning beds pose the same dangers as the sun: They emit ultraviolet (UV) radiation, which causes skin cancer. Don't believe anyone who tells you that because tanning booths emit only UVA rays, they're not hazardous. One study suggests that visiting a tanning booth ten times in a year can *double* your chances of developing melanoma—one of the deadliest types of cancer.

If the threat of skin cancer doesn't frighten you, consider the possibility that lying in a tanning booth can raise your body temperature to a level that may be hazardous to your baby. Having an elevated body temperature during pregnancy—that is, above 102°F (which can happen in a tanning bed, a hot tub, or a sauna)—is associated with spinal malformations in developing babies. And after the middle of your pregnancy, then there's the concern that lying on your back for too long might restrict blood flow to your heart and thus to your baby.

Finally, yet one more downside to tanning: Pregnant women with sensitive skin who expose themselves to UV rays (whether from tanning beds or the sun) may be more prone to chloasma, those dark skin splotches that can appear on your face and occasionally your arms during pregnancy.

. . . To Get Your Teeth Cleaned?

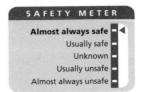

Dr. Thomas Bader, obstetrician: Yes. Don't postpone dental care when you're pregnant. Women with periodontitis (in which a gum infection spreads into the bone and other tissue that support your teeth) are more likely to deliver prematurely. One theory is that gum disease is a marker for cervical or uterine weaknesses; another is that gum disease triggers some sort of inflammatory stimulation in your uterus that causes contractions.

. . . To Get a Tattoo?

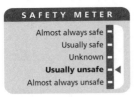

Dr. Deborah Ehrenthal, internist: Tattoos aren't recommended during pregnancy. First of all, your skin changes, and that may change the way the tattoo looks after you deliver your baby. In addition, if the equipment and tattoo ink aren't properly sterilized, there's always the risk you might get a bloodborne infection such as hepatitis B, hepatitis C, or HIV.

Sex: Is It Safe?

. . . To Have Anal Sex?

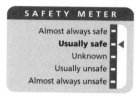

Dr. Gina Brown, obstetrician: Probably. But if you have hemorrhoids, remember that they tend to become larger during pregnancy. And if your hemorrhoids are bleeding and you have anal sex, you can lose a considerable amount of blood, and that can put you and your baby in danger. And just like when you're not pregnant, you should never go from anal to vaginal sex without cleaning up first and changing condoms if you're using one; otherwise, you put yourself at risk for bacterial vaginitis, and there's some concern that this infection can cause preterm labor or make your water break early. Also, unless you're in a monogamous relationship and know that you and your partner are HIV negative, you should use a condom because HIV and other sexually transmitted infections (STIs) are transmitted through broken skin.

. . . To Use a Dildo or a Vibrator?

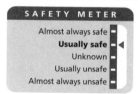

Dr. Gina Brown, obstetrician: It's generally safe, except that you want to be extra careful not to penetrate too forcefully, since plastic is more rigid than flesh. If you're diagnosed with placenta previa, using a sex toy (or, for that matter, having intercourse) could traumatize the placenta and cause heavy bleeding that could jeopardize your pregnancy. If you're at risk for premature labor, having an orgasm could cause contractions. And if your bag of waters is ruptured, there's a risk of infection to the baby because he's no longer protected. In any case, make sure the dildo or vibrator is clean, and don't share it without cleaning it.

. . . To Receive Oral Sex?

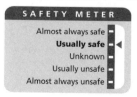

Dr. Deborah Ehrenthal, internist: Licking is okay, but it's not safe to blow into the genital area. Theoretically, if your partner blew hard enough, it could cause an embolism (a bubble of air) to develop in a blood vessel, and that could be lethal for you or the baby.

. . . To Swallow Semen?

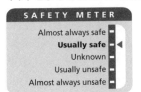

Dr. Gina Brown, obstetrician: There's no danger to the baby from the semen itself. And as long as you're in a monogamous relationship and know that your partner is free of STIs, there's no risk. If your partner is HIV positive, it's not safe because the virus is present in semen, and you and your baby could become infected (whether or not you swallowed it).

. . . To Use a Water-Based Lubricant?

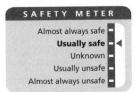

Dr. Gina Brown, obstetrician: That's fine. You may find that you don't actually need lubricant while you're pregnant because the extra vaginal discharge keeps you pretty moist. But there's no danger of the lubricant's getting to the baby because your cervix is tightly closed.

Work: Is It Safe?

. . . To Sit in Front of a Computer for Hours on End?

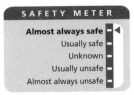

Dr. Lewis Holmes, teratogen specialist: Yes. Because computers are ubiquitous, researchers spent millions of dollars studying whether sitting in front of one causes birth defects or miscarriage—and determined that there's no evidence that it does. Of course, sitting anywhere for hours on end won't do you any good, so get up and walk around every few hours.

. . . To Use a Photocopier?

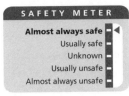

Will Forest, toxicologist: Modern dry-toner photocopiers aren't a hazard. Wet-toner photocopiers that are more than ten years old may pose some risk, but only if you close yourself up in a small, unventilated room and run off thousands of copies.

Travel: Is It Safe?

. . . To Walk through Airport Screening Machines?

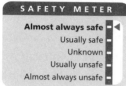

Ann Linden, certified nurse-midwife: Many people mistakenly think these screening machines emit X-rays—they don't. Airport X-ray machines are used only on luggage. The metal detectors that passengers walk through use a low-frequency electromagnetic field to look for weapons. Anything that generates or uses electricity, such as power lines and household appliances, produces an electromagnetic field. At the low levels of a metal detector, this exposure is considered safe for everyone, including pregnant women. The same holds true for the screening wands that are sometimes passed over individual passengers.

. . . To Travel to Developing Countries?

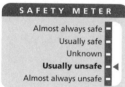

Tekoa King, certified nurse-midwife: It's unsafe if you're within three or four weeks of your due date or if you have problems like hypertension, diabetes, or preterm labor. Many developing countries just don't have the medical resources for mothers or babies with complications. (And obviously, it's best to avoid areas where contagious disease or political unrest is prevalent.)

If you're having a normal pregnancy, the main issue is which immunizations or other preventive treatment you'd need to travel safely in your destination of choice. I don't recommend "live" vaccines (which use a weakened form of the virus they're designed to protect against) because there's a very slight risk of developing a mild form of the disease itself—so some vaccines recommended for exotic travel are safe and some aren't. And I don't recommend medication for pregnant women if it's not absolutely necessary. For instance, if you were traveling to India, where malaria is common, you'd need to take strong antimalarial drugs to prevent infection—not a good idea when you're pregnant.

. . . To Drink the Water?

Dr. Debra Gussman, obstetrician: The best way to ensure that your drinking water is safe overseas is to buy bottled water, now readily avail-

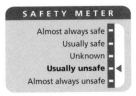

able in most parts of the world. (And if a location is so remote that you can't buy bottled water, you probably shouldn't go there when you're pregnant anyway.) Always avoid tap water in developing countries, which can contain bacteria and parasites that cause traveler's diarrhea or worse. You can get traveler's diarrhea even if the water is perfectly safe for the locals because they've built up immunity to whatever bacteria the water may contain.

Make sure the bottles of water you buy are sealed. And don't worry about offending anyone by insisting that you break the seal yourself. In some countries, unscrupulous merchants and restaurateurs simply fill bottles with tap water and sell it to tourists as "bottled." Don't assume the drinking water in hotels is safe either, unless it comes in sealed bottles. Carbonated water has one distinct advantage: You know it's not from the tap.

Local fruit juices, flavored ices, and drinks with ice pose the same risks as tap water. So does rinsing your toothbrush from the tap or swallowing water when you're showering. If you can't find bottled water when you need it, substitute sports drinks or even canned soft drinks.

. . . To Be Exposed to Radiation on an Airplane?

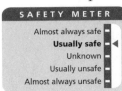

Dr. Natan Haratz-Rubinstein, obstetrician: Few words strike more terror in the hearts of expectant moms than "radiation," but plane travel is generally safe in this regard. Even on land, we're exposed every day to cosmic ionizing radiation, which emanates from the sun and other stars. But on the ground, the earth's atmosphere offers some protection, whereas at high altitudes the atmosphere is thinner and radiation levels are higher. (They can be even higher during solar flares—bursts of radiation caused by disturbances in the sun's atmosphere—but these are rare and last only a short while. To find out if there are solar radiation storms forecast when you're planning to fly—in which case you may want to postpone your trip a day or two—check the National Oceanic and Atmospheric Administration Web site at www.sec.noaa.gov.)

Although some experts think that cosmic radiation could pose a small risk to pregnant pilots, flight attendants, and other frequent fliers, the cosmic ionizing radiation that the average pregnant traveler is exposed to under normal solar conditions isn't considered a problem.

. . . To Get Vaccinated for Travel?

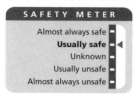

Ann Linden, certified nurse-midwife: It depends on the type of vaccine. Avoid live vaccines, such as those for measles, mumps, rubella, and varicella (chicken pox). Because live vaccines are made from live viruses, there's a very small chance that you—and thus your unborn baby—could actually develop a mild case of the disease the vaccine is designed to protect against.

Some other vaccines, such as those for hepatitis A, hepatitis B, and tetanus, are considered safe and are recommended for pregnant women who are at risk of getting these diseases. The flu vaccine (page 556) is recommended during pregnancy even if you're *not* traveling. For specifics on less common vaccines that may be required for travel to certain countries, talk to your healthcare provider.

The bottom line: If you have the option, don't travel during your pregnancy to countries where the threat of disease is high and a potentially risky shot becomes an issue. In many of these countries, the quality of local health care and the safety of food and water are often questionable as well.

. . . To Visit High Altitudes?

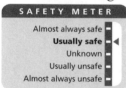

Dr. Mary Lake Polan, obstetrician: It's a question of degree. If you want to go to Denver, it's probably fine. If you want to climb Mount Kilimanjaro, that would not be okay. At high altitudes, you have less oxygen available—and that means your baby gets less oxygen, which can damage her growth and development. It's also harder to get around when the air is thin. It depends on what you can handle and what you're used to. Some women get dizzy or light-headed at 9,000 feet. Some women can tolerate 12,000 feet and feel fine. If you're having difficulty, you can assume your baby is, too. Use common sense. If you're huffing and puffing and getting headaches, then you need to get to a lower altitude—and if you still don't feel well after you descend, seek medical care.

Want a second opinion?
Join **BabyCenter Plus** and get two experts' answers to every one of our 100 pregnancy safety questions, access to our online pregnancy and birth video library, *Consumer Reports* product reviews, and other great benefits. Learn more at http://www.babycenter.com/plus.

RESOURCES

Abuse
If your relationship has become abusive, get help and get out. Talk with friends and family who will support your decision to leave and who may be able to offer you a place to stay. A shelter can also provide you (and your children) a safe haven while you figure out your next steps. Let your healthcare provider know about your situation, and check with the following organizations for other resources in your area.
Family Violence Prevention Fund: www.endabuse.org
National Coalition Against Domestic Violence: www.ncadv.org
National Domestic Violence Hotline: www.ndvh.org
Office on Women's Health of the U.S. Department of Health and Human Services: www.4woman.gov/violence/index.cfm
If you visit these Web sites at home, be sure to clear the memory cache and history files on your computer so your partner won't be able to trace what you're doing online. (The National Domestic Violence Hotline site explains how to do it in detail.)

Allergies
Asthma and Allergy Foundation of America: www.aafa.org

Anemia
March of Dimes: www.modimes.org
National Anemia Action Council: www.anemia.org

Asthma
Asthma and Allergy Foundation of America: www.aafa.org

Babies with Health Problems
There's a vast array of support groups and information sources for families carrying babies with genetic abnormalities and other health problems. A few starting points:
Cleft Palate Foundation: www.cleftline.org
March of Dimes: www.modimes.org
National Down Syndrome Society: www.ndss.org
Spina Bifida Association of America: www.sbaa.org
BabyCenter's Poor Prenatal Diagnosis bulletin board:
http://bbs.babycenter.com/board/1311584

Birth Centers
National Association of Childbearing Centers: www.birthcenters.org

Breastfeeding Help and Advice
La Leche League International: www.lalecheleague.org
See the breastfeeding area at the American Academy of Pediatrics Web site:
www.aap.org/healthtopics/breastfeeding.cfm
The International Lactation Consultant Association can help you find a board-certified lactation specialist: www.ilca.org
BabyCenter's comprehensive breastfeeding area has information galore, photos, bulletin boards, and more: www.babycenter.com/breastfeeding

Breech Babies
American College of Obstetricians and Gynecologists' Breech Baby Patient
Education page: www.acog.org/from_home/websiteBenefits/patient.htm

Cervical Insufficiency
BabyCenter's Cervical Disorders bulletin board:
http://bbs.babycenter.com/board/pregnancy/pregcomplications/1252536

Charting Your Cycle
Sample basal body temperature and cervical mucus chart:
www.babycenter.com/general/preconception/gettingpregnant/7252.html
Download your own chart: www.babycenter.com/general/preconception/
gettingpregnant/7069.html

Childbirth Education
Lamaze International: www.lamaze.org
American Academy of Husband-Coached Childbirth (Bradley Method):
www.bradleybirth.com
Hypnobirthing: www.hypnobirthing.com
International Childbirth Education Association (ICEA): www.icea.org

Childbirth Stories
BabyCenter's Birth Stories bulletin board:
http://bbs.babycenter.com/board/pregnancy/childbirth/3500

Circumcision
American Academy of Pediatrics: www.aap.org

College Savings Plans
www.savingforcollege.com
www.collegesavings.org

Cord Blood Storage
If you're interested in donating your baby's cord blood, visit the site of the National
Marrow Donor Program: www.marrow.org
If you want to store your baby's cord blood for your family's own use, visit the Umbil-
ical Cord Blood Education Alliance: www.parentsguidecordblood.com

Credit Cards
Cardweb publishes a monthly survey of credit card rates: www.cardweb.com
Bankrate keeps a list of the best deals, divided into categories, such as low-interest
cards and airplane mileage cards: www.bankrate.com

Diabetes
American Diabetes Association: www.diabetes.org
National Diabetes Information Clearinghouse: http://diabetes.niddk.nih.gov
BabyCenter's Pregnant with Diabetes bulletin board:
http://bbs.babycenter.com/board/pregnancy/pregcomplications/1143961

Doulas
Doulas of North America: www.dona.org
Doula Network: www.doulanetwork.com

Emergency Birth Assistance
The American College of Nurse-Midwives' Guide to Emergency
Preparedness for Childbirth: www.acnm.org/focus/inplace.cfm

Epilepsy
Epilepsy Foundation: www.epilepsyfoundation.org
National Institute of Neurological Disorders and Stroke: www.ninds.nih.gov

Gestational Hypertension
Preeclampsia Foundation: www.preeclampsia.org
BabyCenter's Pregnancy Complications bulletin board:
http://bbs.babycenter.com/board/pregnancy/pregcomplications/1703

Hepatitis B
Hepatitis B Foundation: www.hepb.org
Hep B information page of the Centers for Disease Control and Prevention:
www.cdc.gov/ncidod/diseases/hepatitis/b/faqb.htm

High-Risk Pregnancies
Sidelines National Support Network: www.sidelines.org
BabyCenter's Pregnancy Complications bulletin board:
http://bbs.babycenter.com/board/pregnancy/pregcomplications/1703

Home Births
American College of Nurse-Midwives: www.midwife.org.
Midwives Alliance of North America: www.mana.org.

Hydramnios
March of Dimes: www.modimes.org
BabyCenter's Amniotic Fluid Disorders bulletin board:
http://bbs.babycenter.com/board/pregnancy/pregcomplications/1202046

Insurance
Insurance page of the Consumer Federation of America:
www.consumerfed.org/backpage/insurance.html

Intrauterine Growth Restriction (IUGR)
BabyCenter's Pregnancy Complications bulletin board:
http://bbs.babycenter.com/board/pregnancy/pregcomplications/1703

Job Safety
Tips for protecting yourself and your baby-to-be while you're on the job:
Occupational Safety and Health Administration: www.osha.gov
National Institute for Occupational Safety and Health: www.cdc.gov/niosh
Organization of Teratology Information Services: www.otispregnancy.org

Lupus
Lupus Foundation of America: www.lupus.org

Maternity Leave Rights
National Partnership for Women and Families: www.nationalpartnership.org
U.S. Department of Labor FMLA fact sheet:
www.dol.gov/esa/regs/compliance/whd/whdfs28.htm

Department of Labor FMLA compliance advice page: www.dol.gov/esa/whd/fmla/
Department of Labor guide comparing state family leave laws with FMLA:
www.dol.gov/esa/programs/whd/state/fmla/index.htm

• •

Maternity Clothes for Special Occasions
Maternity Treasures: www.maternitytreasures.com
Mom's Night Out: www.momsnightout.com
A Pea in the Pod: www.apeainthepod.com

• •

Midwives
The American College of Nurse-Midwives' Find a Midwife tool:
http://find.midwife.org
Check your insurance plan's or HMO's provider list. Most are available online.
The National Association of Childbearing Centers' (NACC) Birth Center Directory:
www.birthcenters.org/fabc
North American Registry of Midwives: www.narm.org
National Association of Childbearing Centers: www.birthcenters.org

• •

Migraine Headaches
National Headache Foundation: www.headaches.org
National Migraine Association: www.migraines.org

• •

Moms-to-Be in Cyberspace
When you're craving reassurance or advice—or just need to vent—there's always the
Internet. And nothing beats a flood of empathetic responses at 3 A.M. for reminding
you that you're not alone in your concerns.
BabyCenter Pregnancy Community: http://bbs.babycenter.com/boards/bbs-preg

• •

Moms-to-Be of Multiples
National Organization of Mothers of Twins Clubs: www.nomotc.org
Triplet Connection: www.tripletconnection.org
BabyCenter's Multiples: Pregnancy Concerns bulletin board:
http://bbs.babycenter.com/board/pregnancy/carryingtwins/3367

• •

Multiple Sclerosis
Multiple Sclerosis Foundation: www.msfacts.org
National Multiple Sclerosis Society: www.nmss.org

• •

Obstetricians/Gynecologists
American College of Obstetricians and Gynecologists' physician finder tool:
www.acog.com/member-lookup
Society for Maternal-Fetal Medicine (an organization for perinatologists) physician
locator tool: www.smfm.org/index.cfm?zone=search&nav=doctor

• •

Oligohydramnios
March of Dimes: www.modimes.org
BabyCenter's Amniotic Fluid Disorders bulletin board:
http://bbs.babycenter.com/board/pregnancy/pregcomplications/1202046

• •

Online Ovulation Calculator
If you know the day of your last period and the length of a typical menstrual cycle,
BabyCenter's ovulation calculator can run the numbers for you:
www.babycenter.com/calculators/ovulation

Overseas Health Updates
Traveler's Health page of the Centers for Disease Control and Prevention:
www.cdc.gov/travel

Paternity Leave
Family and Medical Leave Act: www.dol.gov/esa.whd/fmla
U.S. Department of Labor FMLA factsheet:
www.dol.gov/esa/regs/compliance/whd/whdfs28.htm
National Partnership for Women & Families: www.nationalpartnership.org
Families and Work Institute: www.familiesandwork.org

Placental Abruption
March of Dimes: www.modimes.org
BabyCenter's Placental Disorders bulletin board:
http://bbs.babycenter.com/board/pregnancy/pregcomplications/1232290

Placenta Previa
March of Dimes: www.modimes.org
BabyCenter's Placental Disorders bulletin board:
http://bbs.babycenter.com/board/pregnancy/pregcomplications/1232290

Plus-Size Maternity Wear
Baby Becoming: www.babybecoming.com
Jake and Me: www.jakeandme.com
JC Penney: www.jcpenney.com
Maternity Clothes Online: www.maternity-clothes-online.com
Maternity Mall: www.maternitymall.com
Old Navy: www.oldnavy.com
Pickles & Ice Cream: www.plusmaternity.com

Postpartum Depression
If you have PPD, you're not alone, and you can make it through this challenging time
with the right care. Here are some resources to turn to:
Depression After Delivery (DAD): www.depressionafterdelivery.com
Postpartum Support International: www.postpartum.net
The depression info page of the National Institute of Mental Health:
http://www.nimh.nih.gov/publicat/depression.cfm

Preeclampsia
Preeclampsia Foundation: www.preeclampsia.org
BabyCenter's Preeclampsia bulletin board:
http://bbs.babycenter.com/board/pregnancy/pregcomplications/1143206

Pregnancy Discrimination
Pregnancy discrimination info page of the Equal Employment Opportunity
Commission: www.eeoc.gov/facts/fs-preg.html
National Association of Working Women: www.9to5.org/rights

Pregnancy Journals Online
Want inspiration for starting your own journal—or just need a good read? Check out
BabyCenter's pregnancy diaries.
From Here to Maternity: A first-time mom-to-be chronicles her journey to mother-
hood: www.babycenter.com/heretomaternity
Bringing Up Ben & Birdy: The mother of a toddler shares her take on being pregnant

with Baby Number Two: www.parentcenter.com/ben
Jennifer's Journal: A mom of two discovers—surprise!—that she has a third child on
the way: www.babycenter.com/jennifersjournal

Pregnancy Loss
March of Dimes: www.modimes.org
BabyCenter's Miscarriage bulletin board:
http://bbs.babycenter.com/board/pregnancy/pregnancygrief/3376
BabyCenter's Ectopic Pregnancy bulletin board:
http://bbs.babycenter.com/board/preconception/precongrief/1224442
Losing a pregnancy really is like a death in the family, and it takes time to heal. Visit
BabyCenter's bulletin boards for comfort and support.
Share your pregnancy loss story with women who understand:
http://bbs.babycenter.com/board/4298
Find out how others cope with multiple miscarriages:
http://bbs.babycenter.com/board/1202012
Get support from women trying to conceive after a loss:
http://bbs.babycenter.com/board/3359

Preterm Labor and Birth
March of Dimes: www.modimes.org
Preemies.org: www.preemies.org
BabyCenter's Preventing Premature Births bulletin board:
http://bbs.babycenter.com/board/pregnancy/prenatalhealth/1307452

Seafood Safety
Before eating fish or other seafood—especially sport-caught varieties—contact your
local health department or Environmental Protection Agency office (listed in the "local
government" section of your phone book) for a list of safe fish and fishing waters in
your area. Or visit one of these Web sites:
Fish Advisories page of the Environmental Protection Agency: www.epa.gov/ost/fish
Seafood Information page of the FDA: www.cfsan.fda.gov/seafood1.html

Single Parents
BabyCenter's Single Parents bulletin board:
http://bbs.babycenter.com/board/baby/1198
Parents Without Partners: www.parentswithoutpartners.org
National Organization of Single Mothers: www.singlemothers.org
Single Mothers by Choice: http://mattes.home.pipeline.com/index.html

Stepfamilies
BabyCenter's Blended Families bulletin board:
http://bbs.babycenter.com/board/baby/babyfamily/1379857
Stepfamily Association of America: www.saafamilies.org

Thyroid Disease
American Thyroid Association: www.thyroid.org
Thyroid Foundation of America: www.tsh.org

Weight Woes
BabyCenter's Plus-Sized and Pregnant bulletin board:
http://bbs.babycenter.com/board/pregnancy/8404
American Dietetic Association: www.eatright.org
Overeaters Anonymous: http://overeatersanonymous.org
National Eating Disorders Association: www.nationaleatingdisorders.org

● ●

Wills
DoYourOwnWill: For a small fee, this site lets you fill out a quick online questionnaire to create a simple will: www.doyourownwill.com
US Legal Forms: Also for a small fee, this site allows you download will forms for all 50 states: www.uslegalforms.com/last_will_and_testaments.htm
Nolo Press: This respected legal publishing house's site has a free wills and estate area with useful FAQs. You can also order will and estate planning books online: www.nolo.com

● ●

Working Moms
9 to 5, National Association of Working Women: www.9to5.org
BabyCenter's Working Moms Bulletin Board:
http://bbs.babycenter.com/board/baby/babywork/3397
Working Moms' Refuge: www.momsrefuge.com

INDEX

Boldface page references indicate photographs. <u>Underscored</u> references indicate boxed text.